Recent Advances in
OPHTHALMOLOGY

S. I. DAVIDSON FRCS DO
Director of Studies, Department of Ophthalmology,
University of Liverpool; Consultant Ophthalmic
Surgeon, St Paul's Eye Hospital, Liverpool;
Consultant Neuro-ophthalmologist, Walton
Hospital, Liverpool, UK

F. T. FRAUNFELDER MD
Professor and Chairman, Department of Ophthalmology,
The Oregon Health Sciences University, Portland,
Oregon, USA

Recent Advances in
OPHTHALMOLOGY

EDITED BY

S. I. DAVIDSON
F. T. FRAUNFELDER

NUMBER SEVEN

CHURCHILL LIVINGSTONE
EDINBURGH LONDON MELBOURNE AND NEW YORK 1985

CHURCHILL LIVINGSTONE
Medical Division of Longman Group Limited

Distributed in the United States of America by
Churchill Livingstone Inc., 1560 Broadway, New York,
N.Y. 10036, and by associated companies, branches
and representatives throughout the world.

First edition 1985

ISBN 0 443 03103 7
ISSN 0309-2437

British Library Cataloguing in Publication Data
Recent advances in ophthalmology—No. 7
  1. Ophthalmology—Periodicals
  617.7′005 RE1

Printed in Great Britain at The Pitman Press, Bath

Preface

Increasing complexity and subspecialisation in ophthalmology has now made it difficult for the general ophthalmologist to keep fully informed of recent advances in both surgical technique and medical treatment. Thus a book which attempts to cover recent advances is of increasing importance. It also follows that it is equally essential that such a publication should appear at frequent intervals. The interval between this present edition and the last edition has been 3 years but in this edition the interval between receipt of the various contributions and publication has now been reduced to 12 months. Hopefully this will allow the present volume to be considered a true reflection of recent advances.

Because of progress in the specialty, it is not possible to encompass in one volume all the advances that have occurred in the last 3 years. However, we hope that practising clinicians will agree that a reasonable spread of interest has been provided in this edition and that there is something for everyone in the text.

November, 1984   S.I.D.
                                                                 F.T.F.

Contributors

A. C. BIRD MD FRCS
Professor of Clinical Ophthalmology, Institute of Ophthalmology, University of London, and Moorfields Eye Hospital, London, UK

ROLF BLACH MD FRCS
Consultant Surgeon, Moorfields Eye Hospital, London, UK

ROBERT J. COOLING MB ChB FRCS DO
Consultant Ophthalmic Surgeon, Moorfields Eye Hospital, London, UK

S. I. DAVIDSON FRCS DO
Director of Studies, Department of Ophthalmology, University of Liverpool; Consultant Ophthalmic Surgeon, St Paul's Eye Hospital, Liverpool; Consultant Neuro-ophthalmologist, Walton Hospital, Liverpool, UK

F. T. FRAUNFELDER MD
Professor and Chairman, Department of Ophthalmology, The Oregon Health Sciences University, Portland, Oregon, USA

GEORGE EISNER
Professor of Ophthalmology and Chief, University Eye Hospital, Berne, Switzerland

JAMES C. HAYS BS MD
Clinical Assistant Professor of Ophthalmology, McGee Eye Institute, Oklahoma City, Oklahoma, USA

CREIG S. HOYT AB MD
Professor of Ophthalmology and Pediatrics, and Vice-Chairman, Department of Ophthalmology, University of California, San Francisco, California, USA

HERBERT E. KAUFMAN MD
Professor of Ophthalmology and Pharmacology, and Head, Department of Ophthalmology, Louisiana State University Medical Center School of Medicine; Director, LSU Eye Center, Louisiana State University Medical Center School of Medicine, New Orleans, Louisiana, USA

SIDNEY LERMAN MD
Professor of Ophthalmology, Emory University, Atlanta, Georgia, USA

ROY MAPSTONE MD FRCS
Consultant Ophthalmic Surgeon, St Paul's Eye Hospital, Liverpool; Clinical Lecturer in Ophthalmology, University of Liverpool, UK

L. F. RICH MS MD
Associate Professor of Ophthalmology and Chief, Cornea and External Diseases Service, The Oregon Health Sciences University, Portland, Oregon, USA

WALTER J. RICH FRCS FRCSE DO
Consultant Ophthalmologist, West of England Eye Infirmary, Exeter, UK

M. J. ROPER-HALL ChM FRCS
Consultant Surgeon, Birmingham and Midland Eye Hospital, Birmingham, UK

J. JAMES ROWSEY MD
Clinical Professor of Ophthalmology, University of Oklahoma; Director of Corneal Services, McGee Eye Institute, Oklahoma City, Oklahoma, USA

JERRY A. SHIELDS MD
Director, Oncology Service, Wills Eye Hospital; Professor of Ophthalmology, Thomas Jefferson University, Philadelphia, USA

JAMES B. WISE BA MD
Chairman of Ophthalmology, Baptist Medical Center of Oklahoma; Associate Professor of Ophthalmology, University of Oklahoma Health Sciences Center, Oklahoma, USA

Contents

1. Therapy of herpes simplex

H. E. Kaufman

INHIBITORS OF NUCLEIC ACID SYNTHESIS

Before 1961, there was no really effective treatment for virus infections of the cornea, and there were no specific antiviral drugs. Ocular herpetic infections were treated by means of epithelial debridement, which appeared to have some benefit. However, frequently caustic agents were used (Gundersen, 1936) that were capable of denaturing proteins and causing stromal scarring. It was never clear that this treatment was not worse than the disease. Antimetabolites had been considered as possible agents for use in virus chemotherapy, but virtually all that had been tried were drugs that inhibited the cellular production of nucleosides needed for DNA synthesis. These drugs were never effective because the herpes virus DNA polymerase had a greater affinity for the nucleosides than the cellular DNA polymerase; therefore it was virtually impossible to stop virus multiplication without totally destroying all normal cells as well.

Idoxuridine
Since the DNA polymerase of the virus was known to be specifically coded and was known to have different affinities, compared to the cellular DNA polymerase (Herrmann, 1961), it seemed reasonable that effective virus chemotherapy would have to involve a drug that worked specifically on the viral DNA polymerase, either by inhibiting its activity or by being incorporated itself into a false DNA chain, which would no longer code proper genetic material and therefore would not reproduce, so that new virus would not be made. We first tested idoxuridine because it was very similar to thymidine chemically (Kaufman, 1962) (Table 1.1). The van der Waal's radius of the iodine group was similar to that of the methyl group of thymidine, and it was felt that this similarity would allow idoxuridine to interfere with the uptake of thymidine in the synthetic process. The chloro- and bromo-deoxyuridines appeared to be more toxic than the iodinated form of the molecule.

Table 1.1 Possible sites of inhibition of DNA synthesis by antiviral compounds

Steps in normal DNA synthesis:
    Thymidine → thymidine monophosphate → thymidine triphosphate → DNA → replication
With idoxuridine:
    5-Iodo-2'-deoxyuridine (IDU) → IDU-monophosphate → IDU-triphosphate → IDU-DNA → no
    replication

Iodo-deoxyuridine was synthesised by William Prusoff, of the Department of Pharmacology at Yale University, approximately three years before its first use as an ocular antiviral agent (Prusoff, 1959). The compound was developed originally as an anticancer drug but was relatively ineffective. From the biochemical studies that were carried out at that time, it was known that idoxuridine directly inhibited DNA polymerase and was incorporated into a false DNA. For this reason, and because of its lesser toxicity, this compound was tested as a topical antiviral, and it was found to be effective. A series of double-blind studies confirmed the activity of idoxuridine, but a similar drug, 5-fluorouracil, was found to inhibit the synthesis of thymidine, rather than its uptake, and was not an effective in vivo antiviral agent.

The testing of antiviral drugs was a new area. With further work, it became clear that in animal and clinical studies, the use of complex scoring systems that included redness of the eye, iritis, etc. (Draize et al, 1944) clouded the precise measurement of drug efficacy and made the prediction of drug potency difficult. The results were more precisely predictive when we concentrated on the size of the corneal ulcer alone and the improvement in corneal healing during drug administration.

One of the problems with idoxuridine in its original form was its relative lack of solubility. In part because of this, it was necessary initially to administer the drug every hour during the day and every two hours at night; later, a longer-lasting ointment was used at night. However, clearly, idoxuridine was effective and clinically useful in the treatment of ocular herpes (Kaufman et al, 1962).

Mechanism of action
For antiviral drugs to be effective and to interact with DNA polymerase, they must be present in the cell in the triphosphate form. The first phosphate is added to the molecule either by cellular thymidine kinase or by the virus-encoded enzyme; the virus-encoded thymidine kinase is much more active than the cellular enzyme. Two additional phosphates are rapidly added by cellular enzymes and the compound is then able to interact with the DNA polymerase.

All of the metabolite inhibitors have multiple sites of activity, and it is not always certain which is the true rate-limiting mechanism of action. In spite of this, we can hypothesise a mechanism of action for these drugs. DNA is a helix with a backbone of sugar molecules hooked to each other with 3-,5-bonds, forming a long chain. Attached to the backbone are the bases: adenine, thymine, guanine, and uracil. These bases are read by chemical processes to produce messenger RNA that provides the code for protein synthesis. The base pattern is also involved in the duplication of DNA. The bases themselves are not essential to the structure of the backbone although theoretically, they could stereochemically hinder the formation of the helix.

It appears that the nucleoside analogues that have normal sugar moieties and abnormal purine or pyrimidine substituents for some of the bases, probably are incorporated in the formation of DNA, but the mistakes in the base pattern code for products do not permit the replication of the virus. There may be some direct inhibition of DNA synthesis through abnormal attachments and binding to the DNA polymerase, but in general it seems that the nucleosides with normal sugars and abnormal bases act by incorporation and false coding. Those nucleosides with abnormal sugars—especially abnormalities involving the three or five positions on the carbon chain, which are necessary to link up the sugars to make the DNA chain—probably act largely as chain terminators. They are picked up by the DNA polymerase and one bond forms to a normal sugar molecule of the normal DNA chain, but the chain cannot be continued because the sugar is too abnormal to sustain a 3–5 bonding and permit the synthesis of the backbone of the chain. Thus small pieces of DNA are synthesised and the synthesis of a complete DNA chain is interrupted. This explanation is somewhat oversimplified, and some of the mechanisms are still somewhat uncertain, but it does provide enough of an overview to explain how antiviral drugs exert their effects.

Adenine arabinoside

The next topical antiviral to be developed for ophthalmic use was adenine arabinoside (Underwood, 1962). This arabinose sugar probably acts largely as a chain terminator and is an effective topical antiviral. It is as insoluble as idoxuridine. There has been some suggestion that adenine arabinoside is slightly less toxic than idoxuridine on a chronic basis, but there is no good evidence for this (Dresner & Seamans, 1975). Evidence from double blind studies (Pavan-Langston & Dohlman, 1972) indicate that adenine arabinoside has approximately the same potency as idoxuridine (Table 1.2) and also about the same short term topical toxicity (Dresner & Seamans, 1975). It is

Table 1.2 Efficacy of idoxuridine and adenine arabinoside

| Drug | Mean number of days to re-epithelialisation | | | | Number of patients cleared in 4 weeks |
	Dendritic	Geographic	Combined	Total	
Double blind study:					
Idoxuridine (82 patients)	6.97	6.00	11.00	7.24	75 (91.5%)
Adenine arabinoside (82 patients)	6.67	6.80	8.09	6.88	79 (90.8%)
Open study*:					
Adenine arabinoside (82 patients)	8.08	11.90	11.66	10.54	75 (77.3%)

* Generally the severity of the disease and the duration of symptoms were greater in patients entered in the open study (adapted from Dresner & Seamans, 1975).

also clear that neither adenine arabinoside nor idoxuridine is effective as a primary therapeutic agent in the treatment of stromal disease and iritis.

Trifluorothymidine

Trifluorothymidine, like idoxuridine, was synthesised originally as an anti-cancer drug by Gottschling & Heidelberger (1963). However, trifluorothymidine has several unique properties. It is extremely potent, perhaps because it has a dual mechanism of action; it inhibits the de novo synthesis of thymidine (as a thymidylic synthetase inhibitor), and it also acts directly as a substitute thymidine analogue on DNA polymerase (Heidelberger et al, 1962). It is extremely soluble, so that high concentrations can be obtained in drop form, and ointments are not necessary (Kaufman & Heidelberger, 1964). The drops are usually given between five and eight times a day in the treatment of dendritic ulcer (Wellings et al, 1972), and approximately 97% of patients are cured within two weeks. Resistance to trifluorothymidine occurs, but it is very rare, possibly because of the multiple sites of activity. In the few cases where resistance occurs, the older, less effective drugs can be used. Trifluorothymidine is the most effective topical antiviral now available for the treatment of ocular epithelial herpes, and because of the low incidence of viral resistance, is probably the drug of choice for ordinary topical use.

Out work, as well as studies by others, suggests that trifluorothymidine is also the most potent drug now available for counteracting the steroid effect, when steroids are used as a primary therapeutic agent. Epithelial toxicity from trifluorothymidine is seen infrequently, unless the drug is misused and continued at high frequency for a long time. The drops should not be applied on a frequent dosage schedule for a period of many weeks; when the early high frequency applications are reduced rapidly after about five to seven days, corneal toxicity is rare.

All of the topical antivirals can produce epithelial toxicity. Idoxuridine may appear to be somewhat more toxic, since allergy may play a part in this reaction. The eye may become red, the epithelium keratinised, and punctal occlusion also occurs with herpes infections alone, so it is not certain that idoxuridine therapy is implicated in this problem. All of these antiviral drugs — idoxuridine, adenine arabinoside, and trifluorothymidine — may produce typical allergenic reactions, and all of them may cause a punctate epithelial staining and even epithelial erosions if they are used with high frequency for long periods of time, especially in patients with dry eyes. Cross-allergenicity is virtually unknown, so that a patient unable to use one of these drugs is still likely to be able to use the others. Cross-resistance does occur, but it is also uncommon.

Similarly, recurrences of herpes cannot be prevented by any of our drugs. Some patients have specific triggers for recurrent herpetic keratitis such as fever in children, menstruation, etc. When there is a specific trigger, it may be worthwhile initiating antiviral treatment for the few days that the trigger is present and then stop it. I do not continue an antiviral for a prolonged period as a method of preventing recurrences and when it has been tried, it has not only produced toxicity but also has been ineffective in preventing disease.

TREATMENT OF STROMAL DISEASE: ANTIVIRAL DRUGS AND CORTICOSTEROIDS

Disciform oedema heralds itself primarily as a round patch of corneal oedema in a patient with a clear, unscarred cornea. Folds are present in Descemet's membrane and keratic precipitates of varying sizes develop — typically only under the area of abnormal cornea. Sometimes the disc, which usually is central, may be eccentric, and sometimes the whole cornea may become oedematous.

There is no good evidence that this oedema develops as a direct extension of epithelial disease, and I believe that it does not. There is evidence that the mechanism of the development of disciform oedema is not simply viral invasion of the stroma or multiplying virus but rather is immunologically related (Metcalf & Kaufman, 1976; Williams et al, 1965). The exact nature of this mechanism is not clear at present.

One thing that is clear about disciform oedema is that it nearly always responds to corticosteroids. In the typical patient, disciform oedema will clear if corticosteroids are administered about five times a day. This frequency of administration often must be continued for 7–10 days, but then the corticosteroids can usually be tapered, and given only once or twice a day. Since corticosteroids do not cure anything, the only therapeutic effect is an amelioration of the disease symptoms. The corneal appearance becomes normal, the pain disappears, and the patient can see. Scarring seems to be minimized by reducing the corneal inflammation, as does vascularisation.

Generally, I continue low dose corticosteroids for about three months and in my experience about 85–90% of patients can then stop the steroid-antiviral combination. In some, the disease will relapse and the steroids and antivirals will need to be continued for a longer period of time. It appears clinically to be harmful to stop and start steroids often, and the risks associated with giving corticosteroids only once or twice a day are so small that continuing the medication for prolonged periods of time before cessation seems to be relatively safe.

It is clear that when corticosteroids are given to herpes patients without antivirals, there is a significant incidence of epithelial ulceration — this risk is markedly reduced or eliminated by combining corticosteroids plus an antiviral. Unless there is some contraindication, I always administer an antiviral along with the corticosteroids for the treatment of herpes (Kaufman et al, 1963). Trifluorothymidine appears to be the most potent topical antiviral to prevent corticosteroid complications. The antiviral is used with the same frequency as the corticosteroids; I recommend that the patient apply one drop, wait a few minutes, and then apply the other. Even though the risk of epithelial recurrences may be small when steroid administration is reduced to once or twice a day, I have seen this happen. If the patient is not experiencing toxicity or problems, I continue the antiviral. If problems are developing, it seems worthwhile to take the small risk of epithelial recurrences, and discontinue the antiviral.

When antivirals were less potent than trifluorothymidine, or in some cases, where corticosteroids seem to be required more than five or six times a day, I will frequently administer oral corticosteroids in the absence of systemic contraindications. Oral corticosteroids coming through the ciliary body and iris circulation have a powerful effect on quieting iritis and treating disciform oedema, whereas the concentration of corticosteroids that penetrates through to the corneal epithelium is extremely small. This is just the opposite of topical administration where the epithelial concentration is enormous and the concentration in the iris is reduced as the inside of the eye is reached. If there is corticosteroid sensitivity or an antiviral cannot be used, systemic corticosteroids may avoid some of the problems of the topical drug.

Necrotising stromal keratitis responds somewhat unpredictably and far less well to corticosteroid therapy. Also, there are relentlessly progressive cases of necrotising iritis that do not benefit from topical antiviral agents or corticosteroids. The treatment of these two conditions is unsatisfactory at present. Corticosteroids may reduce inflammation, and any epithelial defect should be healed by antiviral drugs and other supportive means, if possible, but still the response may be erratic.

Mixed disease: dry eyes and recurrent erosion
It is common in patients who have herpes simplex infections of the cornea that the eyes tend to be dry and there may be some lagophthalmos. Similarly, when the basement membrane has been damaged, failure to heal may be due to a recurrent erosion mechanism, specifically a failure of reformation of hemidesmosomes to anchor the epithelial cells to the basement membrane (Kaufman, 1964). Dry eyes, exposure, and poor healing are common causes of prolonged ulceration in herpes. In the absence of corticosteroid therapy, any dendritic or geographic ulcer that has been treated for three weeks or more and has not healed should be assumed to be complicated by some

intercurrent problem rather than continued virus multiplication. In my experience, virus multiplication does not continue beyond three weeks in a non-steroid-treated eye.

SYSTEMIC ANTIVIRAL AGENTS AND OCULAR DISEASE

There are a variety of antimetabolites that inhibit viral DNA synthesis in tissue culture, but are either useless or harmful as systemic antiviral agents. Cytosine arabinoside, as well as idoxuridine and trifluorothymidine (Ansfield & Ramirez, 1971), have been tried in humans and proved to be of limited value for systemic use. It has become clear that for an antiviral agent to be systemically useful, it must spare the host immune system. Any antiviral that also acts as an immunosuppressant appears likely to be ineffective or harmful when administered systemically.

The first systemically useful antiviral was adenine arabinoside. Although it is not a truly selective drug in the sense of sparing the DNA of normal cells, it does spare the host immune system (Zam et al, 1976; Steele et al, 1975). It has been shown to be effective in the treatment of herpes encephalitis, to prevent the spread of zoster in immunosuppressed children, and to have some effect on herpes iritis when given systemically (Abel et al, 1975). The effect on iritis, however, was transient and not very great, and generally not worth the risk of administering a non-selective drug which may have to be given by prolonged intravenous infusion over a period of many hours because of its insolubility.

Selective antiviral drugs

Since the development of adenine arabinoside, a number of selective antiviral drugs have been synthesised. Their mechanisms of action all depend on the fact that antiviral antimetabolites are inactive and must be phosphorylated to be activated. These drugs are constructed so that they can bind to and be phosphorylated by the viral thymidine kinase and thereby be activated by the cellular enzymes. Although the differences are relative, and selectivity is not absolute, it is enough to stop virus multiplication with an acceptable level of toxicity to normal cells. Some of the early drugs that depended on specific viral thymidine kinase phosphorylation and incubation were not very potent, but more recently whole families of drugs have been synthesised which are activated only by the thymidine kinase of infected cells. These drugs offer the possibility of extremely safe, selective antiviral therapy that may possibly be used systemically. Some have been approved for other than ocular topical use but most are still in the experimental or investigational stages of development (Table 1.3).

Acyclovir (Elion et al, 1977; Schaeffer et al, 1978), the most studied of these drugs, has been approved for the treatment of primary genital herpes. It is effective in treating ocular epithelial herpetic disease (Jones et al, 1981), although patients with dendritic ulcers seem to develop stromal disease at about the same rate as those treated with other antivirals. In an uncontrolled non-randomised study done by our group, a combination of oral and topical acyclovir seemed ineffective in treating either necrotising stromal keratitis or disciform oedema (Sanitato et al, 1984) even though some laboratory studies indicated an effect on stromal disease in rabbits (Varnell & Kaufman, 1981) and there was some evidence that, in cataract patients, acyclovir

Table 1.3 Selective and non-selective antiviral drugs

Abbreviation		Trade name	
Non-selective drugs			
IDU	idoxuridine	Stoxil	5-iodo-2'-deoxyuridine
Ara-A	vidarabine	Vira-A	9-β-D-arabinofuranosyladenine; vidarabine
AraADA			Ara-A-2',3-diacetate
TFT	trifluoridine	Viroptic	5-trifluoromethyl-2'-deoxyuridine; trifluoridine
PFA		Foscarnet	phosphonoformate cycladrine
Thimidine kinase selective drugs			
ACV	acyclovir	Zovirax	9-(2-hydroxyethoxymethyl)guanine; acyclovir
BVDU			(E)-5-(2-bromovinyl)-2'-deoxyuridine
DHBG			9-(2,3-dihydroxy-2-butoxymethyl)guanine
DHPG			9-(2,3-dihydroxy-2-propoxymethyl)guanine
FIAC			2'-fluoro-5-iodo-arabinofuranosylcytidine
FMAU			2'-fluoro-5-methyl-arabinofuranosyluridine

penetrates into the stroma (Poirier, 1979). Acyclovir is relatively insoluble, so an ointment is needed for topical application, and its potency may be less than that of trifluorothymidine.

Bromovinyl deoxyuridine is a fascinating compound synthesised by De Clercq and others (1979). It is so selective in its ability to bind to thymidine kinase enzymes that it is phosphorylated to a great extent by HSV type 1 thymidine kinase but very little by HSV type 2 (De Clerq & Zhang, 1982). Thus, this drug may be ineffective — or at least less effective than other compounds — in unidentified cases of HSV-2 or mixed infections, and there is therefore some risk in using this drug even in ocular infections where HSV-2 is uncommon. There is some evidence that bromovinyl deoxyuridine may be effective in treating stromal disease and iritis, but these studies are not conclusive and must be repeated; at this time, judgment on the effect of this antiviral on stromal disease must be held in abeyance.

Some of the newer compounds may be better absorbed orally and more easily used than the earlier compounds, but their exact place in our therapeutic armamentarium is as yet unclear.

The problem with all of these thymidine kinase specific antivirals is that, in the laboratory, resistance to them develops very quickly (Field, 1982). Viruses develop that are thymidine kinase deficient and even in a pool of virus that has never been exposed to any of these drugs, thymidine kinase deficient virus that can flourish in the presence of the drug will be found. In the case of acyclovir, resistant virus has already been seen in human patients (Crumpacker et al, 1982), as well as in the laboratory. Viruses also can alter their thymidine kinase so that they no longer have a high affinity for these drugs, but have a relative resistance to them (Field, 1983). Similarly, viruses can alter their DNA polymerase and by that mechanism become resistant to any of the antivirals. These latter mechanisms are less common than alterations in thymidine kinase.

Early evidence indicates that the thymidine kinase deficient mutants are generally less virulent than those that contain thymidine kinase but the degree of protection from this is not certain (Field & Wildy, 1978). Thymidine kinase deficient mutants have been isolated from patients with rapidly progressive clinical herpes and the possibility of creating large populations of resistant virus by the indiscriminate use of these agents seems great.

Are these new antivirals superior to the previous antivirals? At this time, we really do not know. The newer antivirals probably produce a bit less epithelial toxicity than less selective antivirals such as trifluorothymidine. However, clinical toxicity from these drugs is such a minor problem that it certainly would not pay to trade this for an increased incidence of resistant virus and perhaps a pool of virus in the general population that is drug resistant. I therefore think that unless the new agents can be shown to do something that the older agents do not, they should not be used for topical ocular therapy.

It may eventually be possible to treat necrotising stromal disease and iritis with these new modalities, but the evidence is unclear. We are convinced from both initial studies on dendritic keratitis done with acyclovir, as well as our own combined oral and topical study, that these drugs do not benefit necrotising stromal disease and iritis. It may be that more potent drugs, which permit higher concentrations, will have some effect but only the future will tell. Until that time, however, the additional value of these newer drugs remains unclear.

Treatment of recurrent herpetic disease
It is clear that even the newer drugs given systematically and/or in combination do not eradicate virus from the ganglion (Park et al, 1979; Field & De Clerq, 1981). It is not possible, therefore, with a course of antivirals of any sort, to eliminate recurrences of herpes. Studies are presently being conducted to determine if small amounts of continuous, orally-administered drug reduce the recurrence of clinical disease. For example, can you take a pill in the morning along with your vitamin and prevent herpes? It is not clear whether this will be possible. Preliminary experiments in rabbits have been unsuccessful, but work on genital herpes suggests that continued oral administration of acyclovir may be effective (Nilsen et al, 1982; Straus et al, 1984). Similarly, although these drugs are relatively safe and selectively phosphorylated, this selectivity is not absolute and the safety of long-term, continued administration has not been proven.

INTERFERON

Until relatively recently almost all interferon was produced in the laboratory of Dr. Kari Cantell in Helsinki. He took blood from Finnish donors and used plasma-pharesis to separate out the white cells. When these cells were challenged by Sendai virus, they produced a series of proteins called interferons. The interferons we know today were purified from this heterogeneous pool. This complicated and involved process provided virtually the only source of interferon in the western world at that time.

Interferon is a protein made by virus-infected or -challenged cells which can travel to other cells where it induces a phosphorylated oligonucleotide and sets up a general state of resistance in the new cell, not only to the original challenging virus but to a variety of other viruses. Its spectrum is therefore a broad one, and, of course, it is a natural cell product. There are a variety of interferons. Alpha interferon is formed by challenged normal human leukocytes. When the gene for interferon production is obtained from these leukocytes and placed in micro-organisms such as *E. coli*, an alpha interferon can be genetically engineered and produced by these organisms. There are several subsets of alpha interferon and it is not a single homogeneous product.

Beta interferon is produced by fibroblasts, usually grown in culture and challenged in a similar way. The fibroblast interferon is in many ways easier to make but it seems less effective when given systemically — although its topical effect is the same (Varnell & Kaufman, unpublished data).

Gamma interferon, or immune interferon, is the interferon produced in an immune reaction by white cells. These immune interferons again can be produced naturally or by removing the gene from the white cells and placing it into an organism which will become genetically altered and produce this substance. There is some reason to believe gamma interferon may be more effective than some of the interferons and that in fact combinations of interferons may have some advantages over single types, but this remains uncertain.

There seems to be a dissociation between the therapeutic and the prophylactic effect of interferon. In animals it is easy to see that interferon can protect against herpes better than it can treat herpes. Also we have done a study of epidemic haemorrhagic conjunctivitis in man, using a natural alpha interferon; the interferon seemed to be able to abort the epidemic by preventing infection in family contacts even though it did not alter the disease in the person already affected (Stansfield et al, 1984). We have done two studies to try and prevent recurrences of herpetic keratitis with interferon continually administered twice a day, and no beneficial effects were seen, but it is possible that the concentration of interferon used was not as high as is now obtainable and these studies need to be repeated (Kaufman et al, 1976).

The role of interferon as a therapeutic agent also remains unclear. One of the problems is that interferon is only mildly effective. When given to someone with dendritic keratitis, it will improve the disease, just as it will shrink tumours, but this improvement is far less than that seen with most other drugs and is really relatively a minor therapeutic effect. Other virus diseases, for which present antivirals are not effective, such as adenovirus infection, are being investigated, but the therapeutic role of interferon has not as yet been defined.

Also, like all drugs, interferon can be highly toxic. Systemically, it produces pyrogenic reactions (chills) and if continued, liver and kidney damage in some patients. Topically it can cause nose bleeds and damage to the nasal mucosa as well as allergic reactions and local eye irritation.

Numerous laboratory studies have indicated that interferon can potentiate the effect of the antiviral drugs. More recently, Colin et al (1983) have reported a controlled, double-blind, randomised study that indicates that acyclovir plus interferon is more effective than acyclovir plus placebo. The difference in the effect is not enormous, but certainly it is significant. Similar studies have been done by others (De Koning et al, 1982). The exciting thing about interferon in combination with some of the newer antivirals is not the small increased potency, but rather the possibility that interferon might serve to eliminate the small populations of surviving drug-resistant viruses and thereby provide a safer way of using the newer thymidine kinase selective drugs. Whether this will in fact be the case, and what the role of these combinations will be is, as yet, unclear.

REFERENCES

Abel R Jr, Kaufman H E, Sugar J 1975 Intravenous adenine arabinoside against herpes simplex keratouveitis in humans. American Journal of Ophthalmology 79: 659–664

Ansfield F J, Ramirez G 1971 Phase I and II studies of 2′-deoxy-5-(trifluoromethyl)uridine (NSC-75520). Cancer Chemotherapy Reports Part I 55: 205–208

Colin J, Chastel C, Renard G, Cantell K 1983 Combination therapy for dendritic keratitis with human leukocyte interferon and acyclovir. American Journal of Ophthalmology 95: 346–348

Crumpacker C S, Schnipper L E, Marlowe S I, Kowalsky P N, Hershey B J, Levin M J 1982 Resistance to antiviral drugs of herpes simplex virus isolated from a patient treated with acyclovir. New England Journal of Medicine 306: 343–346

De Clercq E, Descamps J, De Somer P, Barr P J, Jones A S, Walker R T 1982 (E)-5-(2-Bromovinyl)-2′-deoxyuridine: a potent and selective antiherpes agent. Proceedings of the National Academy of Science of the USA 76: 2947–2951

De Clercq E, Zhang Z-X 1982 Differential effects of E-5-(2-bromovinyl)-2′-deoxyuridine on infections with herpes simplex virus type 1 and type 2 in hairless mice. Journal of Infectious Diseases 145: 130

De Koning W J, Van Bijsterveld O P, Cantell K 1982 Combination therapy for dendritic keratitis with human leukocyte interferon and trifluorothymidine. British Journal of Ophthalmology 66: 509–512

Draize J H, Woodard G, Calvery H O 1944 Methods for the study of irritation and toxicity of substances applied topically to the skin and mucous membranes. Journal of Pharmacology and Experimental Therapeutics 82: 377–390

Dresner A J, Seamans M L 1975 Evidence of the safety and efficacy of adenine arabinoside in the treatment of herpes simplex epithelial keratitis. In: Pavan-Langston D, Buchanan R A, Alford C A Jr (eds) Adenine arabinoside: an antiviral agent, Raven Press, New York, p 381–392

Elion G B, Furman P A, Fyfe J A, deMiranda P, Beauchamp L, Schaeffer H J 1977 Selectivity of action of an antiherpetic agent 9-(2-hydroxy-ethoxymethyl)guanine. Proceedings of the National Academy of Sciences of the USA 74: 5716–5720

Field H J 1982 Development of clinical resistance to acyclovir in herpes simplex virus-induced mice receiving oral therapy. Antimicrobial Agents and Chemotherapy 21: 744–752

Field H J 1983 A perspective on resistance to acyclovir in herpes simplex virus. Journal of Antimicrobial Chemotherapy 12: 129–135

Field H J, De Clerq E 1981 Effects of oral treatment with acyclovir and bromovinyldeoxyuridine on the establishment and maintenance of latent herpes simplex infection in mice. Journal of General Virology 56: 259–265

Field H J, Wildy P 1978 The pathogenicity of thymidine kinase-deficient mutants of herpes simplex virus in mice. Journal of Hygiene 81: 267–277

Gottschling H, Heidelberger C 1963 Fluorinated pyrimidines XIX. Some biological effects of 5-trifluoro-methyl-2′-deoxyuridine on Escherichia coli and bacteriophage T4B. Journal of Molecular Biology 7: 541–560

Gundersen T 1936 Herpes corneae: with special references to its treatment with strong solution of iodine. Archives of Ophthalmology 15: 225

Herrmann E C Jr 1961 Plaque inhibition test for detection of specific inhibitors of DNA containing viruses. Proceedings of the Society of Experimental Biology and Medicine 107: 142–145

Heidelberger C, Parsons D G, Remy D C 1962 Synthesis of 5-trimethyluracil and 5-trifluoromethyl-2′-deoxyuridine. Journal of the American Chemical Society 84: 3597–3598

Jones B R, Coster D J, Michaud R, Wilhelmus K R 1981 Acyclovir (Zovirax) in the management of herpetic keratitis. In: Sundmacher R (ed) Herpetische augenerkrankungen, J F Bergmann Verlag, Munich, p 295–300

Kaufman H E 1962 Clinical cure of herpes simplex keratitis by 5-iodo-2′-deoxyuridine. Proceedings of the Society of Experimental Biology and Medicine 109: 251–252

Kaufman H E 1964 Epithelial erosion syndrome: metaherpetic keratitis. American Journal of Ophthalmology 57: 983–987

Kaufman H E, Heidelberger C 1964 Therapeutic antiviral action of 5-trifluoromethyl-2′-deoxyuridine in herpes simplex keratitis. Science 145: 585–586

Kaufman H E, Martola E, Dohlman C 1962 Use of 5-iodo-2′-deoxyuridine (IDU) in treatment of herpes simplex keratitis. Archives of Ophthalmology 68: 235–239

Kaufman H E, Martola E L, Dohlman C H 1963 Herpes simplex treatment with IDU and corticosteroids. Archives of Ophthalmology 69: 468–472

Kaufman H E, Meyer R F, Laibson P R, Waltman S R, Nesburn A B, Shuster J J 1976 Human leukocyte interferon for the prevention of recurrences of herpetic keratitis. Journal of Infectious Diseases 133: A165–A168

Metcalf J F, Kaufman H E 1976 Herpetic stromal keratitis — evidence for cell-mediated immunopathogenesis. American Journal of Ophthalmology 82: 827–834

Nilsen A E, Aasen T, Halsos A M, Kinge B R, Tjotta E A L, Wikstrom K, Fiddian A P 1982. Efficacy of oral acyclovir in the treatment of initial and recurrent genital herpes. Lancet ii: 571–573

Park N-H, Pavan-Langston D, McLean S L 1979 Acyclovir in oral and ganglionic herpes simplex virus infections. Journal of Infectious Diseases 140: 802–806

Pavan-Langston D, Dohlman C H 1972 A double blind clinical study of adenine arabinoside therapy of viral keratoconjunctivitis. American Journal of Ophthalmology 74: 81–88

Poirier R H 1979 Aqueous penetration characteristics of three antiviral compounds, trifluridine, Ara-AMP, and acycloguanosine. Ocular Microbiology Group Annual Meeting, San Francisco, November 3, 1979.

Prusoff W H 1959 Synthesis and biological activities of idododeoxyuridine, an analog of thymidine. Biochimica et biophysica acta 32: 295–296

Sanitato J J, Asbell P A, Varnell E D, Kisslingt E, Kaufman H E 1984 Acyclovir in the treatment of herpetic stromal disease. American Journal of Ophthalmology, in press

Schaeffer H J, Beauchamp L, deMiranda P, Elion G B, Bauer D J, Collins P 1978 9-(2-hydroxyethoxy-methyl)guanine activity against viruses of the herpes group. Nature 272: 583–585

Stansfield S K, De La Pena W, Koenig S, Espaillat Cabral A, Kaufman H E, Hatch M H, Hierholzer J, Schonberger L B 1984 Human leukocyte interferon in the treatment and prophylaxis of acute hemorrhagic conjunctivitis. Journal of Infectious Diseases 149, 822–823

Steele R W, Chapa I A, Vincent M M, Hensen S A, Keeney R E 1975 Effect of adenine arabinoside on cellular immune mechanisms in man. In: Pavan-Langston D, Buchanan R A, Alford C A Jr (eds) Adenine arabinoside: an antiviral agent, Raven Press, New York p 275–280

Straus S E, Takiff H E, Seidlin M, Bachrach S, Lininger L, Di Giovanni J J, Western K A, Smith H A, Lehrman S N, Creagh-Kirk T, Alling D W 1984 Suppression of frequently recurring genital herpes: a placebo controlled double-blind trial of acyclovir. New England Journal of Medicine 310: 1545–1550

Sundmacher R, Cantell K, Neumann-Haefelin D 1978 Combined therapy of dendritic keratitis with trifluorothymidine and interferon. Lancet ii: 678

Underwood G E 1962 Activity of 1-β-D-arabinofuranosylcytosine hydrochloride against herpes simplex keratitis. Proceedings of the Society of Experimental Biology and Medicine 111: 660–664

Varnell E D, Kaufman H E 1979 Antiviral agents in experimental herpetic stromal disease. In: R Sundmacher (ed) Herpetische Augenerkrankungen, J F Bergmann Verlag, Munich p 303–308

Wellings P C, Awdry P N, Bors P H, Jones B R, Brown D C, Kaufman H E 1972 Clinical evaluation of trifluorothymidine in the treatment of herpes simplex corneal ulcers. American Journal of Ophthalmology 73: 932–942

Williams L E, Nesburn A B, Kaufman H E 1965 Experimental induction of disciform keratitis. Archives of Ophthalmology 73: 112–114

Zam Z S, Centifanto Y M, Kaufman H E 1976 Failure of systemically administered adenine arabinoside to affect humoral and cell-mediated immunity. American Journal of Ophthalmology 81: 502–505

2. Anterior segment surgery*

L. F. Rich

INTRODUCTION

Anterior segment surgery of the eye can be a broad, extensive topic including all forms of ocular surgery performed on the front portion of the eye for the purpose of altering its health or cosmetic characteristics. This discussion will be limited to surgical alterations of the cornea, iris, sclera, limbus, and conjunctiva.

As concepts of the function of an organ evolve, surgical approaches and techniques change as well. Technological advance helps us devise manipulations of ocular structures not previously possible. Furthermore, as new materials and tools become widely available, certain surgical procedures become commonplace in clinical practice and are no longer limited to the research laboratory.

Some tool and surgical modalities deserve special attention and will be considered outside the scope of this chapter, for example, the myriad variations of intraocular lens implant design.

A dominant trend of anterior segment reconstruction in this decade is the growing realisation that we have the capacity to manipulate visual function through alterations of corneal structure. Not only are we able to treat diseases, such as bullous keratopathy, in a highly refined and successful manner, but we can now address ourselves to conditions heretofore considered unapproachable. An obvious example is the field of refractive corneal surgery, which is developing rapidly.

In keeping with the theme of recent advances in eye care, therefore, we will explore in this chapter the contribution of newer technology on anterior segment surgery. Of course, man's experience with these new tools and concepts is equally important.

PENETRATING KERATOPLASTY

Availability of donor tissue

Throughout the world, penetrating ketatoplasty is being performed more frequently now than ever before. Greater numbers of full-thickness corneal transplants are performed for a wider variety of reasons. Public awareness of organ transplantation is increasing through the educational efforts of governmental and volunteer organisations, and the lay press popularises the idea of organ transplantation by publicising stories of how a particular individual's life has been saved or sight restored. Consequently, the availability of donor tissue continues to improve.

However hard-earned, increased availability of donor tissue does not produce a surplus, since the demand is also greater. Perhaps having more donor material allows

* This study was supported by a grant from Research to Prevent Blindness.

researchers to contrive new ways of using ocular tissue, but there is no doubt that transplantation of ocular tissues has more widespread clinical application today than ever before. The networking of eye banks through communication channels extending over long distances is responsible for much of the growth spurt in corneal transplantation. Preservation and longer term storage of corneae permit greater utilisation of donated eyes, for we are now able to transport tissue to areas where the most immediate need exists.

Evaluation of corneal endothelium

Corneal surgeons are becoming increasingly aware of the role of the endothelial cell in corneal health. Although not all aspects of corneal endothelial cell metabolism and function are known, there is no doubt that corneal clarity is in large part dependant on this cell layer. The influence of intraocular inflammation, pressure, and chemical factors circulating in the aqueous are recognised as sources of endothelial dysfunction (Fraunfelder, 1982). Drugs, whether topically applied or systemically absorbed, can readily alter the metabolic efficiency and morphology of the endothelium (Rich, 1983). Recent interest has centred on the interaction of chemicals and light, specifically ultraviolet light (Lerman, 1982), on the health of the cellular transparent media of the eye, the lens and cornea.

An increasing recognition of the role of the endothelium is responsible for certain advances in surgical techniques. Protection of the corneal endothelium with viscous agents, such as sodium hyaluronate, is an example which cataract and corneal surgeons now utilise daily. These agents afford protection to the endothelium by providing a mechanical barrier to friction, maintaining anterior chamber space between surfaces, and lubricating points of contact should they occur (Polack, 1983). Viscous agents greatly increase the safety and success rate of certain intraocular procedures, such as penetrating keratoplasty and intraocular lens implantation.

Documentation of endothelial cell changes has become possible in a clinical setting with specular endothelial microscopy. This non-invasive photographic technique, first used in laboratory research (Maurice, 1968), has been improved and adapted into a clinical tool. An understanding of diseases, such as aphakic bullous keratopathy, has been gained from use of this and other modalities of in vivo corneal evaluation.

Some newer edothelial cameras have the capacity for photographing corneal endothelium without touching the ocular surface, thereby eliminating or minimising patient apprehension. Wide-field specular microscopy permits assessment of the endothelium over a large area (Koester et al, 1980); localised areas of endothelial damage or disease can be identified and compared with more normal areas on the same photograph. Statistical evaluation with wide-field specular microscopy is not as prone as earlier types of specular microscopes to errors of sampling. A higher degree of accuracy in following endothelial changes is therefore possible (Koester et al, 1980).

The functional capacity of the corneal endothelium relies not only on the numbers of cells per square millimetre but is related to the pleomorphism and metabolic state of the cells (Kaufman et al, 1965). The major task of the endothelium is corneal deturgescence, and an estimation of corneal thickness is helpful in quantifying the ability of this cell layer to do its job. New ultrasonic pachometers are highly accurate tools for measuring corneal thickness. These instruments can provide precise and reproducible measurement of total corneal thickness which correlates well with the state of corneal dehydration and endothelial cell capacity (Rao et al, 1979).

Surgical advances

A recognition of the role of the endothelium in corneal health and these newer methods of assessing it have influenced corneal surgery dramatically in recent years. Ophthalmic surgeons alter what they do based on measurements of these factors, and results tend to improve concomitantly. For example, use of chemicals during surgery, such as intraocular irrigating solutions, becomes of prime concern. Ultraviolet filters are being inserted in operating microscope lights to minimise damage to the cornea as well as deeper structures.

An ophthalmologist's surgical judgement is potentially influenced by these tools which permit endothelial assessment. In the future, rotational autografts may be utilised more frequently for displacement of a corneal opacity if endothelial assessment shows a relatively healthy state of functional capacity in the area outside the scar. Such autografts eliminate the possibility of rejection and minimise surgical damage because the manipulated tissue is not subjected to storage or as much trauma and potential exposure to infectious agents.

Suture materials and suturing techniques have been improved over the past two decades with tremendous impact on anterior segment surgery. Non-absorbable suture materials of nylon or prolene in diameters as small as 16 microns are used frequently today. Epithelialisation occurs over the surface of these small calibre sutures which effectively buries the stitch, providing minimal foreign body sensation. Retention of the suture for months or years is possible because these relatively inert materials have little tendency to stimulate corneal neovascularisation. When employed as interrupted sutures, titration of astigmatic postoperative curvatures can be accomplished by selectively removing sutures in the steeper axis of the cylinder.

In penetrating keratoplasty, surgeons are still debating the advantages of interrupted versus running sutures. Interrupted sutures permit rapid healing of a corneal graft, but many corneal surgeons employ continuous sutures in 'double-running' fashion in which two continuous sutures are placed (Troutman, 1974; McNeill & Kaufman, 1978).

Many suture manufacturers are concentrating on variations in the calibre or shape of ophthalmic surgery needles. Use of a 'bi-curve' or 'fishhook' needle is advocated as a means of expressing open the wound while the suture is placed, thereby permitting deeper placement in the tissue. Closer apposition of posterior corneal surfaces promotes wound healing and decreases complications related to posterior wound gape.

In penetrating keratoplasty, data have been collected which point to the importance of a uniform, symmetrical incision in both donor and recipient toward minimising postoperative astigmatism (Olson, 1981). Mathematical theory and experimental data support the necessity of performing trephination as perpendicular to the surface as possible. Maintaining adequate fixation on the recipient eye during this process is paramount for minimising distortion on the globe at the time of trephination. Fixation rings, to date, offer the best chance of distributing pressure in a relatively uniform fashion. These fixation devices, such as metal straps or wire circular rings, can be sutured to the globe at several points and have the added advantage of supporting the globe once the eye is opened. Many surgeons emphasise that placement of the ring must be symmetrical with regard to the limbus to avoid distortion of the cornea during or after trephination (Olson, 1981). Others claim that symmetrical placement of the ring makes little or no difference, since after suturing the graft and removing the ring the globe retains its original shape (Fine, 1980).

Several new corneal trephination systems have been devised to minimise distortion induced by the cut itself. The Hessburg trephine attaches to the surface of the cornea by suction, and the cutting blade (which is separate from the suction device) places little pressure on the globe during trephination. Motorised trephines have also been advocated because they too allow the surgeon to place less pressure on the globe during the cutting process.

Anterior segment procedures combining penetrating keratoplasty with cataract extraction, with or without an intraocular lens implant, are becoming more common (Troutman & Gaster, 1980). Planned extracapsular cataract extraction in combination with perpetrating keratoplasty has the theoretical advantage of supporting the vitreous and hopefully minimises the incidence of cystoid macular oedema postoperatively in graft patients. Indeed, when the vitreous is not violated in aphakic penetrating keratoplasty, the incidence of cystoid macular oedema is less than when mechanical vitrectomy is performed (Kramer, 1981). With the posterior capsule intact, there should be an equal or lower incidence of these macular changes.

Penetrating keratoplasty has been combined with glaucoma procedures, although this practice is not widespread. In aphakic penetrating keratoplasty, the same problems exist for glaucoma control as with aphakes in general, namely the maintenance of the filtration opening and prevention of corneal damage through anterior chamber collapse in the immediate postoperative period. For this reason, there is still a controversy as to whether cyclocryotherapy is the procedure of choice in glaucoma patients who have had penetrating keratoplasty. It is advisable, wherever possible, to control the glaucoma medically with as low a level of drug therapy as possible to maintain a margin well below maximal medical therapy so glaucoma surgery in the immediate postoperative period will not be necessary (Troutman & Gaster, 1980).

Revision of the pupil during penetrating keratoplasty, and to a lesser degree during cataract surgery, has become an acceptable practice and is of obvious cosmetic value. Sector iridectomies should be closed with non-absorbable sutures in attempting to prevent forward displacement of the iris in the postoperative period, which might jeopardise the graft. Postoperative photophobia is minimised if the pupil is made round (Troutman, 1977). The potential for peripheral anterior synechiae formation is decreased if the iris is sutured to make a round pupil. Sphincterotomy in cases of corectopia enlarges the pupillary aperture, which is necessary in many cases, but has the disadvantage of weakening sphincter action.

REFRACTIVE AND LAMELLAR KERATOPLASTY

Refractive keratoplasty is a term used to describe surgical manipulations on the cornea for the purpose of altering its refractive power. Refractive keratoplasty comprises a number of surgical techniques which will be discussed, although not in depth, in this chapter.

Astigmatism control

Soon after Fyodorov revived Sato's original work on radial keratotomy for the reduction of myopia, investigators began utilising keratotomy techniques to alter corneal astigmatism. Variations in placement of keratotomy incisions along a given axis can be combined with radial keratotomy for myopia or may be performed separately for astigmatism reduction alone.

Following penetrating keratoplasty, relaxing incisions can be made in the graft-host wound to flatten the steeper axis (Troutman, 1977). An incision of three clock hours length is made in the circular wound perpendicular to the steeper corneal meridian. These incisions must be made deep in cornea nearly to Descemet's membrane and will correct between two and seven diopters of post-penetrating keratoplasty astigmatism. Although surface healing is rapid, stabilisation of the astigmatic error may take weeks after such incisions are made. If a contact lens is desired, a wait of up to two or three months may be required before the lens can be fitted because a significant graft-host wound override is present while remodelling of the wound occurs.

The Ruiz technique for astigmatism control incorporates a series of corneal incisions perpendicular to the steeper axis combined with four radial incisions. This technique has the ability to correct larger degrees of astigmatism than relaxing incisions. It can be used following penetrating keratoplasty, following cataract extraction or to correct primary astigmatism (Nordan, 1983).

Corneal wedge resection was introduced by Troutman (1977) in the early part of the 1970s. It has gradually gained acceptance as a method for correcting large degrees of astigmatism following cataract or corneal surgery. Rarely is it used for the correction of primary astigmatism. It is reserved for those cases in which the astigmatism is greater than 8–10 diopters. In this technique, a crescentic wedge of corneal tissue, triangular or 'wedge-shaped' in cross section, is removed perpendicular to the flatter meridian. When the remaining edges of the wound are sutured, the chord length of the globe in that meridian is shortened and the overlying corneal curvature thereby steepened (Troutman, 1977). The axis perpendicular to the meridian which is being steepened is made flatter, but there is a shift in the refractive error toward the myopic side. This operation has the disadvantage of long recovery time, for the corneal wound must heal sufficiently to permit suture removal without separating. As much as four to six months may transpire before the patient's refractive error stabilises after the procedure.

Generally speaking, in all of these techniques, the closer the incision is to the centre of the cornea, the greater its influence on astigmatism. Nevertheless, incisions made near the limbus during cataract surgery can greatly alter corneal contour (Jaffe, 1981). With absorbable sutures and a cataract incision in the superior sector of the limbus, against-the-rule astigmatism is usually produced. With non-absorbable suture materials, induced astigmatism is dependent on the tension of the suture. If interrupted sutures are used, the steeper axis can be flattened postoperatively by cutting the suture in that axis, thereby increasing the chord length of the globe in that meridian and flattening the corresponding corneal curvature. Intraoperatively, adjustable knots can be tied and the corneal curvature measured with an operating room keratometer to identify the steeper axis, while adjustment of tension is done to produce a more desirable contour.

Keratomileusis

The term keratomileusis is derived from Greek roots meaning 'to grind' or 'chisel' the cornea. In this technique, the cornea is hardened by freezing, and a new curvature is generated on a cryolathe. The particular curvature produced determines the refractive power of the cornea following this treatment, and the total refractive power of the eye can be altered predictably (Barraquer, 1970). The procedure can be done as an autoplastic procedure, in which case the patient's cornea is sectioned with a microelectrokeratome (a carpenter's plane-like device capable of cutting sections of 0.05 mm accuracy). The resected portion of the patient's corneal tissue is then frozen on the cryolathe, reshaped with the lathe cutting tool, and replaced on the recipient's cornea by suturing. In the homoplastic procedure, donor tissue previously prepared according to the patient's refractive requirements is sutured in place of the resected recipient cornea.

That corneal tissue could be treated in this manner and remain clear was established by Barraquer. Thus, keratomileusis and its sister procedure, keratophakia, are considered 'Barraquerist' refractive techniques. Keratomileusis may be used to correct hypermetropia or myopia depending on the curve generated on the resected tissue (Barraquer, 1981). In both cases, if done as an autoplastic procedure on the patient's own cornea the postoperative cornea is always thinner than it was preoperatively. This is thought to be in part responsible for a mild but significant regression in the degree of correction over time in the case of myopic keratomileusis.

Keratophakia

Keratophakia is limited to correction of high degrees of hypermetropia, such as aphakia. In this procedure, the patient's cornea is resected with the microelectrokeratome, but an intracorneal convex lens fashioned from donor cornea is inserted between the resected halves of recipient cornea, which are then resutured. This 'lenticule sandwich' steepens central cornea, inducing the refractive change (Fig. 2.1). The lenticule is made from donor tissue, and its precise parameters of curvature and diameter are determined by the patient's refractive requirement (Barraquer, 1970). The lenticule may be produced at the time of surgery or prepared preoperatively and stored until needed (Friedlander et al, 1980). Keratophakia is therefore a homoplastic procedure.

Epikeratophakia

Epikeratophakia is a technique in which a corneal lenticule is sutured onto rather than into the recipient cornea. In this technique, a microelectrokeratome is not used and there is very little disturbance of recipient cornea. Only a small 1 mm ring of Bowman's membrane and superficial stroma is removed from recipient cornea outside the visual axis, and the preprepared lenticule of donor tissue is sutured onto the groove (Kaufman, 1980). Recipient keratocytes migrate through the mid-peripheral rim where Bowman's membrane is absent and repopulate the donor tissue. The resultant cornea contains two Bowmans' membranes, one donor and one recipient, with stroma between (Fig. 2.2). Since stromal healing occurs only in the mid-peripheral ring, rapid re-epithelialisation is critical (Rich, 1981).

Both myopia and hyperopia of small or large degrees can be corrected by this

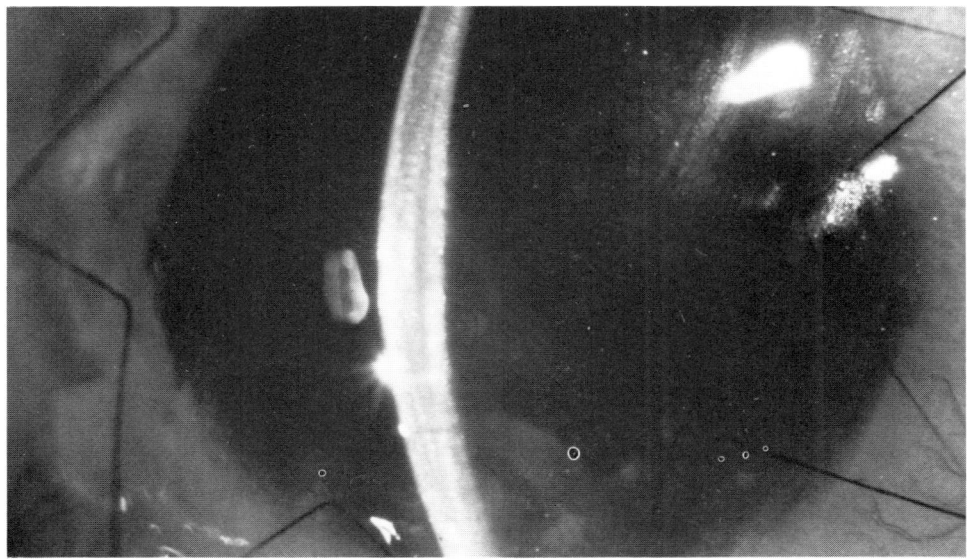

Fig. 2.1 One day postoperative corneal appearance of a patient who has had keratophakia. Note intralamellar lenticule which increases the radius of corneal curvature.

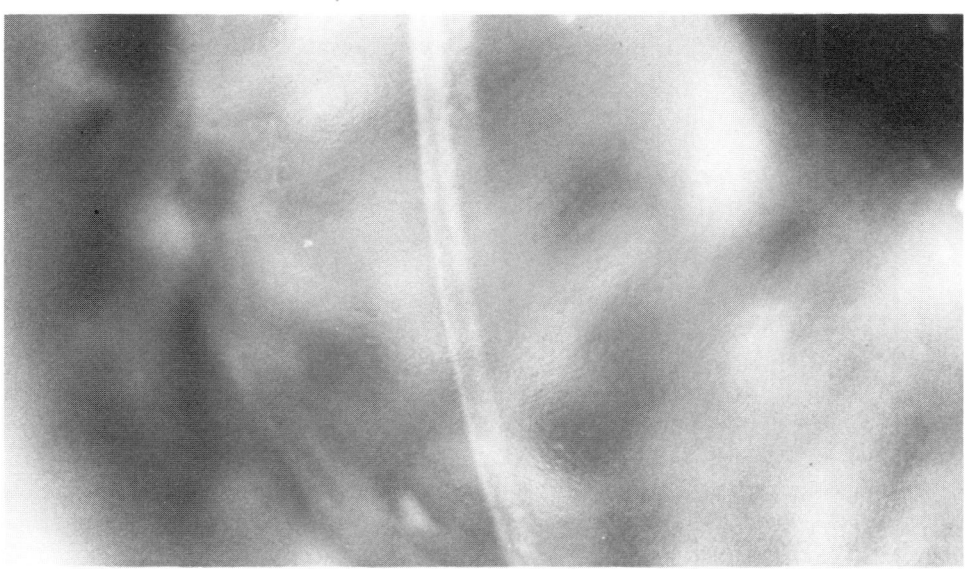

Fig. 2.2 Biomicroscopic corneal photograph of a patient who has had epikeratophakia. The corneal reflections indicate two Bowman's membranes, donor on the left, recipient in the middle, and recipient Descemet's membrane on the right.

method. The particular refractive error correction desired is presented to a computer which determines the curve to be generated on the donor tissue to provide a lenticule of the desired power.

The greatest advantage of epikeratophakia is its simplicity. Lenticules can be prepared in advance in a wide range of powers. Transplanting the tissue into a small ring of resected Bowman's and stroma is neither difficult nor time consuming. If for some reason the graft fails to clear or does not heal properly, it can be removed, and the recipient cornea regains a clear optical zone once re-epithelialised. Only the 1 mm mid-peripheral stromectomy ring outside the visual axis becomes scarred. The procedure can be repeated.

Alloplastic implants
Research is being conducted on the potential for alloplastic materials to affect changes in corneal contour when implanted in the stroma after corneal resection with the microelectrokeratome. Newer hydrogel materials, similar to those used in soft contact lens manufacturing, can be retained in the stroma with high degrees of clarity. Long-term retention of these materials appears promising, and with improved manufacturing techniques and testing of a wider variety of materials, it is quite possible that alloplastic materials will be an important part of refractive keratoplasty in the future.

THERAPEUTIC ANTERIOR SEGMENT REVISION

Optical lamellar
Although keratomileusis is often thought of as a technique used only for the correction of refractive errors, the procedure may be adapted for therapeutic use. In patients whose disease process requires lamellar keratoplasty, the donor tissue may be prepared using keratomileusis which incorporates the refractive error of the patient in the donor tissue. For example, patients with a history of corneal ulceration or penetrating injury in which the corneal scar is in anterior stroma may need a lamellar corneal graft, and the donor tissue can be cryolathe-treated to correct the pre-existing refractive error. In some cases, the microelectrokeratome can be used to remove anterior corneal stromal pathology, but in some cases, the distortion of the cornea is so extensive that free-hand dissection is required for safe removal of pathological structures.

Monocular aphakes occasionally are encountered who have no recourse for correction of their refractive error but a refractive corneal procedure. A significant number of these patients were made aphakic as a result of perforating corneal injury. Often, there has been distortion of other anterior segment structures or glaucoma has been induced. These patients may be intolerant to contact lenses, and secondary intraocular lens implantation may be contraindicated. In such cases, correcting the aphakic refractive requirement with a keratorefractive procedure accomplishes a two-fold goal: removal of corneal scar while providing alteration of the ocular dioptric power.

The following case illustrates this approach. An elderly gentleman who wore soft contact lenses developed a bacterial corneal ulcer in his right eye. The resultant corneal scar was limited to the anterior half of the stroma. He did not wish to have an intraocular lens implant and disliked aphakic spectacles. A lamellar keratoplasty was required to remove the anterior portion of the corneal scar in the visual axis so the donor tissue was prepared with plus power rather than as a plano, parallel-faced disc (Fig. 2.3). This procedure is called homoplastic hypermetropic keratomeliseus, but since it corrects for the corneal scar as well, it is really a combined therapeutic and refractive technique.

Corneoscleral grafting

Not infrequently, tumours and other disease processes in the anterior segment of the eye invade more than one structure. Replacement of corneoscleral defects with donor material may be necessary after the pathological material is removed. In the case of tumours of the iris or ciliary body, a pupillary defect may result from excision of the lesion and resuturing the iris may be necessary.

Corneoscleral tissue is best taken from a whole donor eye at the time of surgery rather than preparing it in advance, since the size of the patch graft required may not be known before the extent of pathology is recognised. Whenever possible, the cornea and sclera to be resected from the recipient eye should be outlined with a trephine so donor tissue can be prepared with the same instrument and satisfactory coaptation of cut edges obtained. Undermining the edges of recipient cornea and sclera helps to seat the donor tissue (Christensen, 1964). Trephination may be performed across limbal borders on donor and recipient eyes. Such dissection can be either full-thickness or partial-thickness lamellar procedures. If full-thickness, care must be taken to prevent loss of intraocular contents, and scleral support rings are required. For example, a tumour of the ciliary body may be removed following full-thickness corneoscleral resection, but the surgeon must be prepared for extensive bleeding, loss of vitreous or damage to the lens. Wet-field (radio frequency current) cautery or laser photocoagulation intraoperatively are excellent methods of controlling bleeding and produce less shrinkage and distortion of tissue than heat cauterisation. Mechanical vitrectomy instruments must be available in such cases, and the surgeon should be prepared for the necessity of lens extraction should it dislocate or appear cataractous. In cases of suspected malignancy, cryotherapy to the edges of the wound helps destroy microscopic extensions of tumour tissue and may prevent recurrence.

Some disease processes extend through the anterior segment with irregular borders and are not amenable to trephination. The diseased tissue may either be too large for standard trephine diameters or so irregular that round trephination is not possible if the entire lesion is to be removed through a single hole. In these cases, free-hand dissection is possible (Christensen, 1964). As the surgeon gains experience with this technique, induced distortion can be minimised to a level where it is no more disruptive than when the dissection was outlined with a trephine. This procedure has been advocated for marginal ulceration, repair of perilimbal areas in recurrent pterygium dissection, and repair of traumatic injuries or tumours near the limbus (Christensen, 1964).

Large 'cap' or 'crown' grafts incorporating cornea and sclera can be used in cases where there is such extensive anterior segment degradation that conventional procedures cannot be done because the recipient tissue cannot provide enough support to maintain the integrity of the globe (King & Wadsworth, 1981). Extreme ectasias of the eye, such as keratoglobus, or advanced melting processes require

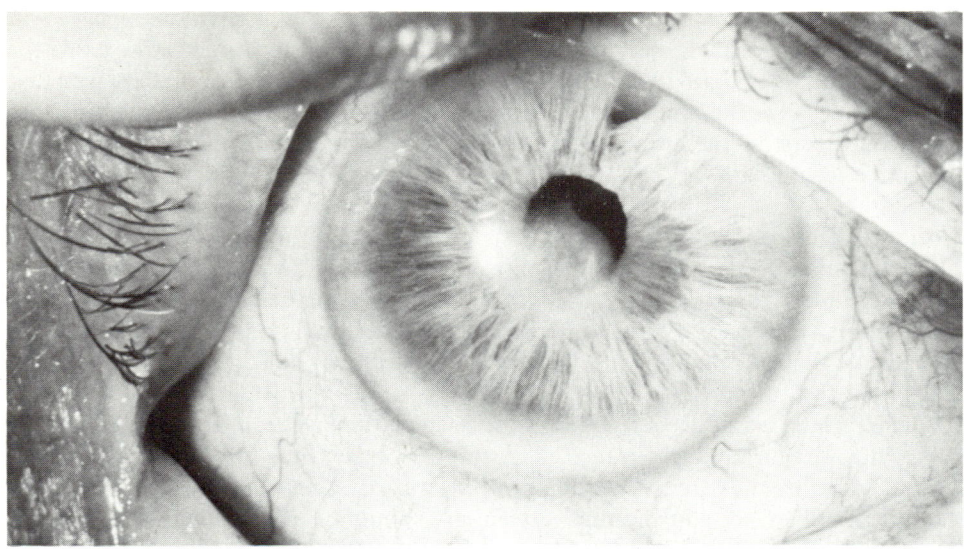

a

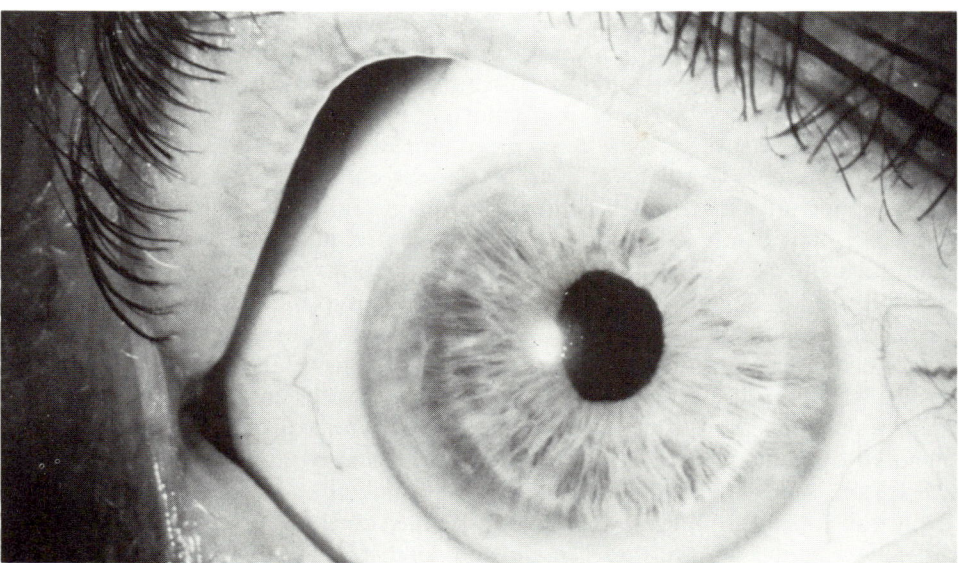

b

surgery in multiple stages if the eye is to be saved and recovery of vision is to be at all possible. In these situations, a corneoscleral graft measuring 14 or 15 mm in diameter, either partial or full-thickness, can be temporising but eye-saving, setting the stage for a later procedure designed at recovering visual function (Fig. 2.4). Usually, full-thickness corneoscleral grafts become cloudy from rejection but a penetrating kerato-plasty can be performed one year later, a clear graft obtained, and vision restored. In such cases, compromised aqueous humour outflow is a possibility and measure-

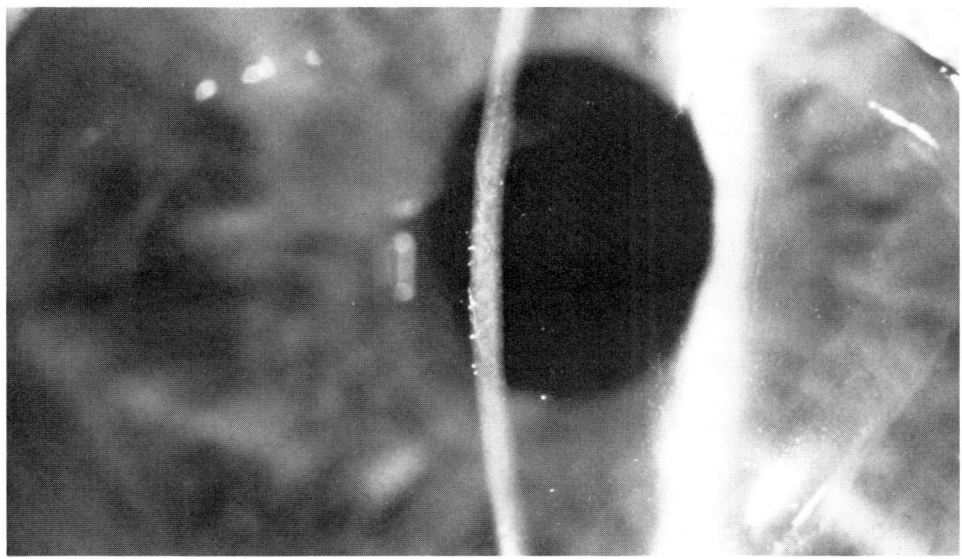

c

Fig. 2.3   a, photograph of a corneal scar in anterior stroma following a bacterial corneal ulcer.
b, photograph of same patient after homoplastic hypermetropic keratomileusis has been performed.
c, postoperative slitlamp view of the same patient.

ment of intraocular pressure at each postoperative visit is necessary if treatment is to
succeed.

Pterygium surgery

The problem of how best to treat pterygium is ubiquitous, although in certain areas of
the world the frequency of this disorder is much higher. In the tropical and
subtropical areas of the world, ophthalmologists have much greater experience in
dealing with pterygium than surgeons in the more temperate zones and colder areas.
Pterygium is most often a cosmetic blemish but can threaten sight. Restriction of
ocular motility can interrupt binocularity.

Earlier in the century, ophthalmic surgeons argued the advantage of one surgical
technique over another in the removal of pterygium. Perhaps because recurrence rates
vary in different parts of the world or possibly because statistical analyses in one study
are not comparable to those of another, no one surgical technique has become
dominant. Nevertheless, some principles have been established which diminish the
chances of a pterygium recurring.

Most ophthalmic surgeons who deal with pterygia recognise the need to smooth the
area of excision as much as possible to avoid leaving irregularities near the limbus
(Paton, 1975). Some advocate use of a motorised rotating burr for this purpose, but
this increases the potential for perforation. Elimination of feeder vessels by cauterisation or laser therapy is necessary. Application of beta irradiation with a strontium 90
applicator, either at the time of surgery or in three successive treatments following
surgery, is advocated by many pterygium surgeons. Some reserve radiation for
treatment or recurrent pterygia only and do not apply it when removing a primary
pterygium.

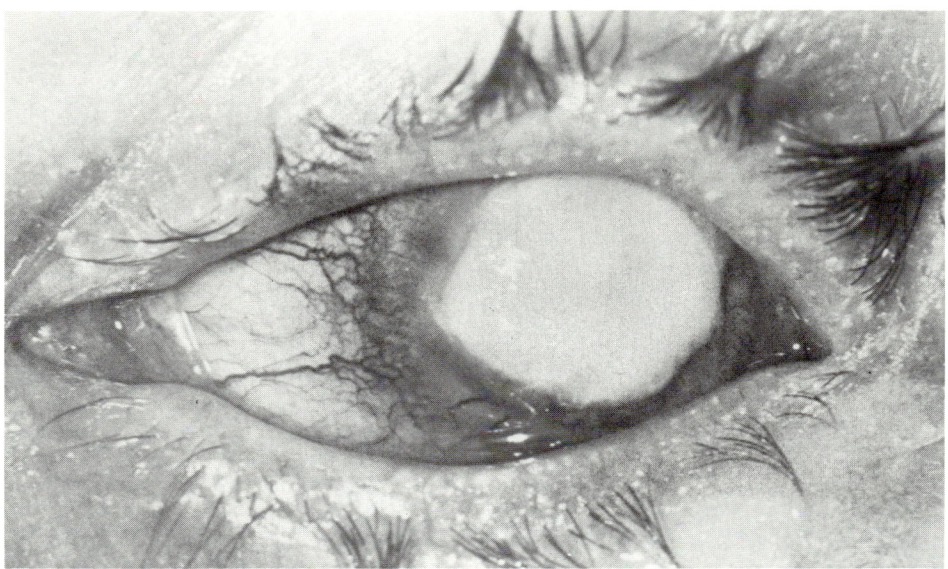

a

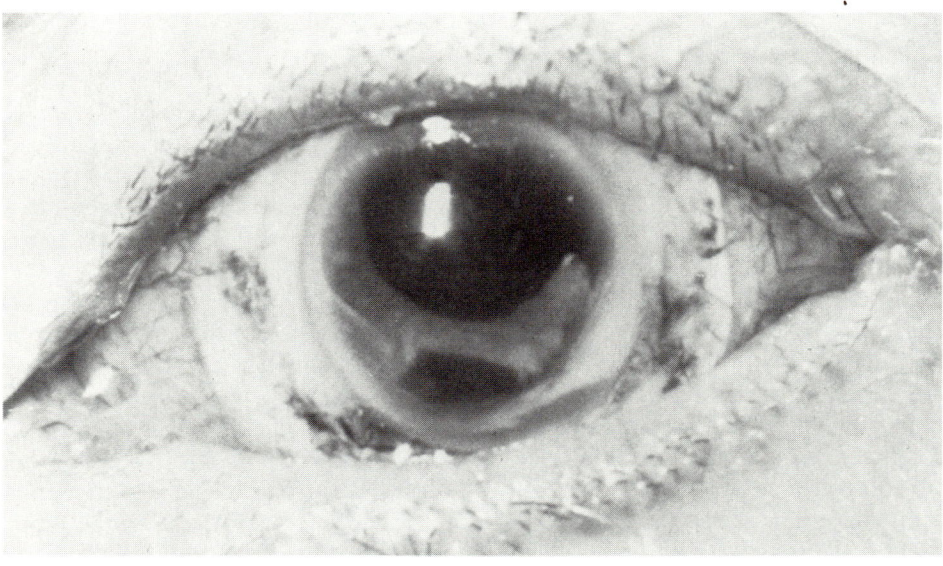

b

Fig. 2.4   a, photograph of the eye of a patient in which a severe bacterial ulceration has destroyed nearly all corneal tissue. **b,** photograph of the same eye 10 months following corneoscleral 'cap' or 'crown' graft, lens extraction and iridectomy. Note the scleral host-graft incision site 3–4 mm beyond the limbus.

Recurrent pterygia are difficult to manage. Often, the scarring resulting from a primary excision may be made worse if exposure to wind, dust or sunlight continues. The cicatricial mass may tether the globe and restrict abduction or other ocular movements. Malposition of eyelids can occur and exposure changes develop. In a high percentage of cases, surgery in this situation is followed by yet another recurrence, and the patient may be worse off than if a second surgery had never been attempted.

A newer technique that is gaining acceptance involves a multi-faceted approach recognising currently accepted concepts of the genesis of pterygium. First, the pterygium is removed and corneal contour smoothed. If there has been extensive scarring, as with most recurrent pterygia, removal of as much of the cicatrix as possible is accomplished. Scarring may involve the medial rectus, so care must be taken to avoid disinserting its attachment to the globe. Isolating the insertion with a muscle hook and separating if from scar facilitate this manoeuvre. Decreasing the mass of the scar is essential, but wherever possible the conjunctiva should be retained; perhaps only 1–2 mm of the pterygium head will be excised from the conjunctiva. Bleeding is controlled with wet-field (radio frequency) cautery. Beta irradiation to the bare sclera during the operation is advisable. Then, a section of conjunctiva from the same eye or the opposite eye, preferably from a portion of the globe near the limbus, is transplanted into the area of the excised pterygium. Edges of this conjunctiva are sutured to the recessed edges of excised pterygium on one side and to the limbus on the other. This provides a normal barrier to regrowth of the pterygium and frees the restriction of ocular motility from the scar, and the cauterisation and radiation inhibit feeder vessels and further cicatrisation. Advantages of this approach are its relatively low recurrence rate and potential for producing an excellent cosmetic result (Fig. 2.5).

Some ophthalmologists have advocated corneoscleral grafts produced by either free-hand dissection or trephination to bridge the area of pterygium excision and replace that tissue destroyed or removed from previous excisions. Production of a more normal limbal contour is thought to be a barrier to pterygium regrowth (King & Wadsworth, 1981). This technique is best reserved for cases where corneal thickness has been reduced to less than one-half of normal following previous surgeries.

Conjunctival surgery

Surgery of the conjunctiva is being revived by oculoplastic surgeons and ophthalmologists who deal with anterior segment reconstruction. As mentioned above, autoplastic conjunctival grafting is often necessary for treatment of conditions where there has been focal loss of conjunctival tissue. Movement of conjunctiva as a flap can be accomplished without completely severing it, which has the advantage of leaving its blood supply intact. There is often insufficient tissue, however, to permit such translocation without significantly interfering with the structure of function elsewhere. In such cases, a free graft of conjunctiva may be severed from its original blood supply and placed in a new location with a high probability that the graft will survive (Thoft, 1983). These grafts can be taken from one eye and moved to the other of the same patient with equally high degrees of success.

The advantages of conjunctival transplantation are several. First, a defect can be repaired and tissues brought back to a more normal configuration than if they were left to epithelialise. Transplanted conjunctiva contains goblet cells which contribute mucus, so an eye with transplanted conjunctiva has improved surface lubrication. In

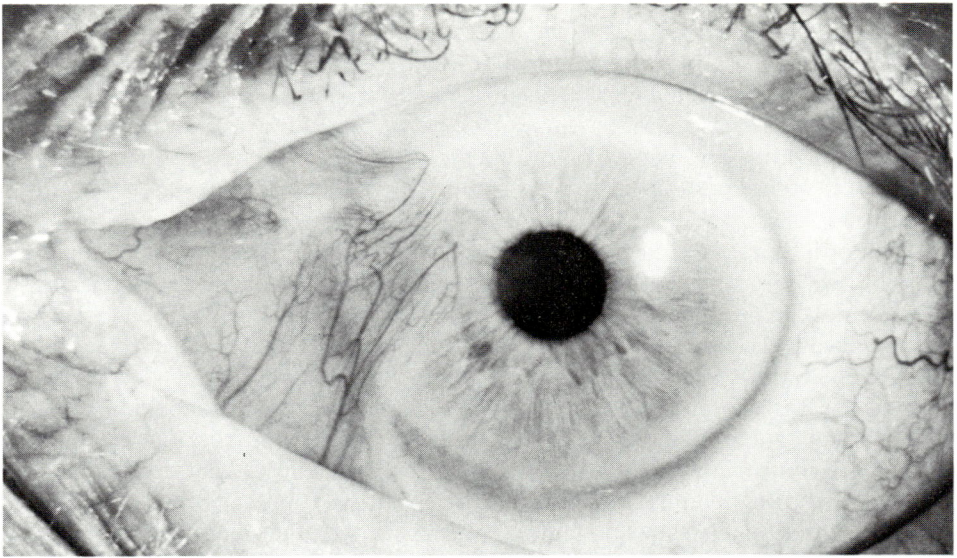

a

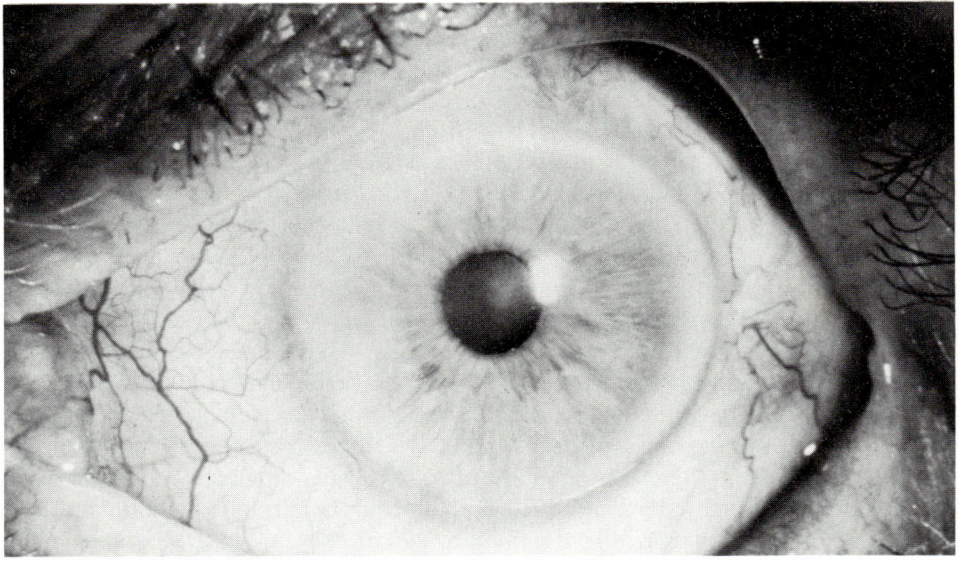

b

Fig. 2.5   a, photograph of a patient with a recurrent pterygium. **b,** photograph of the same patient 7 weeks following pterygium excision combined with beta irradiation and conjunctival graft.

such conditions as alkali burns, this is extremely important and conjunctival transplantation therefore becomes a valuable tool (Thoft, 1983).

Conjunctival banking has made homoplastic conjunctival transplantation possible. Although tried in the past, it is being revived with greater success using new ocular tissue preservation techniques (Thoft, 1982).

Recession of conjunctival tissues, for example, to reform a fornix in ocular pemphigoid, has advantages. Often, these patients may be improved, and the health of the ocular suface maintained for years by retarding the formation of ankylosing symblepharon. Covering the cut edges of conjunctiva with a barrier, such as thin cellophane wrap, may inhibit the formation of scar between cut surfaces while epithelialisation is occurring.

THE INFLUENCE OF NEW INSTRUMENTS AND TECHNOLOGY

Tissue adhesives

Manufacturers of surgical materials have recently investigated the possibility of substituting tissue adhesives for sutures in certain types of wound closure. This has not become popular, however, and tissue adhesives have not become widely distributed. Nevertheless, cyanoacrylate tissue adhesive has been found useful in many anterior segment ocular problems.

Cyanoacrylate is irritating to intraocular structures; contact with uveal structures and the lens should be avoided. The adhesive, once dry and hardened, becomes a barrier to inflammatory cell infiltration and may be retained on surface ocular structures for weeks or months (Kenyon et al, 1979). It is particularly helpful in this regard for patching areas of corneal melting, as in rheumatoid arthritis patients. The cyanoacrylate adhesive also has antimicrobial properties and inhibits the spread of microbes in cases of corneal ulceration (Hyndiuk et al, 1983).

Should a hole develop in the cornea, cyanoacrylate adhesive can be applied to temporarily close the defect (Kinyoun et al, 1974). This has many potential advantages. In patients who are unable to withstand surgery, sealing a tissue defect can re-establish a watertight intraocular atmosphere and prevent serious complications or loss of the eye. Performing penetrating keratoplasty on a soft open eye is difficult and prone to irregularities in the trephination process; sealing the leak with cyanoacrylate adhesive permits reformation of intraocular pressure, and trephination is therefore easier. In cases of corneal melting, application of cyanoacrylate to a small perforation may be followed in 6–10 weeks by healing behind the plug of adhesive, and surgery may not be required. As fibrovascular tissue grows beneath the adhesive, the material spontaneously sloughs leaving a sealed wound which is often re-epithelialised.

In nearly every case of tissue adhesive application, the surface of the dried material is extremely hard and irritating. A bandage soft contact lens must be applied to cover the cornea so the patient can tolerate the glue.

Cutting devices

In the past decade, great advances have been made through technological improvements in manufacturing knives and cutting devices. Available to a limited degree in the past, diamond and ruby knives are now more accessible and widely used in surgical practice. Both are extremely hard materials which retain their sharpness, but ruby has the advantage of being less expensive and can be manufactured in a larger variety of shapes. Diamond blades are manufactured as straight knives or are attached to a footplate and micrometer advancement gauge which permits accurate adjustment of the cutting depth desired. These knives are particularly useful in radial ketatotomy or in making corneal or scleral incisions, particularly those for refractive purposes. Motorised knives are advocated by several anterior segment surgeons. Rotary trephines attached to an electrical motor drive unit permit the surgeon to apply less pressure on an eye during the trephination process. Several of those presently manufactured, however, are bulky and interfere with the surgeon's view of the eye during trephination, which is seen by many to be a disadvantage and an unnecessary added danger.

The microelectrokeratome, as discussed above in the section on keratomileusis, is a tool based on the principle of the carpenter's plane but must be used in conjunction with a suction ring fixation device. The suction ring has one or two dovetail grooves through which the microkeratome slides. Suction rings of various heights allow a greater or lesser amount of cornea to vault through its central opening, and the diameter of the corneal resection can thereby be controlled. The microelectro-keratome head itself cointains an oscillating knife which protrudes beneath its surface. A spacer is placed between the microkeratome head and the blade to vary the amount of protuberance of this blade, which determines the thickness of the tissue resected from the cornea. Thus, a corneal resection of precise thickness and diameter can be produced with this combination of instruments (Barraquer, 1970).

The microelectrokeratome has disadvantages and is dangerous in inexperienced hands. Although the suction ring is applied for a few seconds or minutes only, intraocular pressure increases to 65 mm Hg in the process. To date, there have been no serious consequences, such as central retinal artery or vein occlusion, resulting from suction ring use. Errors in preparing the microkeratome head or selection of the proper ring may result in perforation into the anterior chamber or irregular resections. For these reasons, practice with the suction and microelectrokeratome in the laboratory is advocated before utilising it on patients.

Corneascopes

The photokeratoscope was devised over a decade ago for evaluating corneas when fitting contact lenses. This instrument was designed to measure corneal curvature over an area much larger than the 3–4 mm of central cornea covered by standard keratometry and permitted determination of mid-peripheral corneal curvatures to aid in prescribing intermediate and peripheral bevels on a contact lens. However, it met with limited acceptance and its role was not expanded for purposes other than contact lens fitting.

As research and application into the various refractive corneal procedures expand, an understanding of the role of peripheral corneal curvature becomes essential. The corneascope is designed to satisfy this need and is, to date, one of the best clinical tools for evaluating corneal topography (Rowsey et al, 1981). Similar to the photokerato-scope, the corneascope projects a series of concentric rings of light onto the cornea and their reflection from the corneal surface is photographed. Using a computer, the examiner may determine the radius of curvature of the cornea in a specific meridian and position relative to the central cornea or limbus. The image is somewhat like that produced by a placido disc but can be photographed for later reference. Corneal distortion in positions not measured with standard keratometry can be detected. This tool is valuable for evaluating the course of healing following corneal refractive surgery and for determining, in a research sense, the changes produced by a given procedure. In addition, the cataract or corneal surgeon can determine which sutures are distorting the corneal contour and selectively remove the offending stitch. Corneal astigmatism may therefore be titrated to a minimal amount.

Computers

Analysis of anterior segment contour, even with corneascopes and photographs, can be a time consuming process. When computers are applied to analyse data of corneascope photographs, an evaluation of corneal topography is more rapid and can be projected onto a television screen in simulated three-dimension display. The image can then be rotated and viewed from various angles. Furthermore, a statistical comparison of changes in corneal contour in a given patient or in a series of patients is possible in a relatively easy fashion using the computer.

Rapid computation of data using a printer-calculator or computer has made the Barraquer cryolathe procedures possible. In the operating room, the surgeon enters the parameters of the patient's refractive requirements, and the computer quickly provides the new corneal curvature to which the resected disc must be modified to provide this power change. In a matter of seconds, the surgeon can resect a portion of the patient's cornea, freeze it on the cryolathe, and generate a new curvature, but this is possible intraoperatively only if the computer is available.

Predictive data for determination of intraocular lens power has become possible and easier by using computers of one form or another. Of course, A-scan ultrasonic biometry is an essential part of the intraocular lens power determination process, but computers have refined accuracy and precision. Given axial length and corneal curvatures, the computer can quickly provide the surgeon with the information necessary to insert an anterior or posterior chamber lens of proper power.

Thus, computers have influenced anterior segment surgery to a great degree. They have provided the means for widespread use of operations which would not be possible otherwise.

Now, computers are utilised not only for predicting and determining certain parameters preoperatively and data analysis post-operatively but are being adapted for diagnostic uses in a clinical sense as well. Use of computers has become firmly entrenched in modern ophthalmic practice and will continue to play an even more important role in the future. The anterior segment surgeon would do well therefore to become familiar with the mechanics and use of computers in his practice.

REFERENCES

Barraquer J I (ed) 1970 Queratoplastia refractiva. Volume I. Instituto Barraquer de America, Bogotá
Barraquer J I 1981 Keratomileusis for myopia and aphakia. Ophthalmology 88: 701–708
Christensen L 1964 Corneoscleroplasty with scalpel. Transactions of the Pacific Coast Oto-Ophthalmological Society 45: 323–345
Fine M 1980 Graft astigmatism: prevention and correction. In: Symposium on medical and surgical diseases of the cornea. Transactions of the New Orleans Academy of Ophthalmology, C V Mosby, Saint Louis, p 562–570

Fraunfelder F T (ed) 1982 Drug-induced ocular side effects and drug interactions, 2nd edn, Lea and Febiger, Philadelphia

Friedlander M H, Rich L F, Werblin T P, Kaufman H E, Granet N 1980 Keratophakia using preserved lenticules. Ophthalmology 87: 687–692

Hyndiuk R A, Nassif K F, Burd E M 1983 Infectious diseases. Bacterial diseases. In: Smolin G, Thoft R A (eds) The cornea, Little, Brown and Company, Boston, p 147–167

Jaffe N S 1981 Cataract surgery and its complications, 3rd edn. C V Mosby, Saint Louis, p 92–110

Kaufman H E 1980 The correction of aphakia. American Journal of Ophthalmology 89: 1–10

Kaufman H E, Robbins J E, Capella J A 1965 The endothelium in normal and abnormal corneas. Ophthalmology 69: 931–936

Kenyon K R, Berman M B, Hanninen L A 1979 Tissue adhesive prevents ulceration and inhibits inflammation in the thermal burned rabbit cornea. Investigative Ophthalmology Visual Sciences 18 (Suppl): 1196–1199

King J H, Wadsworth J A C 1981 An atlas of ophthalmic surgery, 3rd edn, J B Lippincott, Philadelphia, p 314–320

Kinyoun J L, Hyndiuk R A, Hull D S 1974 Treatment of corneal perforations with cyanoacrylate. Wisconsin Medical Journal 73 (Suppl): 117–119

Koester C J, Roberts C W, Donn A, Hoefle F B 1980 Wide field specular microscopy. Clinical and research applications. Ophthalmology 87: 849–860

Kramer S G 1981 Cystoid macular edema after aphakic penetrating keratoplasty. Ophthalmology 8: 782–787

Lerman S 1982 Direct and photosensitized UV radiation and the eye: experimental and clinical observations. Metabolic, Pediatric and Systemic Ophthalmology 6: 27–32

Maurice D M 1968 Cellular membrane activity in the corneal endothelium of the intact eye. Experientia 24: 1094–1095

McNeill J I, Kaufman H E 1978 Early visual rehabilitation after keratoplasty: a double running suture technique. Annals of Ophthalmology 10: 652–655

Nordan L T 1983 Current status of refractive surgery, C L Printing, San Diego, p 49–52

Olson R J 1981 The effect of scleral fixation ring placement and trephine tilting on keratoplasty wound size and donor shape. Ophthalmic Surgery 12: 23–26

Paton D 1975 Pterygium management based upon a theory of pathogenesis. Transactions of the American Academy of Ophthalmology and Otolaryngology 79: 603–614

Polack F M 1983 Atlas of corneal pathology, Masson, New York, p 28

Rao G N, Shaw E L, Arthur E J, Aquavella J V 1979 Endothelial cell morphology and corneal deturgescence. Annals of Ophthalmology 11: 885–899

Rich L F 1981 Epikeratophakia. Transactions of the Pacific Coast Oto-Ophthalmological Society 62: 161–169

Rich L F 1983 Toxic drug effects on the cornea. Journal of Toxicology 1: 267–297

Rowsey J J, Reynolds A E, Brown R 1981 Corneal topography corneascope. Archives of Ophthalmology 99: 1093–1100

Schachar R A, Black T D, Huang T 1981 Understanding radial keratotomy, LAL Publishing, Denison

Thoft R A 1982 Indications for conjunctival transplantation. Ophthalmology 89: 335–339

Thoft R A 1983 Conjunctival surgery for corneal disease. In: Smolin G, Thoft R A (eds) The cornea, Little, Brown and Company, Boston, p 465–476

Troutman R C 1974 Microsurgery of the anterior segment of the eye. Volume I. Introduction and basic techniques, C V Mosby, Saint Louis, p 194

Troutman R C 1977 Microsurgery of the anterior segment of the eye. Volume II. The cornea: optics and surgery, C V Mosby, Saint Louis, p 266–283

Troutman R C, Gaster R N 1980 Combined keratoplasty techniques. In: Symposium on medical and surgical diseases of the cornea, Transactions of the New Orleans Academy of Ophthalmology, C V Mosby, Saint Louis, p 284–312

3. The use of viscous and viscoelastic substances in ophthalmology

G. Eisner

SURGICAL TACTICS IN OPHTHALMIC MICROSURGERY

The development of modern microsurgery has changed ophthalmic surgery in many ways. Microsurgery is not confined to the use of higher magnification and miniaturised instruments; it requires entirely new surgical tactics. A manipulation formerly executed with great skill in a straightforward manner is now subdivided into multiple micromanipulations which allow much better control over the tissues to be treated. But the increasing number of surgical actions also involves a greater risk of involuntary tissue damage. The field of microsurgical strategy therefore is not only the desired action on the tissue ('offensive strategy'), but also the prevention of undesired side effects ('defensive strategy') on the surrounding tissue.

The offensive tactics can be summarised as tissue-tactics and comprise classical surgery with forceps, knives and sutures. The more recent defensive tactics can be subdivided into surface- and space-tactics. *Surface-tactics* is a passive defence of tissue surfaces against touch by instruments, implants or other tissues and is accomplished by covering the surfaces with protecting agents (e.g. plastic sheets or viscous layers). *Space-tactics* is a more active protection against touch by providing sufficient space for manipulations within the eye. It is accomplished by space maintaining or enlarging devices such as hydrodynamic flow systems, gas, oil or viscoelastic substances (Figs. 3.1 and 3.2).

CRITERIA FOR THE SELECTION OF VISCOUS OR VISCOELASTIC MATERIAL

Physical properties

Optical properties
Substances suitable for intraocular use should not impair the visibility of the operation field. Transparency, therefore, is a primary prerequisite. Further, the index of refraction should not deviate much from that of aqueous in order to avoid distortion and changes of spatial orientation in the field. A colour slightly different from aqueous is useful for easier distinction between the injected substance and the transparent contents of the eye.

Surface tension
If there is a difference in phase (e.g. gas) or water solubility (e.g. silicon oil) surface tension phenomena occur at the interface between the injected material and aqueous. The surface acts as a membrane which can be used as a surgical tool for sealing pathways or separating tissue layers. The enclosed material tends to assume the shape

Surgical tactics in ophthalmology		Tactical goals	Targets of surgical action	Instruments
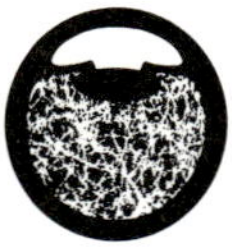 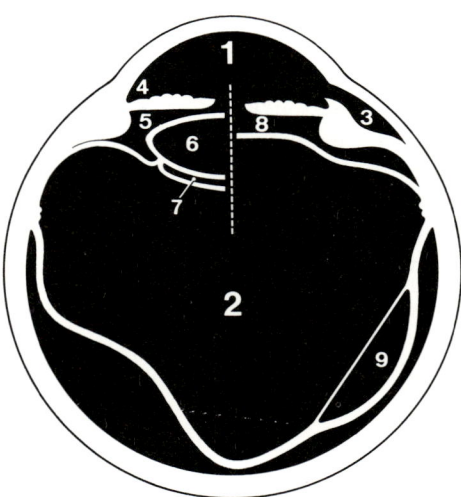	Tissue tactics	Sectioning Removal } of tissue Uniting	Cornea Iris Lens Vitreous Retina	Knives Forceps Sutures
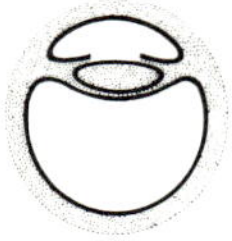	Surface tactics	Protection of surfaces	Endothelium Lens capsule Anterior hyaloid Inner limiting membrane	Viscous fluids Plastic sheets
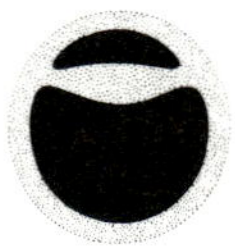	Spatial tactics	Maintenance or expansion of intraocular compartments Blockade of connecting pathways	Intraocular chambers and subcompartments (see Fig. 3.2)	Hydrodynamical flow systems Viscoelastic fluids Bubbles with surface "membranes" (gas, oil)

Fig. 3.1 Surgical tactics in ophthalmology.

Fig. 3.2 The intraocular spaces and their subcompartments: 1 Anterior chamber; 2 Vitreous space; 3 Sclero-uveal interspace; 4 Irido-corneal sinus ('chamber angle'); 5 Irido-capsular space; 6 Intercapsular sinus; 7 Hyalocapsular interspace; 8 Irido-hyaloidal space; 9 Vitreoretinal interspace.

of a sphere which can be used to form or to restore spherical shapes of the surrounding tissues. The specific weight of the injected material determines whether the bubble will raise or descend in aqueous and whether it can be used to elevate or to depress the surrounding tissue. Otherwise, the chemical composition of the bubble content is of interest only in as far as the time of absorption is concerned, that is, whether the injected material will have short or long lasting effect. Based on these principles, specific tactics can be developed for surgery with bubbles; but this is beyond the scope of this paper that is confined only to the tactical use of materials without surface tension effects.

Viscosity

Watery fluids and viscous fluids differ in their internal friction and, hence, in their velocity of flow. Their action as surface or space tactical tools is based on the relation between the rate of inflow and outflow. The higher the velocity of flow, the more demanding is the control of the flow system by the surgeon (Fig. 3.3a). Conversely, slow flow velocity is a stabilising factor in surgery. Viscous fluids are ideal surface tactical tools, since layers deposited on to tissue or implant surface will remain there. As space tactical tools, however, their usefulness depends on the outflow resistance that for a given viscosity in turn depends on the size of the outflow orifice (Fig. 3.3b). In other words: As space tactical tools viscous fluids are suitable in walled off cavities

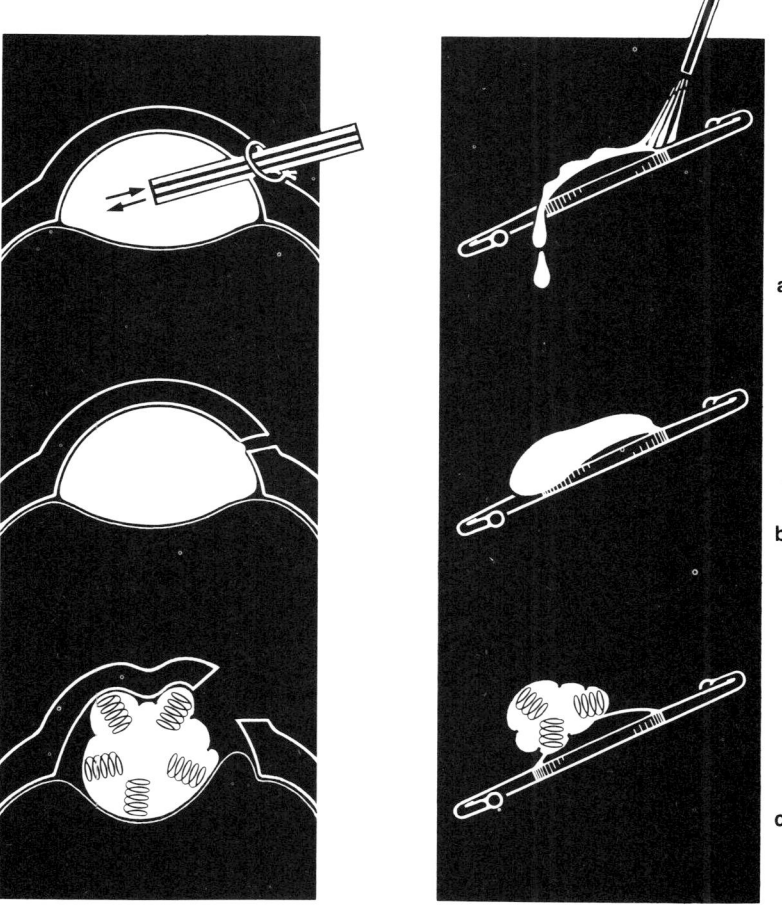

Fig. 3.3 Surface and space tactical use of liquids, viscous and viscoelastic substances. Left = space tactics; right = surface tactics. **a** Liquids. The efficiency of liquids as space tactical tools depends on a strict control of inflow and outflow (closed chamber, monitoring of in- and outflow volumes). In surface tactics a continuous flow is necessary. **b** Viscous material. In space tactics viscous material is efficient when the outflow orifice is small enough to build up sufficient resistance. In surface protection it forms even layers on tissue surfaces or implants and is an ideal coating agent. **c** Viscoelastic material. As a space expander viscoelastic material is independent of outflow conditions and hence suitable even in open chambers or subcompartments. Applied on surfaces it maintains a stable irregular shape and is easily wiped off when touching an obstacle.

with small orifices (e.g. anterior chamber) but they are inefficient space expanders in open intraocular subcompartments.

Elasticity

Elastic materials are resistant against deformation and therefore stable as to their shape. They are ideal space tactical tools since their action is independent of flow conditions. They are excellent space expanders in open cavities and subcompartments, actually, wherever they are applied. Conversely, they are less useful as surface tactical tools. On account of the stability of their shape, they do not spread into covering layers but remain prominent plugs that are easily ripped off a surface (Fig. 3.3c).

Viscoelasticity

While viscous and elastic materials belong to two different physical categories (Fig. 3.4) and have therefore different modes of action (Fig. 3.5), in many substances both

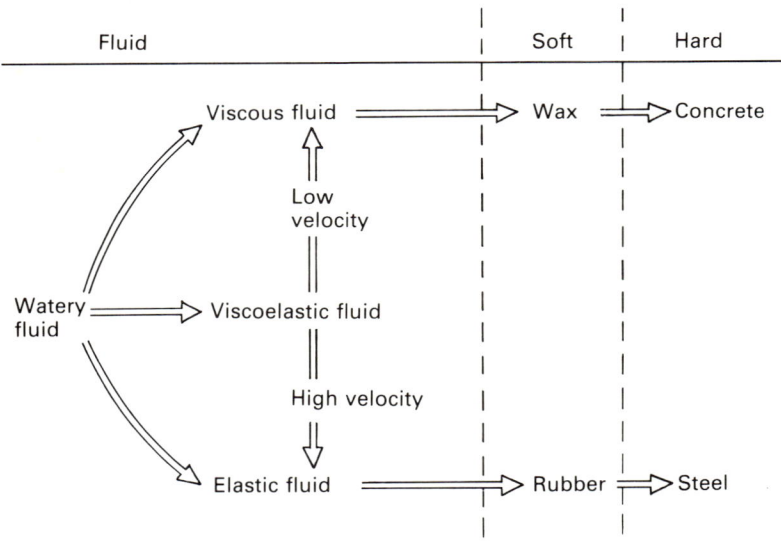

Fig. 3.4   Simplified schema of viscous and elastic behaviour.

properties occur concomitantly. In viscoelastic solutions, the viscous and elastic responses to a mechanical force depend on the velocity of the impact. At slow velocities the molecules can rearrange their configuration and respond with viscous flow. At high velocity of impact, the rearrangement cannot occur, the molecular chains deform, and the mechanical energy is stored as elasticity. The optimal solution for surgical purposes is a substance with a transition from viscous to elastic behaviour at relatively low velocities. However, if solid bodies are moved through such substances above the critical velocities, forces are transmitted to surrounding tissue surfaces which may disrupt cellular connections. Therefore, abrupt motions of tissue, instruments or implants near surfaces covered with viscoelastic material should be avoided.

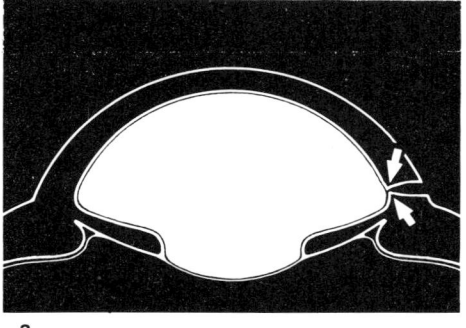
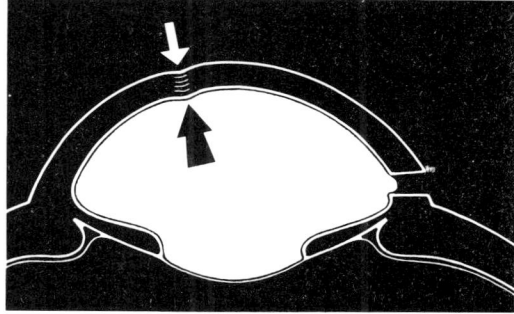

a   b

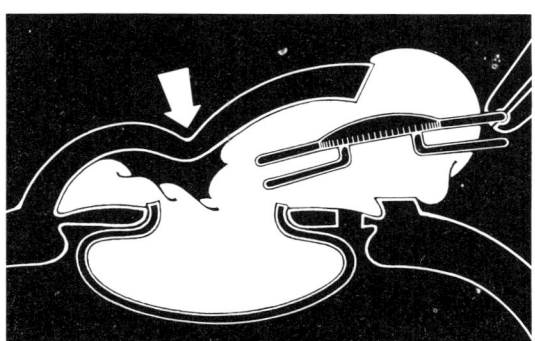

c

Fig. 3.5 The viscous and the elastic mode of preserving anterior chamber depth against vitreous pressure. **a** The viscous mode. The counterpressure against the vitreous is determined by the outflow resistance at the orifice (arrows) and this in turn by the degree of viscosity. **b** The elastic mode. The counterpressure is determined by the resistance against the deformation of the cornea through the hinge fold. The formation of this fold is a prerequisite for the gaping a limbal incision (see Eisner, 1980). The force against the deformation of the cornea is provided by the elasticity of the corneal tissue in case of a chamber containing aqueous. This natural resistance is reinforced by the elasticity of the viscoelastic bolus (broad arrow). **c** Preventing the elastic mode of 'wound closure'. If, conversely, viscoelastic material is used for the purpose of keeping an incision open (e.g. for introduction of an implant without touching the wound edges with instruments), no viscous material should be deposited (arrow) where the cornea is going to form the hinge fold (that is, underneath the imaginary line connecting the two ends of the limbal incision).

Chemical properties

As far as surface or space tactical purposes are concerned, the usefulness of a substance depends mainly on its physical properties. The chemical composition is of interest only with regard to the tolerance within the eye: non-toxic, non-allergenic, reabsorption without inflammation, and no interference with wound healing.

General considerations

Generally speaking one may assume that natural compounds of human tissue such as sodium hyaluronate or chondroitin sulphate will meet the criteria for biological tolerance better than artificial compounds (e.g. methylcellulose). When reviewing clinical reports on favourable results, one has to bear in mind, however, that some of the criteria are dose dependent; when used at low concentrations or in small amounts, clinical safety may look satisfactory for substances that perhaps would not stand highly elaborate tests.

The lower the concentration of molecules used to obtain high viscosity the better the tolerance, because osmolarity is low. Viscous material with a high concentration and hence high osmolarity has been shown to dehydrate the adjoining tissue (McRae et al, 1983).

Hyaluronic acid

Hyaluronic acid is a natural compound of connective tissue. In the ocular cavities it is a major component of the vitreous and occurs as a covering layer on the tissue surfaces of the anterior segment (Laurent, 1982). Therefore, when hyaluronic acid is used as a surgical tool, the condition of the eye deviates from normal only in a temporarily increased concentration of hyaluronic acid at a specific location.

Hyaluronic acid is not metabolised or degraded within the eye. Most likely it passes unaltered through the trabecular meshwork as a large molecule (still being smaller than blood cells), and is transported then with the blood flow to the liver (Frazer et al, 1981). Hyaluronic acid is a linear polysaccharide composed of sodium glucuronate and N-acetyl-glucosamine. The chain is unbranched and contains no covalent inter-molecular bridges. In physiological salt solution the molecules form very flexible long random coils that contain much water in their spongelike interstices. As the concentration is increased, the molecular coils start to overlap and are compressed. Chain-chain interactions occur, and the viscosity increases steeply (e.g. a five fold increase in concentration cause a 1000 fold increase in viscosity). Concomitantly, the elastic properties of the solution increases.

HEALON

Healon^R is a 1% solution of highly purified sodium hyaluronate from rooster combs. First introduced in 1965 as a vitreous substitute (Balazs & Sweeney, 1965) it had stood the test of time and clinical trial for years when in the seventies the need for surface and space tactical tools for the anterior segment arose. (Miller & Stegmann, 1980; Eisner, 1980, 1981). Healon consists of very large hyaluronic acid chains with molecular weights between 2 to 5×10^6, and has a viscosity as high as 100 to 300×10^3 centistokes. One of its great advantages is that the transition from viscous to elastic behaviour occurs yet at low concentrations and at low velocities. Owing to its elasticity, Healon can be injected easily through a 30-gauge cannula but still retains its original shape in aqueous.

Besides the physical action in surgical tactics there are also biological effects, based on chemical properties: The random coil molecule is highly hydrated. Small molecules can penetrate it but larger molecules (such as fibrinogen, collagen, proteoglycons) are excluded. In vitro, solutions inhibit migration of lymphocytes, granulocytes and macrophages (Comper & Laurent, 1978). Also inhibited is phagocyte activity and the synthesis and release of prostaglandins by macrophages during phagocytosis (Sebag, Balazs & Eakins et al, 1984). However, the movement of fibroblasts and epithelial cells is not inhibited and there is no interference with wound healing (Arzeno & Miller, 1982).

OTHER PREPARATIONS OF HYALURONIC ACID

Other preparations of hyaluronic acid from rooster combs or umbilical cord differ from Healon in the length of the molecular chain. Hence, their viscosity, elasticity and osmolarity is different and accordingly their application as either space or surface tactical tools.

Chondroitin sulphate

Chondroitin sulphate from shark cartilage was introduced in 1980 as a coating for intraocular lenses by Soll et al (1980). Chondroitin sulphate is a natural compound of connective tissue and one of the major glycosaminoglycans of the corneal stroma.

The molecular structure is quite similar to hyaluronic acid with the main difference in the presence of sulphur and double negative charges per molecular subunit (Fig. 3.6).

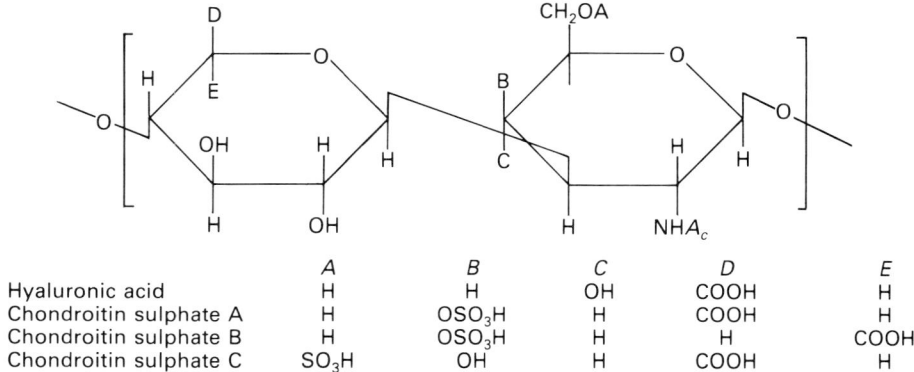

	A	B	C	D	E
Hyaluronic acid	H	H	OH	COOH	H
Chondroitin sulphate A	H	OSO_3H	H	COOH	H
Chondroitin sulphate B	H	OSO_3H	H	H	COOH
Chondroitin sulphate C	SO_3H	OH	H	COOH	H

Fig. 3.6   Related molecular structures of mucopolysaccharides (from Harrison et al, 1982).

This double negative charge is considered advantageous by the promoters, because it might better counter electrostatic fields of instruments or implants. The molecular size of the chondroitin sulphate preparation CDS™ Cilco is 5 to 100×10^3. The molecule thus being much smaller than hyaluronic acid, the concentrations needed to obtain similar viscosities are much higher and so are the resulting osmolarities.

Twenty per cent of CDS has a viscosity of 150 centistokes and an osmolarity of 636 m Osm; 50% solution of CDS has 3.100 centistokes and an osmolarity of 1666 m Osm. Yet 20% solutions produced reduction in corneal thickness and lens opacities in monkeys (McRae et al, 1983). Being less elastic than hyaluronic acid, 20% chondroitin sulphate needed extremely high pressure to be injected through a 30-gauge cannula and 50% could not pass at all (McRae et al, 1983). Chondroitin sulphate is more a surface than a space tactical tool. Its biological disadvantages may be minimised when using only small quantities for coating.

Methylcellulose
Two per cent Hydroxypropylmethylcellulose (brand name: Methocel E4 premium) was introduced by Fechner in 1976 for coating of intraocular lenses. It is an artificial compound in the eye and there is no experimental analysis as to its biological activity or elimination from the eye and the body. Clinically, however, in a more recent report on 400 implant operations, Fechner did not observe any side effects, beside the pressure increases known to result from all viscous substances.

The main advantage of Methocel is its availability at a low cost. It can be prepared by every pharmacist according to the prescription given by Fechner, and can be autoclaved. It is highly hydrophilic and easily diluted — and therefore easily irrigated from the eye. Being mainly· viscous and barely elastic it is predominantly a surface tactical tool.

INDICATIONS FOR THE USE OF VISCOUS SUBSTANCES

For the protection of tissue surfaces, viscous layers can be applied on to the tissue directly (e.g. endothelium, lens capsule, anterior hyaloid etc.) or, conversely, upon the source of potential damage (e.g. instruments or implants).

The difference between the two methods is the size of surfaces to be coated and hence the quantity of viscous material required for sufficient protection. For covering instruments or implants, only small amounts are necessary. Used in this way, therefore, viscous substances that might be harmful when injected in large quantities, still may turn out to be safe enough.

INDICATIONS FOR THE USE OF VISCOELASTIC MATERIAL

Expansion of intraocular spaces and their subcompartments

Figures 3.7–3.16 show the use of viscoelastic substances as space expanders. Their purpose is to provide sufficient freedom of movement during surgical manoeuvres. In

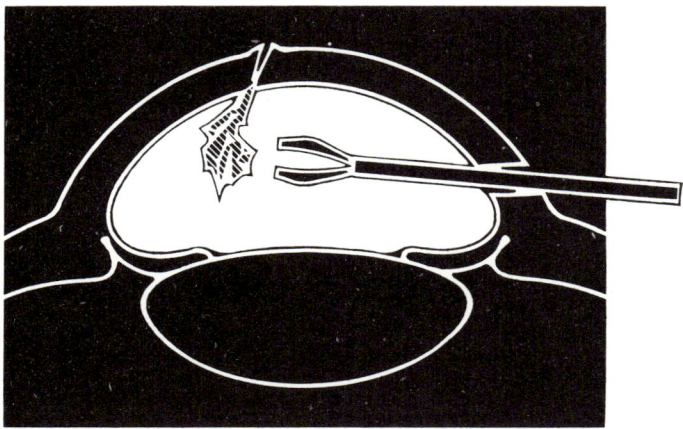

Fig. 3.7   Indications for the expansion of the entire anterior chamber. Protection of endothelium while operating at the iris/lens diaphragm, protection of iris and lens while cutting or trephining the cornea. Overall protection is necessary when extracting a sharp foreign body from the chamber.

this way they protect the surrounding tissue and increase the safety margins for delicate procedures.

Further, the expansion of an intraocular compartment may be used to create counterpressure against a pressure increase in the vicinity. For example, in the pseudophakic eye, viscoelastic material injected into the anterior chamber prior to intravitreal injection of air prevents shallowing and consequent endothelial touch.

Blockade of pathways

Figures 3.17–3.20 show the use of viscoelastic material as obstructing agents. Their purpose is to prevent the shifting of intraocular fluids. On the one hand, they are indicated for preventing the invasion of specific ocular compartments by foreign material (e.g. blood, fluid, lens material, Figures 3.17 and 3.18); on the other hand, the blockade is used to retain the fluids within their original compartment in order to

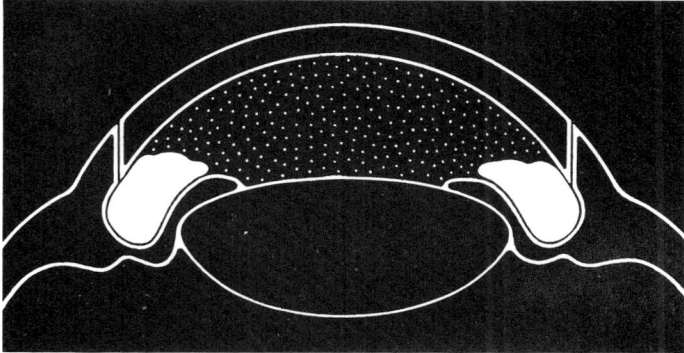

Fig. 3.8 Indications for the expansion of the iridocorneal angle. Removal or prevention of anterior synechiae in keratoplasty with large sized graft or in trauma with peripheral lacerations of the cornea.

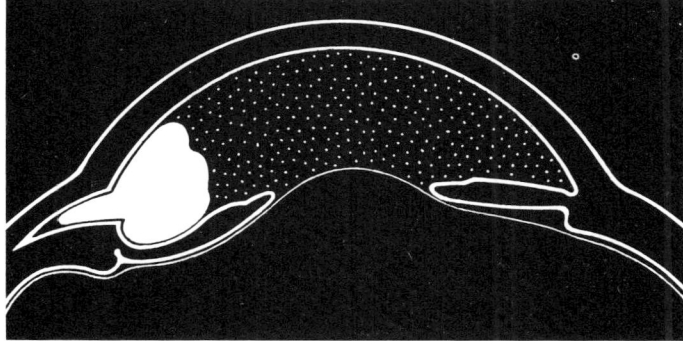

Fig. 3.9 Indications for the expansion of the sclero-uveal interspace. Maintaining patency of cyclodialysis and prevention of haemorrhage.

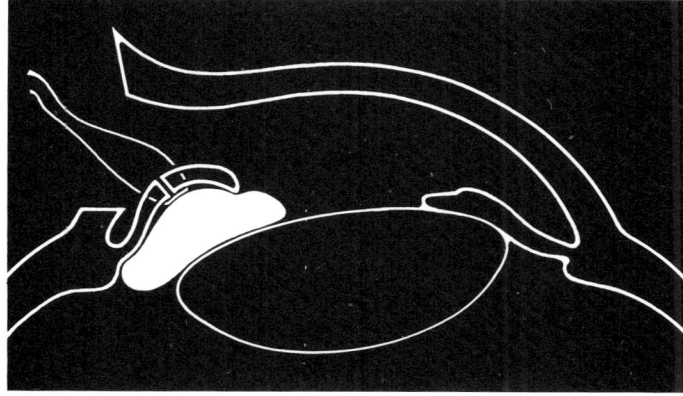

Fig. 3.10 Indication for the expansion of the iridocapsular space. Protection of intact lens during suturing the iris.

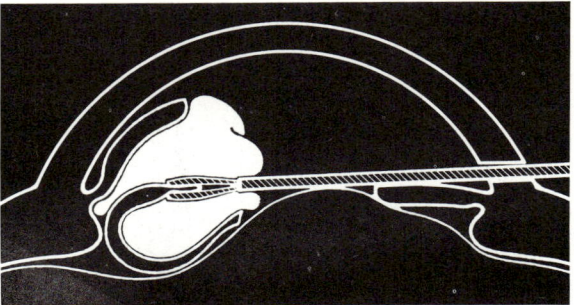

Fig. 3.11   Indications for the expansion of the iridocapsular space and intercapsular sinus. Protection of iris and anterior hyaloid during grasping and removal of capsular remnants.

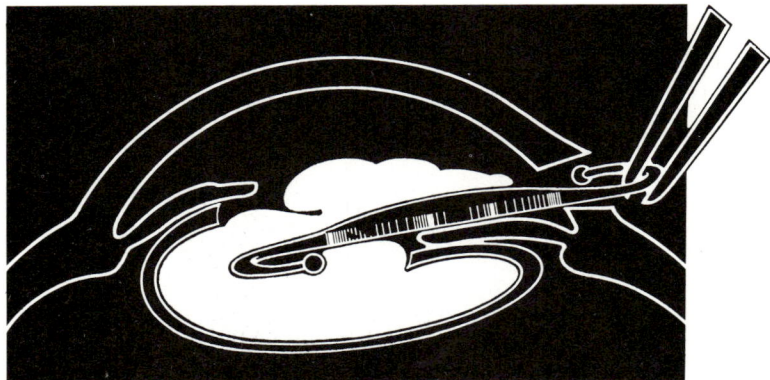

Fig. 3.12   Indications for the expansion of the intercapsular sinus. Facilitating the insertion of implant loops 'into the bag'.

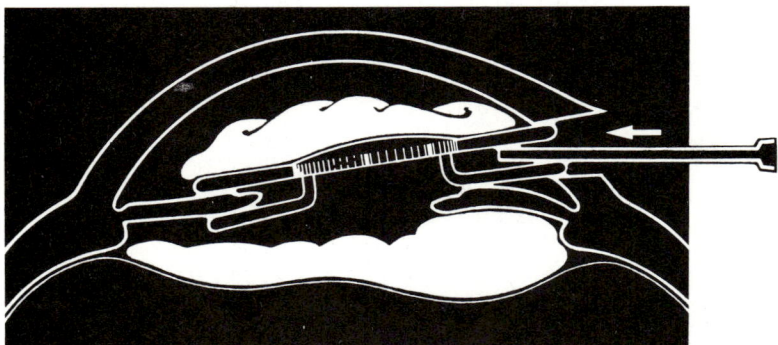

Fig. 3.13   Indications for the expansion of the iridohyaloidal space. Protection of the anterior hyaloid during insertion of implants after intracapsular cataract extraction or during suturing of the iris in aphakia.

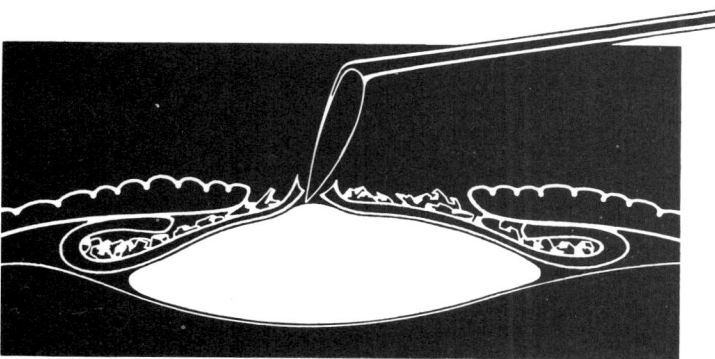

Fig. 3.14 Indications for the expansion of the capsulo-hyaloidal interspace. Protection of the anterior hyaloid during posterior capsulotomy or discision of a secondary cataract.

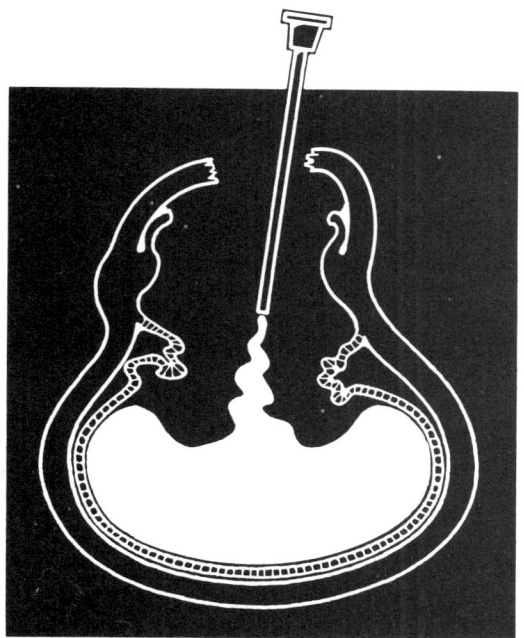

Fig. 3.15 Indications for the injection into the vitreous space. Reshaping of posterior segment and repositioning of folded retina in a collapsed globe.

secure sufficient tension there (e.g. aqueous, vitreous, cortex of the lens, Figures 3.19 and 3.20).

Blockade of the trabecular outflow increases the intraocular pressure. Therapeutically this can be used in various conditions of acute or chronic hypotony. Further, it can be used for a pressure increase prior to enucleation for malignant melanoma. According to Sudarsky et al (1981) pressures about 100 mmHg provoke collapse of the veins within the tumour and prevent the escape of malignant cells from the globe during the surgical manoeuvres.

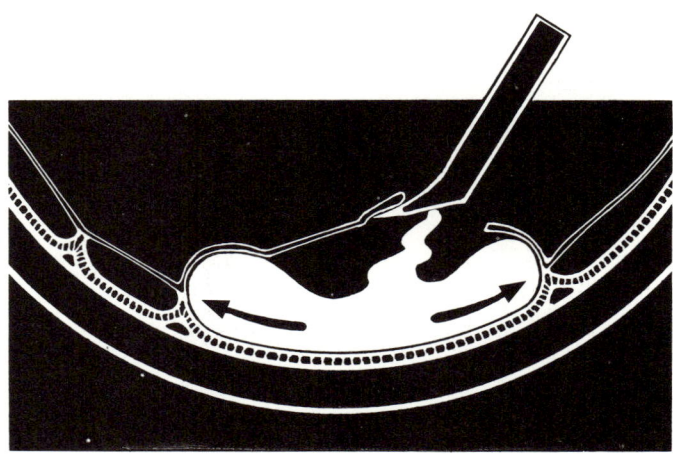

Fig. 3.16 Indications for the expansion of the vitreoretinal interspace. Increasing the distance of membranes from the retinal surface in order to facilitate their identification and dissection. *Note.* The main direction of forces applied for lifting the preretinal membranes is parallel to the retinal surface and therefore traction on the retina is minimal.

Irrigation

In contrast to watery fluids, the kinetic energy of viscoelastic material is low, and the control of fluid movements therefore easy. An example for irrigation with slow velocities (Fig. 3.21) is the dislocation of tissue particles or foreign bodies from hidden places behind the iris towards the pupil. There they can be grasped mechanically under visual control and removed safely without risking damage of the surrounding tissue.

Viscoelastic material as a soft spatula

Viscoelastic material can be used to extend or translocate mobile tissue in a very delicate way. It is efficient, however, only when working against low resistance. In case of high resistance the material tends to bypass if there is any way of escape with a lower resistance. For example: Viscoelastic material is ideal for repositioning a dislocated iris or flattening a wrinkled retina. However, it will not break strong fibrinous or fibrous connections. Only after these are broken by other means, viscoelastic material is useful to keep them separated (space expanding effect).

Viscoelastic substances as buffer

The high internal friction of viscous fluids decreases the velocity of movements. The danger of damage by involuntary movements of instruments or implants hence is decreased.

In an intraocular cavity, foreign bodies remain suspended free and stable, once removed from their original site. There they can be grasped, changed in orientation and regrasped until the optimum position for the evacuation through the incision is obtained.

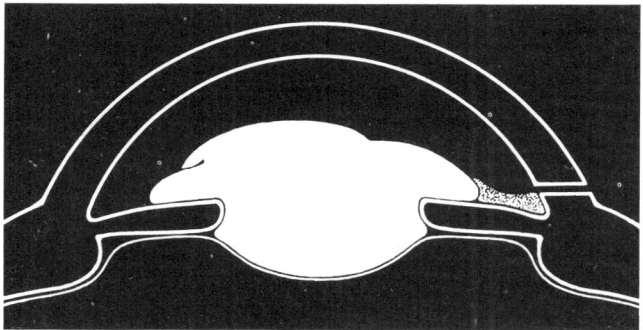

Fig. 3.17 Blockade of intraocular haemorrhage. Blockade of haemorrhage at its source or blockade of pathways through pupil.

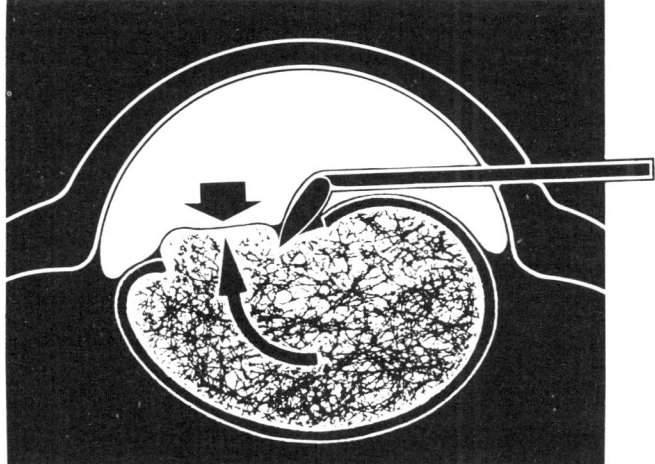

Fig. 3.18 Blockade of capsular incisions in cataracts with fluid cortex. The prevention of a prolapse of fluid cortex through a capsular incision attains two tactical goals: maintaining the tension of capsule necessary for easy dissection and preserving visual control of the operative field.

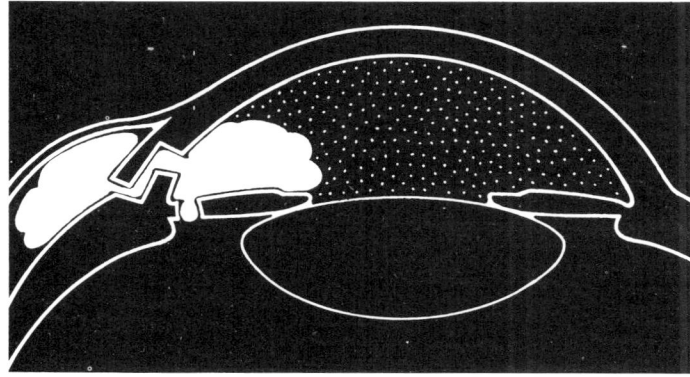

Fig. 3.19 Blockade of early aqueous outflow through filtration fistula in glaucoma in order to maintain anterior chamber postoperatively.

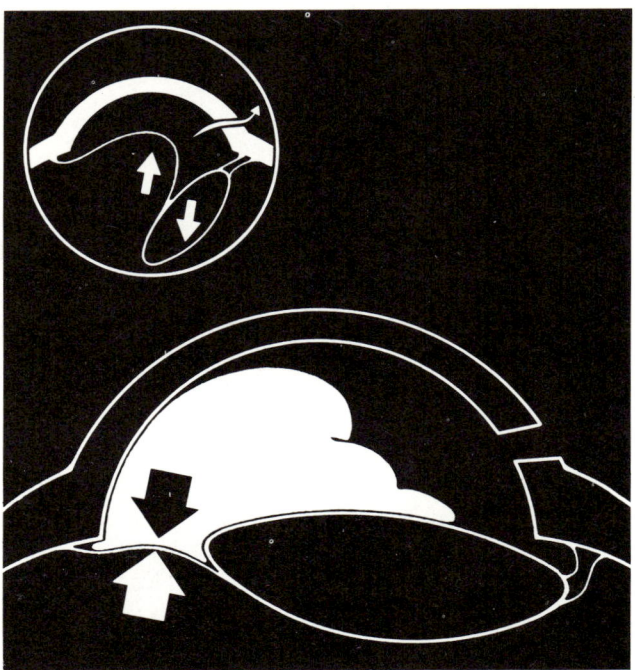

Fig. 3.20   Blockade of vitreous prolapse in case of subluxation of the lens. If on opening the anterior chamber the vitreous prolapses forward through a gap in the zonule, the lens may fall backwards (inset). Blockade of the zonular gap with viscoelastic material is used to prevent the vitreous prolapse and subsequent dislocation of the lens.

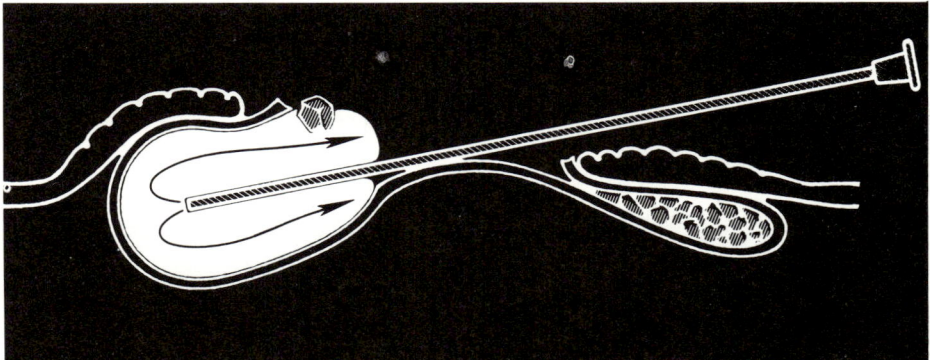

Fig. 3.21   Slow-flow irrigation with viscoelastic material. Foreign body is removed from retroiridal space towards the pupil with well controlled slow irrigation in order to be grasped there under visual control.

Implants that cannot be brought straightforward into their destination on account of an unforeseen obstacle will remain stable in a provisional position. There they can be regrasped, reorientated and then inserted into their final position once the pathways have been cleared.

Further, the decrease in mobility can be exploited for fixation of movable tissue without forceps; iris sutures, for example, can be placed easily through the delicate

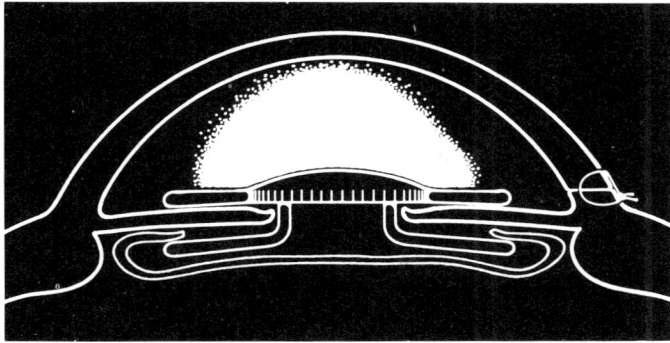

Fig. 3.22   Viscoelastic buffer in front of an implant. Protection of the endothelium in case of postoperative flattening of the anterior chamber. *Note:* The chamber angle has been flushed clean with fluid in order to permit aqueous outflow.

tissue immobilised merely by viscoelastic material. Remnants of anterior capsule flaps can be immobilised in a suitable position for sectioning with microscissors. The buffering action is useful also for stabilising gas or silicon oil. The mobility of the bubbles is decreased and their position is less prone to change with every movement of the patient's head.

The buffering effect can be extended into the postoperative period when a viscoelastic bolus is left in proper position at the end of surgery. Such longlasting buffers may protect the cornea against touch of an implant in unreliable patients (Fig. 3.22) or prevent anterior synechiae in keratoplasty and peripheral corneal wounds (Fig. 3.8).

One has to keep in mind, however, that the chamber angle (or at least the major part of the circumference) should be cleaned of viscoelastic material at the end of the operation in order to prevent an increase in intraocular pressure.

Other indications

Besides intraocular application, viscoelastic substances can be used on the outer eye. The goal again is the coating of tissue surfaces and maintaining patency of interspaces and pathways. Chemical effects such as inhibition of inflammatory reaction are desirable adjuncts.

Healon was used by the author in various conditions of the conjunctiva prone to develop symblepharon (such as Steven-Johnson syndrome, chemical burns), in chronic disease of the corneal surface (such as recurrent erosions, chronic ulcers, dry eye complications) and in obstructions of the lacrimal pathways (recurring adhesions after probing of large stenoses). The results were generally favourable and sometimes even astonishing. But for obvious reasons, no reliable statistical comparisons can be made. We have to rely on clinical impressions and the confirmation of these by others (Reim & Lenz, 1983).

Statistical evaluation is possible only in experimental work. Saric & Reim (1983) studied chemical burns in animal eyes and confirmed the beneficial effect of Healon on the prevention of symblepharon.

TECHNIQUE OF APPLICATION

The application of viscoelastic material differs from that of watery fluids. The latter will spread evenly throughout the whole cavity wherever they are injected, and they are easy to reaspirate. Viscoelastic fluids will stay exactly where put, and if injected to the wrong site they are hard to remove. Examples of specific techniques of application are shown in Figures 3.23–3.29.

Generally speaking, the surgeons should:

— avoid blockading the compensatory outflow of the fluids occupying the space to be filled with viscoelastic substance (Fig. 3.23)

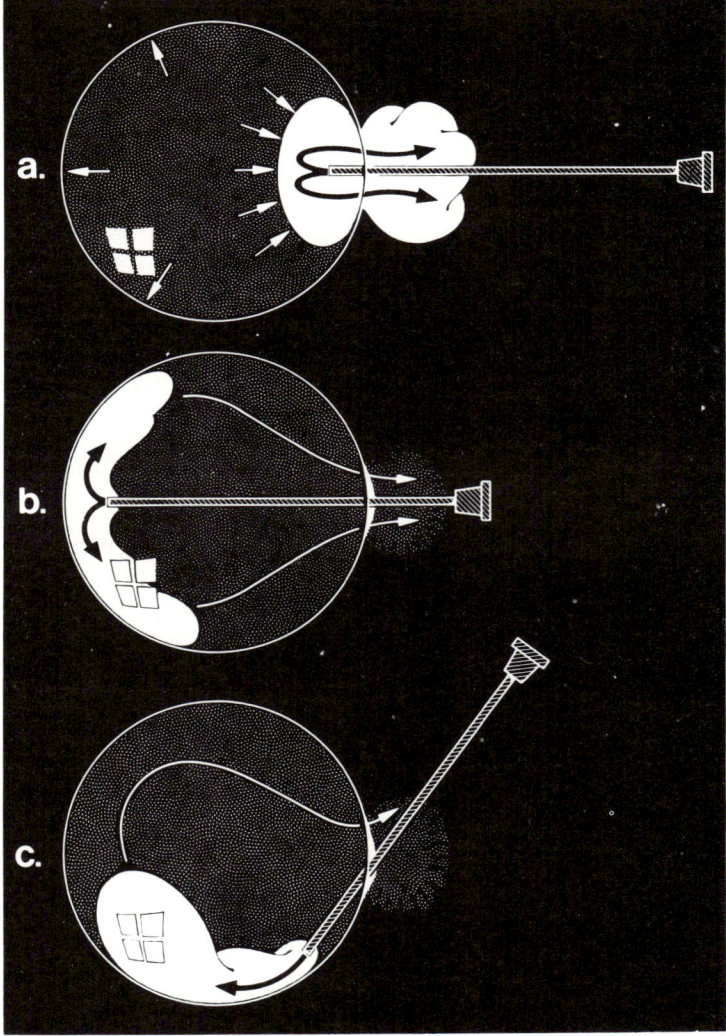

Fig. 3.23   Technique of injection into the anterior chamber through a small orifice. **a** Problem: deposited at the entrance, the viscoelastic bolus obstructs the compensatory outflow of aqueous. If one tries to introduce more viscoelastic material the intraocular pressure will rise and prevent further injection.
b and **c** Solution: beginning the injection opposite the entrance (**b**) or laterally (**c**), leaves the pathways for the outflow of aqueous open.

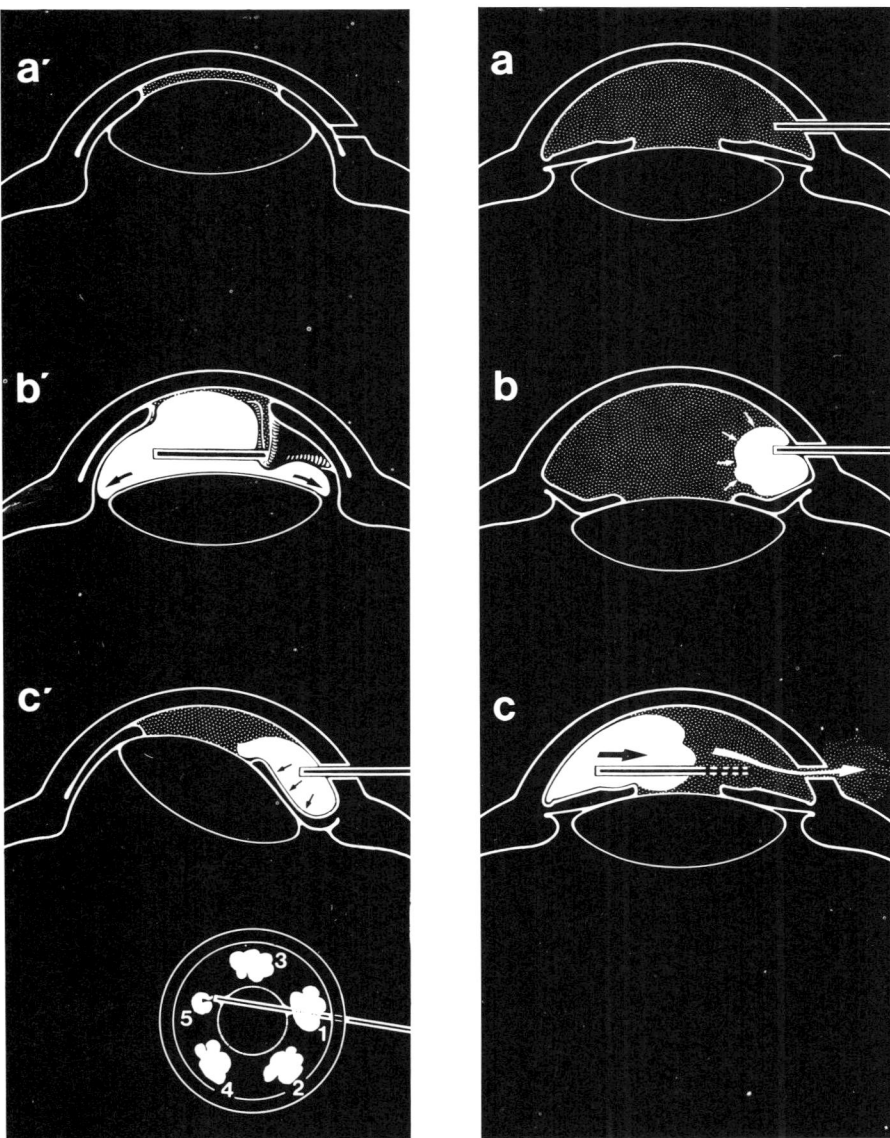

Fig. 3.24   Technique of injection into an empty anterior chamber

Left. **a** Initial situation before injection. **b** Problem: when injecting opposite the entrance — as would be appropriate in a deep chamber — viscoelastic material may penetrate through the pupil behind the iris where it will be difficult to remove later on. **c** Solution: in an empty chamber the injection starts at the entrance since no aqueous outflow is to be provided for. In order to obstruct the pathway into the retro-iridal space, the iris is depressed with a viscoelastic bolus against the lens, starting near the entrance and then continuing with the deposition all around the circumference (1–5). Only then the viscoelastic material is injected directly at the pupil.

Right. Juxtaposition with the injection into a deep chamber in order to show the contrast between the two situations. In the deep chamber it is the injection at the entrance that creates problems (**b**), and the solution is to begin opposite the orifice (**c**).

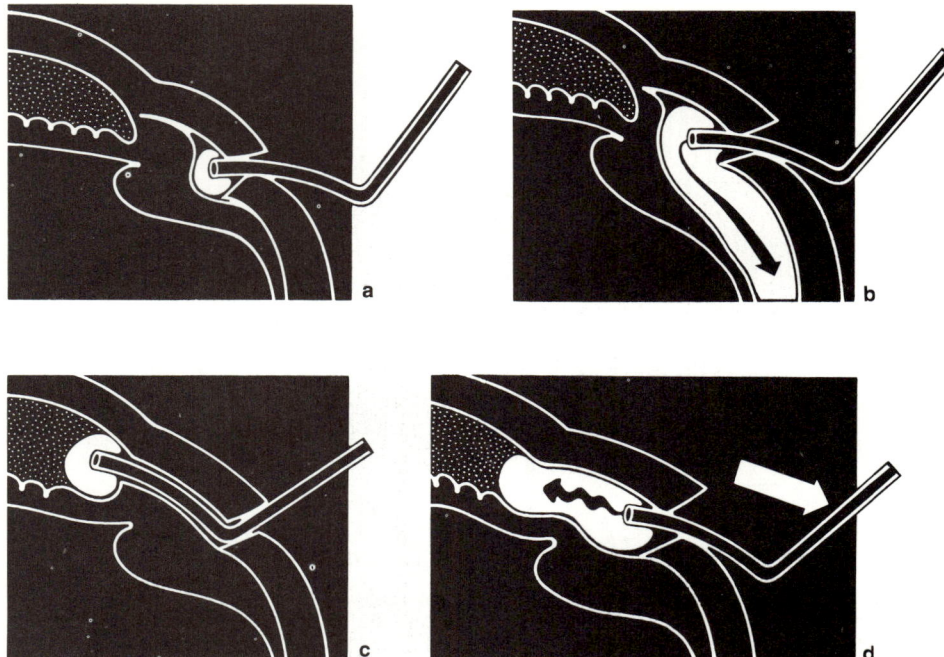

Fig. 3.25   Technique of injection into a cyclodialysis cleft. **a** and **b** Problem: when viscoelastic material is injected through a cyclodialysis cannula while progressing towards the scleral spur (**a**) there is a risk of the material escaping backwards — following the lower resistance — and detaching the posterior choroid (**b**). **c** and **d** Solution: viscoelastic material is not injected while progressing but only when retracting the cannula. The resistance at the scleral spur then already has been overcome and the injected viscoelastic bolus will expand forward through the cleft towards the anterior chamber (**d**).

— blockade the compartments that must not be filled (Fig. 3.24) in order to prevent inadvertant penetration of viscoelastic material

— avoid inflating adjacent regions that might compress the compartment to be filled (Fig. 3.26).

SIDE EFFECTS OF VISCOELASTIC SUBSTANCES

The same properties of viscoelastic material that are valuable in one situation may be adverse side effects in another situation.

Side effects during surgery

Figures 3.30–3.35 show some of these side effects and demonstrate methods of circumventing them.

The blockade of orifices may prevent rapid wound closure in case of emergency (Fig. 3.30). The space expanding effect may cause compensatory shifting of tissue that can put at risk the tactical goal (Figs. 3.31–3.33). The high resistance may cause deviation of movements away from the viscous containing space towards regions of lower resistance (Figs. 3.34 and 3.35).

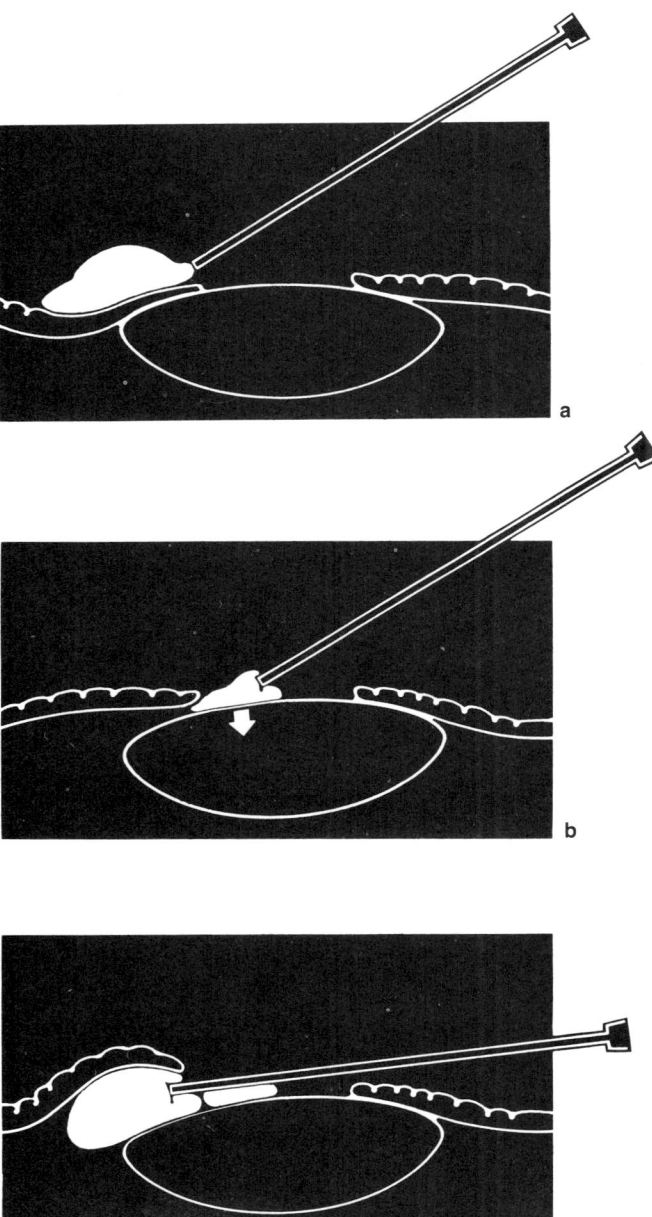

Fig. 3.26   Techniques of injection into the iridocapsular space. **a** Problem: when injecting directly towards the pupillary margin, there is risk of viscoelastic material being deposited onto the iris surface, compressing thus the iridoscapsular space instead of opening it. **b** and **c** Solution: to prevent this, the injection is directed first against the lens. This is depressed by the bolus (**b**), the iridocapsular cleft expands and thus permits the injection of more material into the iridocapsular space (**c**).

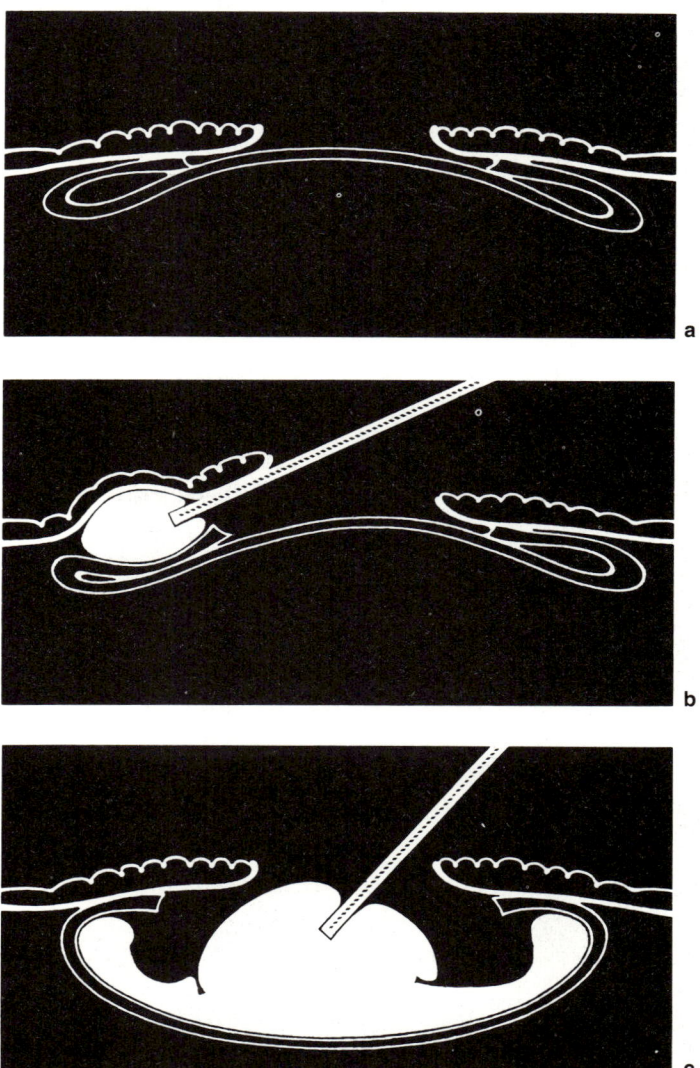

Fig. 3.27   Technique of injection into the iridocapsular space or into the intercapsular sinus in extracapsular cataract extraction. **a** Problem: in case of a narrow pupil, the borders of the anterior capsulotomy are invisible and the differentiation between iridocapsular and intercapsular space is difficult. **b** and **c** Solutions: the iridocapsular space is enlarged by lifting the iris slightly with the tip of the cannula while injecting (**b**). The intercapsular space is unfolded by starting the injection at the centre of the posterior capsule (**c**). The viscoelastic material then will spread towards the periphery and thereby expand the intercapsular sinus.

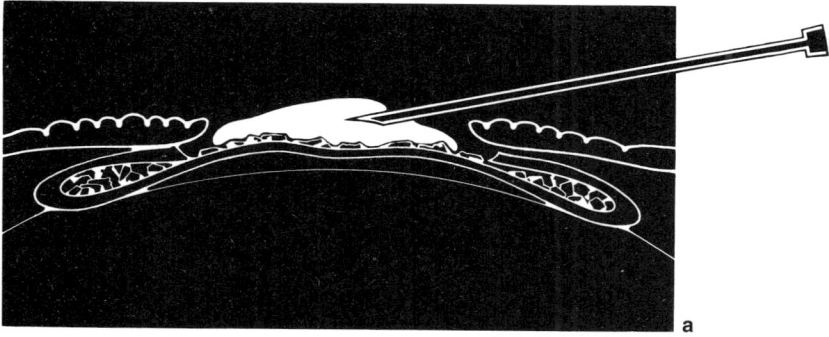

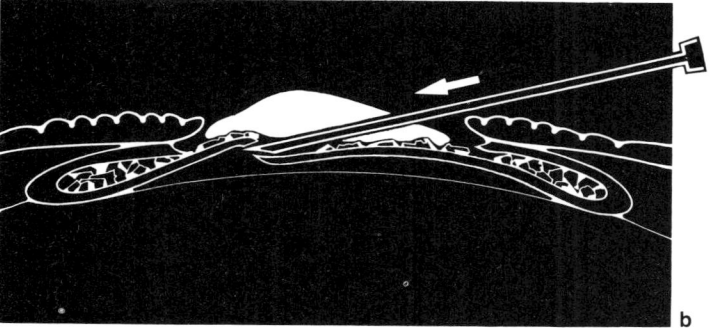

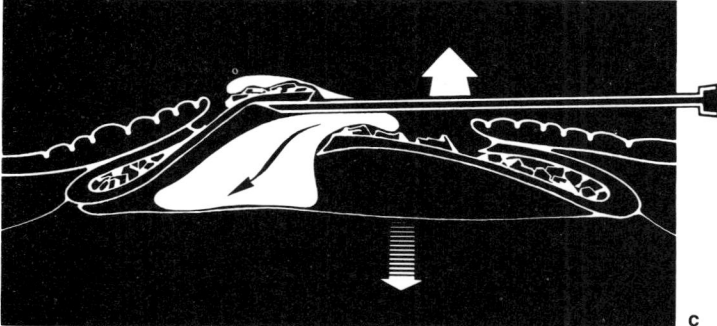

Fig. 3.28 Technique of injection into the hyalocapsular interspace. Problem: the extremely vulnerable anterior hyaloid is so close to the posterior capsule of the lens, that it is hardly possible to insert an injecting cannula into the interspace without damaging the vitreous. Solution: only a minute gap in the posterior capsule is made with the tip of the cannula and then the viscoelastic material aspirated into the interspace by creating a vacuum there. **a** First, viscoelastic material is injected above the posterior capsule. **b** The capsule is opened by mere touching with the tip of the cannula. **c** By raising the cannula, the capsule then is lifted, so that vacuum is produced in the interspace which aspirates the viscoelastic material from above. Once the interspace is enlarged slightly, further injection of viscoelastic material is easy.

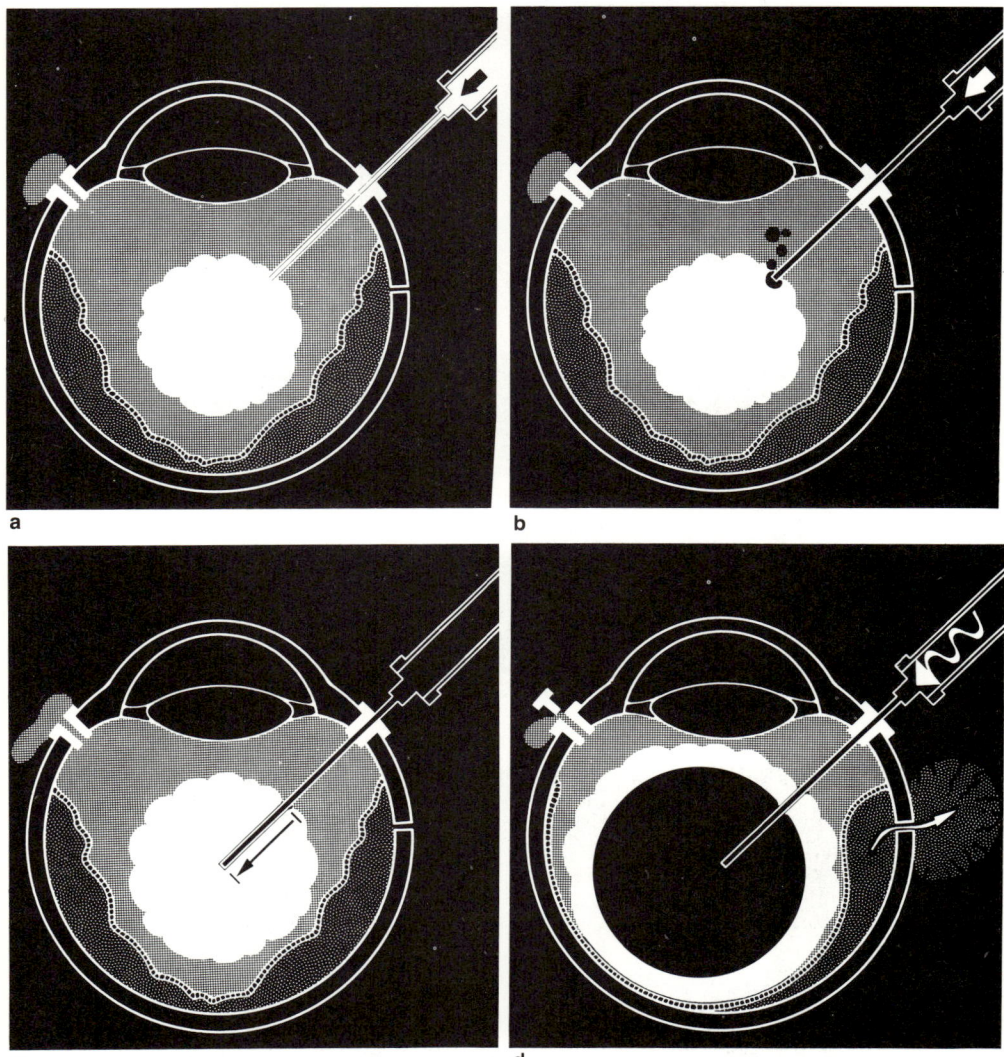

Fig. 3.29   Technique of the injection of gas into a viscoelastic bolus. **a** and **b** Problem: if after injecting the viscous bolus the cannula is maintained in its initial position (**a**) while trying to inject the gas bubble, the latter will follow the lower resistance. It escapes into the surrounding fluid (**b**) instead of penetrating into the more resistant viscous medium. **c** and **d** Solution: before the injection of gas the cannula is pushed forward into the centre of the bolus (**c**) and only then is the bolus inflated with gas (**d**).

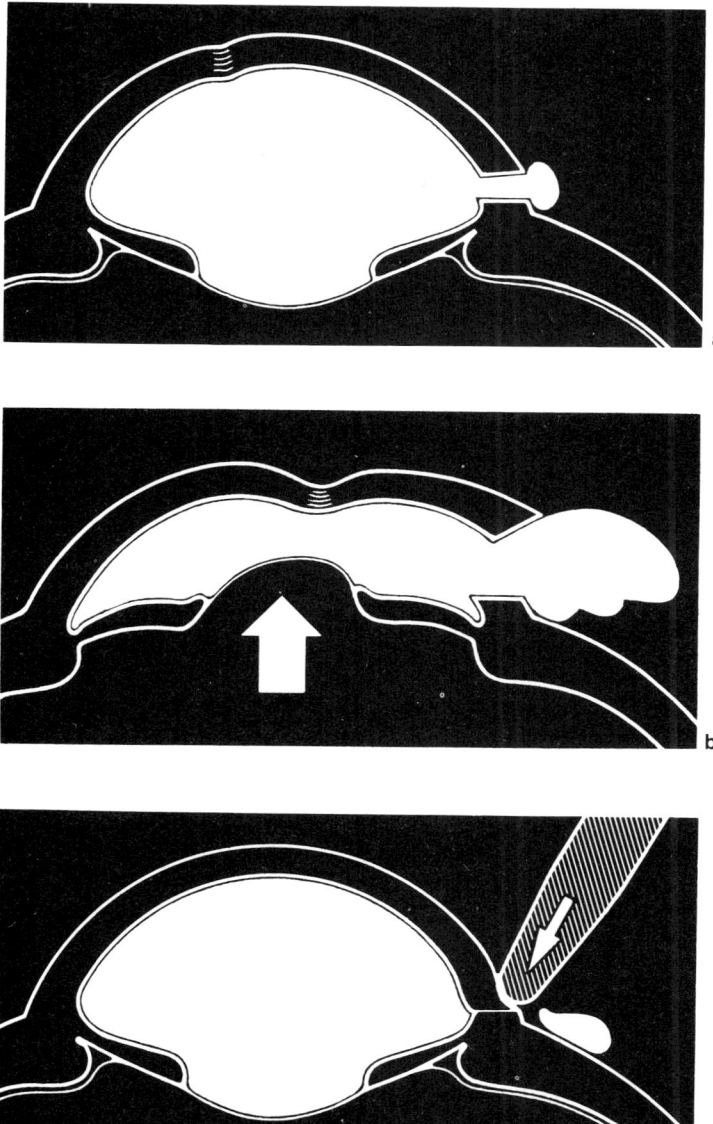

Fig. 3.30 Complications from viscoelastic material. Blockade of the valve closure of a corneoscleral incision. **a** and **b** Problem: a viscoelastic bolus between the wound lips prevents closure of the valve (**a**). In case of an increase of the vitreous pressure the valve will gape instead of close more tightly. The way is free for the injected viscous bolus and intraocular tissue to prolapse (**b**). **c** Solution: the edges of the wound are kept free from viscous material during all manipulations, except those where gaping with the help of a bolus is intended as part of the tactical plan (see Fig. 3.5c).

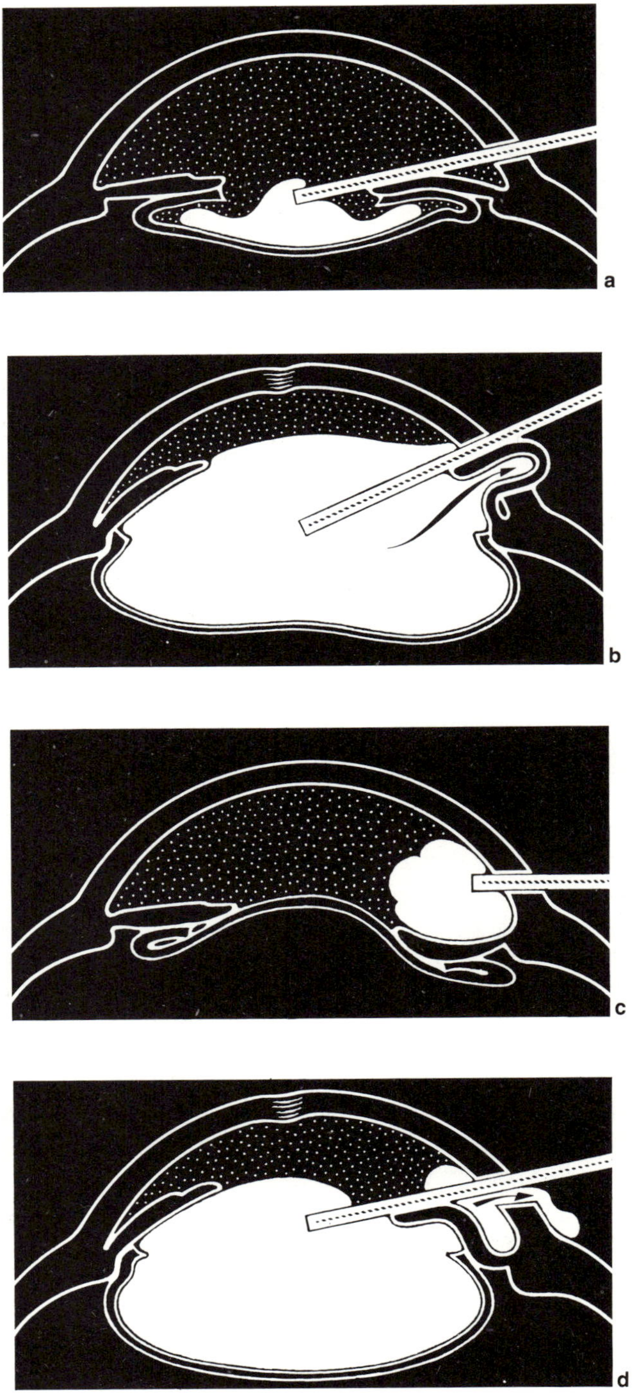

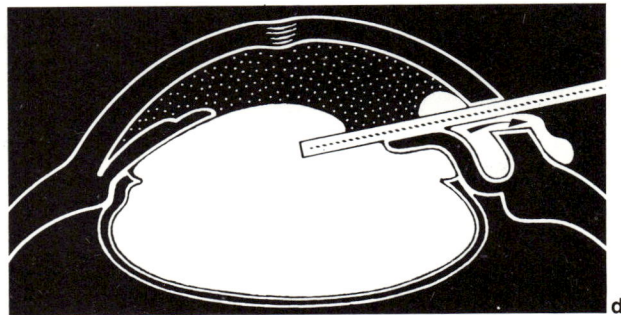

The decrease of thermal convection may produce increased effects on cold or heat application. Cryoprobes, therefore, must be carefully isolated in order to avoid oversized ice balls. Similarly, endodiathermy probes need sufficient cooling through irrigation with watery fluid in order to prevent overheating of tissues.

The decreased flow velocity prevents the rapid spreading of drugs injected into the eye (for instance acetylcholine or alphachymotrypsin). To obtain full efficiency, the viscoelastic material must be flushed away from the target and then the drug applied close to the receptors.

The decreased mobility of the iris prevents repositioning of a distorted pupil or an iris prolapse through elasticity of the tissue or muscular action. In order to restore the shape of the iris diaphragm in a viscous medium, the high resistance must be overcome by the direct action of mechanical instruments, e.g. spatula, or hooks.

Side effects in the postoperative period

The main problem caused by viscoelastic material in the postoperative phase is the increase in intraocular pressure. This rise being rapid in onset and dependent on dilution is considered to be caused by mechanical obstruction of the trabecular outflow channels (McRae et al, 1983; Pape & Balazs, 1980). Surprisingly, in experiments with sodium-hyaluronate the injected sample with the lowest viscosity caused the highest intraocular pressure (Denlinger et al, 1980). This was explained by the high coherence of highly viscous solutions which consequently are washed out more slowly by aqueous; the fluid passing through the outflow channels then contains only little hyaluronate and is not very viscous.

As a general rule, the magnitude of the pressure increase and its duration depend on the quantity of material left in the eye and its viscosity, or in other words: On the mode of application (filling of spaces, covering of large surfaces or merely coating of an implant) and on the chemical nature of the substance (molecular size and entanglement).

Differences in opinion among various authors as to the occurrence and the severity of the pressure rise may be explained by technical particularities in their use of viscoelastic material.

Residual transparent viscoelastic material (e.g. Healon) cannot be visualised directly. But its presence can be presumed from the immobility of particles suspended in a cavity and the coalescence of blood into small droplets. With the disappearance of the viscoelastic substance mobility of particles is restored and the blood droplets are resolved.

Since the delay necessary for viscoelastic material to vanish from the anterior chamber depends on technical details of the surgical procedure, no general rules can be given.

Every surgeon should learn from experience the 'normal' duration of absorption from the anterior chamber following his own surgery. Any unusual prolongation is

---

Fig. 3.31 Complications from viscoelastic material. Prolapse from overdose in the retroiridal space. **a** and **b** Problem: in case of injection behind the iris (**a**) an overdose may produce a prolapse of iris or tissue from the retroiridal space (**b**). **c** and **d** Solution: in case of a commencing prolapse the material immediately behind the orifice protrudes first. If this is aqueous, the surgeon may be unaware of the extrusion. Therefore, viscoelastic substance is injected behind the entrance (**c**). In case of a commencing prolapse, the bolus will escape first and is a warning sign easily recognized by the surgeon (**d**).

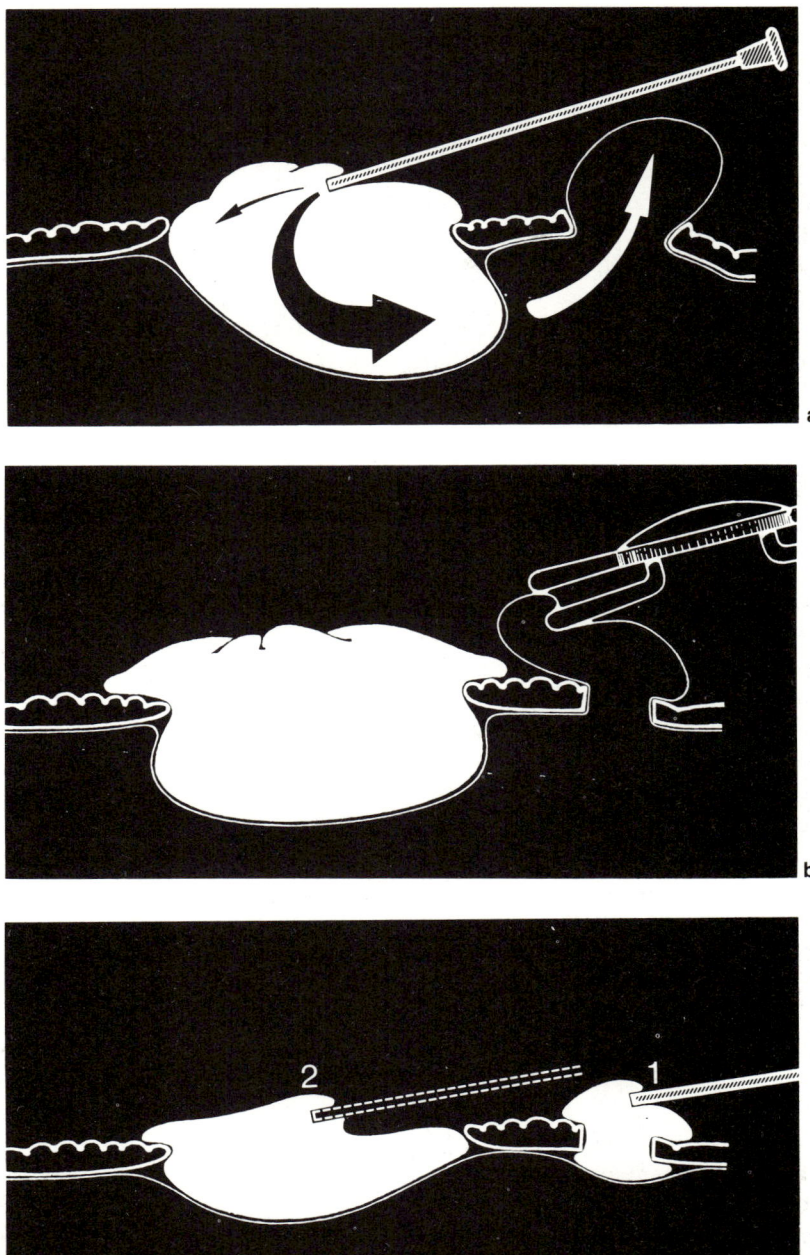

Fig. 3.32 Complications from viscoelastic material. Compensatory shift of vitreous in the pupillary area after intracapsular extraction. **a** and **b** Problem: when depressing the anterior hyaloid at the pupil, there is a compensatory bulge at the peripheral iridectomy (**a**), compromising the access to the anterior chamber (**b**). **c** Solution: in a first step, the iridectomy is obstructed by a viscoelastic bolus (1) before injecting at the pupil (2).

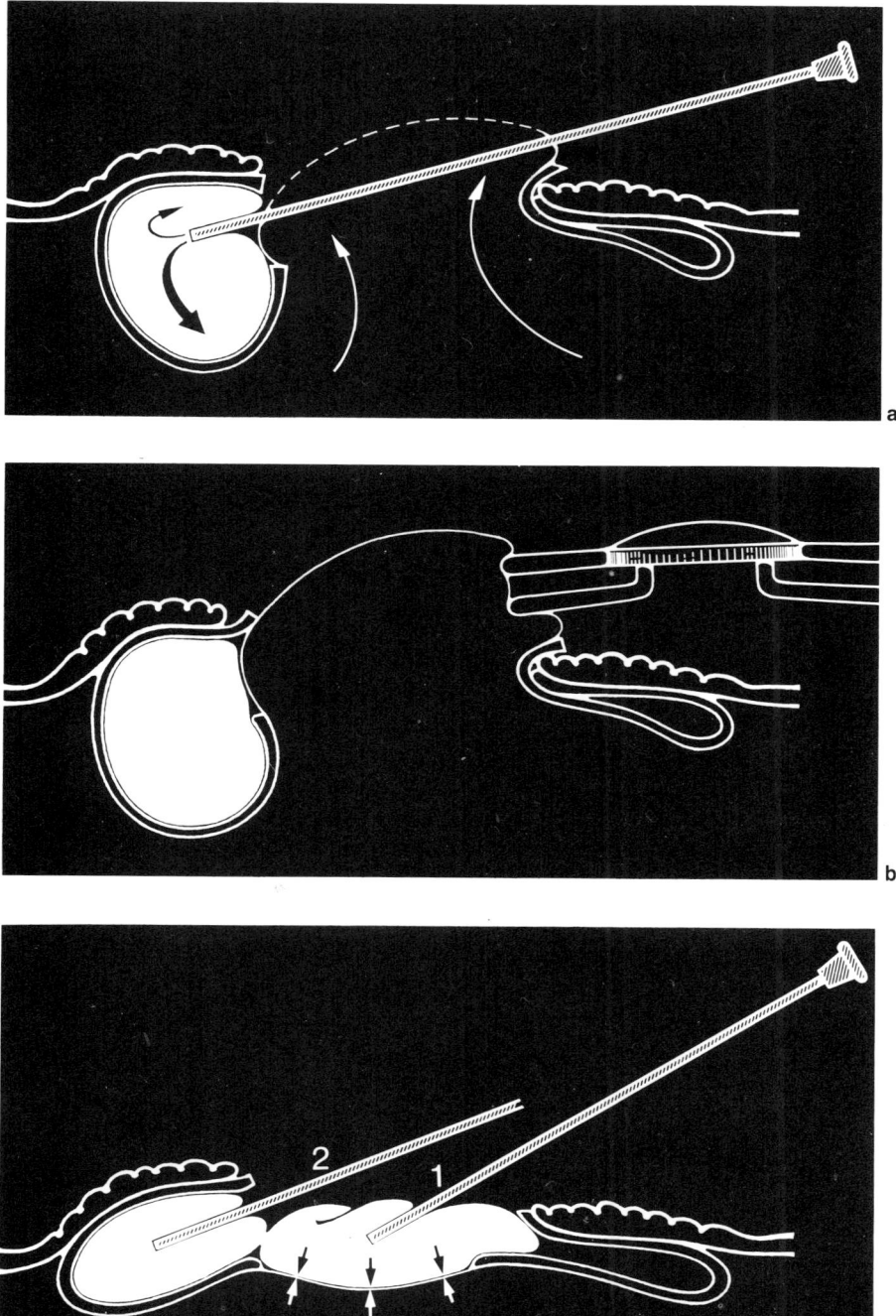

Fig. 3.33   Complications from viscoelastic material. Compensatory shift of vitreous in case of a ruptured posterior capsule. **a** and **b** Problem: when injecting behind the iris, there is a compensatory bulge of the anterior hyaloid (**a**) that will prevent the access into the expanded space (**b**). **c** Solution: in a first step, the tear in the capsule (1) is obstructed, and only then is the retroiridal space expanded (2).

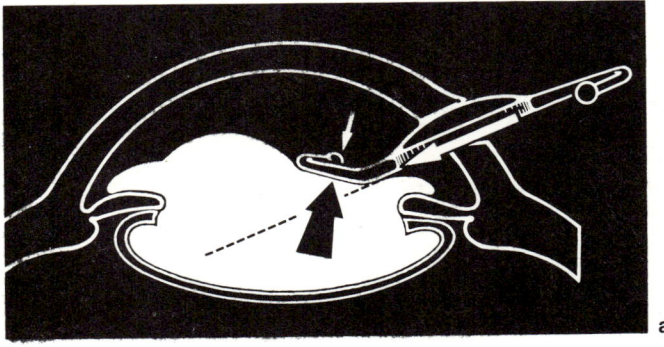

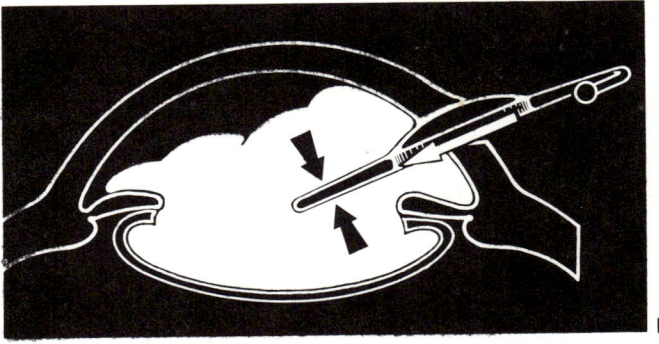

Fig. 3.34   Complications from viscoelastic material. Sliding layer preventing the insertion of loops into the retroiridal space. **a** Problem: if viscoelastic material is injected onto the iris surface and into the capsular bag, this layer of higher density offers a higher resistance (broad arrow) than the overlying liquid (thin arrow). It deflects deformable loops and prevents their insertion behind the iris. **b** Solution: if dense material is continuous from the incision to the target, the high resistance is overcome at insertion into the anterior chamber. During further travel through the chamber the resistance on both sides of the loop are equal (arrows) and hence the loops can be brought to the intended site without deviation.

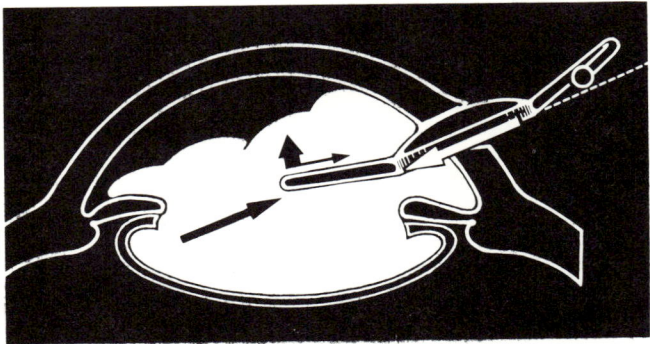

Fig. 3.35   Complications from viscoelastic material. Deflection of angled loops. Problem: when angled loops proceed through viscoelastic medium the resistance (medium arrow) has a vector component that increases the deflection (broad arrow). This may prevent the insertion of loops behind the iris while directing the body of the implant straight to the desired position (arrow in implant). Solution: an additional depressing force must be applied at the loop (e.g. with a spatula) in order to overcome the high resistance of the medium and to reduce the deflection.

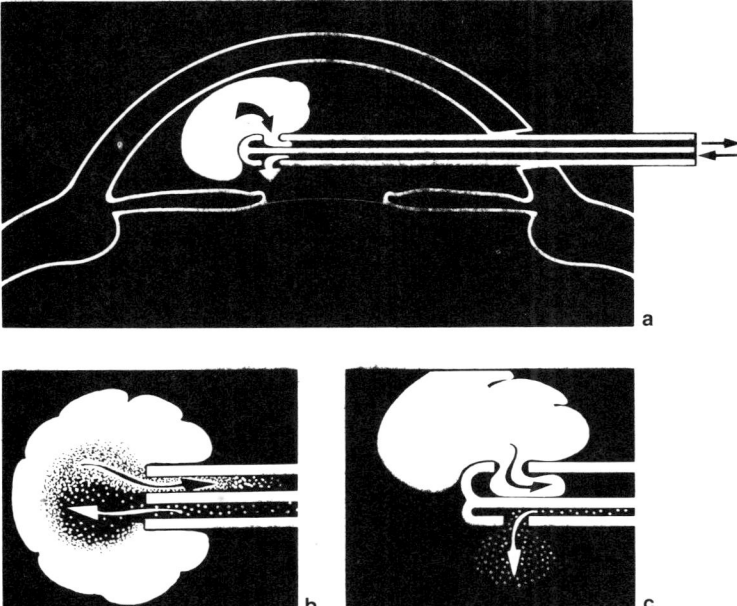

Fig. 3.36   Technique of removal of viscoelastic material by aspiration. **a** Double aspiration/infusion cannula permits replacement of evacuated volume while aspirating. **b** Aspiration of viscoelastic material by dilution. Infused watery fluid dilutes viscous material in front of the cannula. The outflow pathways can be made narrow because the aspirated material is diluted and hence less viscous. The infusion port is directed forward in order to bring the diluting watery fluid into vicinity of the aspiration port. **c** Aspiration of viscoelastic material in bulk: The diameter of outflow pathway (orifice and lumen of cannula) should be large enough for passage of material with high flow resistance. The infusion port is situated laterally, as far away from the aspiration port as possible in order to prevent watery liquid from interfering with the aspiration of the material with high flow resistance.

indicative of decreased production of aqueous if the tension is low; or if tension is high, one has to suspect obstacles in the trabecular meshwork, either a pre-existing glaucoma, or the presence of enzyme digests, haemorrhage or inflammation. The latter possibility should always be borne in mind since delayed disappearance of viscoelastic material is an important early warning sign of abnormal inflammatory reaction.

REMOVAL OF VISCOELASTIC MATERIAL

Removal of viscoelastic material from the anterior chamber is indicated in order to prevent pressure rise in the postoperative period.

There are two ways to evacuate the material: Removal in bulk or removal by dilution. Both methods can be performed either by aspiration (Fig. 3.36), or by irrigation (Fig. 3.37). Removal in bulk allows easy control of the completeness of the evacuation. But since a large volume leaves the globe at one time a sudden collapse of the chamber may occur. Removal by dilution, conversely, is a slow process with easy

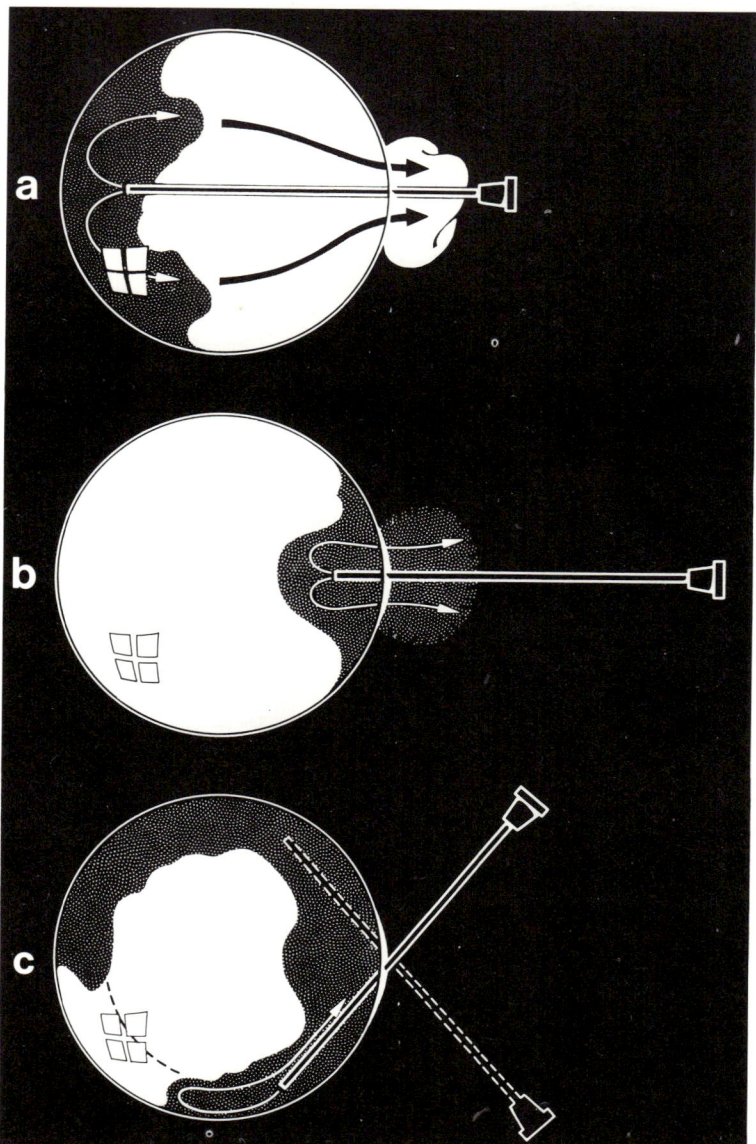

Fig. 3.37   Technique of removal of viscoelastic material from the anterior chamber by irrigation.
a Irrigation in bulk. If the evacuation of the complete bolus is planned, the irrigating fluid is injected
opposite the entrance orifice. The bolus will blockade the outflow of the irrigating fluid and is extruded with
increasing pressure. Similarly air can be used instead of fluid as an expelling agent. Irrigation by dilution:
b Fluid injected directly behind the entrance orifice will flow out again. Only the adjacent area of viscous
material will be diluted and removed by the irrigation. **c** If irrigation of the entire chamber angle is
planned, the entrance is kept free from viscous material during the whole process of irrigation. The viscous
material in the angle is diluted by continuous irrigation, starting from the entrance and slowly progressing
around the whole circumference.

monitoring of the chamber. However, the completeness of evacuation is difficult to assess.

CONCLUSION

The modern viscous and viscoelastic substances are new and very effective tools for solving surface and space tactical problems. Viscous material is better suitable for surface tactical use, viscoelastic material for space tactics. While both substances are applied with the same instrument as watery liquid — that is, through cannulae — the technique of application is quite different. Watery fluids can be injected anywhere within an intraocular space in order to fill it, because they will spread evenly throughout all compartments and their connecting pathways. Viscous material is similar but will spread more slowly. Therefore, to speed up the surgical action, the injection is applied as near as possible to the target. Viscoelastic material, conversely, will stay where put. It can be compared to a mechanical instrument rather than to a liquid. It must be applied directly at the target when needed and removed later on when it has accomplished its task.

There is no doubt that in the future the ophthalmic surgeon will be provided with new substances varying in viscosity and elasticity. Among these he may choose the most appropriate substance for every specific purpose — similar to classical solid surgical instruments that exist in various shapes and are selected step by step according to the various surgical procedures contemplated.

REFERENCES

Arzeno G, Miller D 1982 Effect of sodium hyaluronate on corneal wound healing. Archives of Ophthalmology 100: 152

Balazs E A, Sweeney D B 1965 The injection of hyaluronic acid and collagen preparations in eye surgery. In: Schepens C L, Regan C D (eds) Controversial aspects of the management of retinal detachment, p 200–202

Comper W D, Laurent T C 1978 Physiological function of connective tissue polysaccharides. Physiology Review 58: 255–315

Denlinger J L, Schubert H, Balazs E A 1980 Na-hyaluronate of various molecular sizes injected into the anterior chamber of owl monkey; disappearance and effect on intraocular pressure. Proceedings of the International Society for Eye Research 1: 88

Eisner G 1981 Der raumtaktische einsatz Einer viskösen Substanz (Healon[R]). Klin Mbl Augenheilk 178: 32–39

Eisner G 1980 Eye surgery, Springer-Verlag, Heidelberg, p 97–100

Forrester J V, Balazs E A 1980 Inhibition of phagocytosis by high molecular weight hyaluronate. Immunology 40: 435–446

Fraser J R E, Laurent T C, Pertoft H, Baxter E 1981 Plasma clearance, tissue distribution and metabolism of hyaluronic acid injected intraveinously in the rabbit. Biochemical Journal 200: 415–424

Harrison S E, Soll D B, Shayegan M, Clinch T 1982 Chondroitin sulfate: A new and effective protective agent for intraocular lens insertion. Ophthalmology 89: 1254–1260

Laurent U B G 1982 Studies on endogenous sodium hyaluronate in the eye. Abstracts of Uppsala Dissertations from the Faculty of Medicine 428

McRae Scott M, Edelhauser H, Hyndiuk R et al 1983 The effects of sodium hyaluronate, Chondroitin sulfate and methylcellulose on the corneal endothelium and intraocular pressure. American Journal of Ophthalmology 95: 332–341

Miller D, Stegmann R 1980 Use of Na-hyaluronate in anterior segment eye surgery. American Intraocular Implant Society Journal 6: 13–15

Pape L G, Balazs E A 1980 The use of sodium hyaluronate (Healon) in human anterior segment surgery. Ophthalmology (Rochester) 87: 699–705

Reim M, Lenz V 1983 Behandlung von schweren Verätzungen mit hochpolymerer Hyaluronsäure (Healon). (in press)

Saric D, Reim M 1983 Behandlung von Verätzungen des vorderen Augenabschnittes mit hochpolymerem Na-Hyaluronat (Healon) (in press)

Sebag J, Balazs E A, Eakins K E et al 1984 The effect of hyaluronic acid on prostaglandins synthesis and phagocytosis by mononuclear phagocytes in vitro (in press)

Soll D B, Harrison S E, Arturi F C, Clinch T 1980 Evaluation and protection of corneal endothelium. American Intraocular Implant Society Journal 6: 239–242

Sudarsky R D, Jakobiec F A, Rodriguez-Sains R, Poole T A 1981 Induced ocular hypertension prior to enucleation for chorioidal melanoma. American Academy of Ophthalmology 88: 31A–33A

4. Radial keratotomy*

J. J. Rowsey   J. C. Hays

INTRODUCTION

The lessons of radial keratotomy surgery produce ambivalent feelings in the ophthalmic community. We would like to review the historical insights of this surgery and our current surgical results and recommendations.

Sato analysed the combination of posterior and anterior corneal incisions to reduce myopia and astigmatism (Sato, 1950; Sato et al, 1953). He was able to obtain an average of 3.00 diopters of myopic correction with radial keratomy with a large range of refractive change of 1.50–7.00 diopters. The magnitude of the potential myopic correction and significant complications from the preliminary studies were not well recognised until the renewed interest and research of Fyodorov & Durnev (1979). Fyodorov was able to accomplish reduction of myopia of 2.65 diopters ± 0.2 diopters with a 3 mm optical zone, and 1.25 ± 0.13 diopters of myopia reduction with a 4.5 mm optical zone. Subsequent extensive study by several investigators in the United States has confirmed the effectiveness of radial keratotomy in reducing myopia and the lack of predictability of this procedure.

Hoffer et al (1981) reported an average decrease in myopia following radial keratotomy of 3.4 diopters ± 2.2 in 52 patients in a preliminary study. Cowden (1982) reported on an additional 25 eyes undergoing radial keratotomy with a 16-incision procedure. Only 1.18 diopters of refractive change was observed with this technique with a preoperative myopia of 1.6–9.25 diopters.

Bores et al (1981) reported their early experience in the United States with the comment that 'over-enthusiasm of patient and physician, especially in marginal cases, must be avoided.' Four hundred eyes of 223 patients underwent radial keratotomy with a 16-incision procedure. Preoperative myopia was −2.00 to −11.00 diopters in this population. Although up to 3.12 diopters of residual myopia was observed in the early patients presented, a residual myopia of only 1.18 diopters was seen in the later patients studied. Bores noted that incisions with razor blades, while adequate, did not cut to the full set depth. Razor blade knives were therefore extended to compensate for this shallow cut. An additional blade length of approximately 40 microns was required to produce an adequate incision. Although the predictability and surgical accuracy of the procedure were not provided, Bores suggested that patients 'in the 2–6 diopter range have an excellent prognosis for vision without glasses — particularly those with initially steep keratometer readings.'

Cowden & Bores (1981) subsequently reported 20 patients who underwent radial keratotomy between January and April of 1980. In 6 months, they noted an average

*This work was supported by an unrestricted grant from Research to Prevent Blindness, the Louise and Gustavus Pfeiffer Foundation, and the private philanthropy of the citizens of Oklahoma.

63

decrease in myopia of 3.10 diopters, with a range of 0.37–5.37 diopters refractive change. Maximum surgery with peripheral corneal re-deepening was attempted in patients with high degrees of myopia of −4.00 to −8.37 diopters. The average decrease in myopia in these patients was 3.76 diopters, with a range of 1.50–5.37 diopters. The degree of corneal flattening was best correlated to the size of the optical zone, with smaller optical zones producing larger refractive changes. Cowden and Bores (1981) commented on Cowden's paper (Cowden, 1982), suggesting that 'a retrospective study previously reported by the author indicated that the lower the initial keratometer readings were, the lesser the amount of correction obtained. Also, eyes with higher degrees of myopia tended to obtain a greater change of the corneal curvature. Data from the prospective patients reported in this paper failed to support that previous finding.' Cowden noted, however, that the 'time required for stabilisation of the corneal curvature appears to be about 3 months in most cases; however, gradual deterioration continued to occur in one-third of the cases followed.'

Definitive animal studies with keratometric and histologic data were subsequently provided by Jester et al (1981b). The effect of radial keratotomy was examined in the owl monkey. A 16-incision or 8-incision radial keratotomy was performed, and the eyes were studied with histologic and ultrastructural analysis. The authors stated that 'the loss of initial corneal flattening following radial keratotomy corresponded with the contracture of the wound as demonstrated by histopathologic and ultrastructural study.' The main variability in the operative result related to the variability in surgical incision depth, although adequate counter pressure at the corneoscleral limbus was obtained with fine-toothed forceps. The use of a broken razor blade chip or a Beaver 76-A blade may have accounted for some of the histologic depth variation. As measured by the Terry keratometer, a significant corneal flattening of 4.00 diopters, range 1.25–8.50 diopters, was noted keratometrically with a 16-incision radial keratotomy incision, and 3.25 diopters of keratometric corneal flattening, range 1.25–5.00 diopters, was observed with 8 incisions. Marked regression of the corneal flattening was noted so that at the end of 6 months, only 0.5 diopter of residual corneal flattening was observed in the 16-incision group, and 1.00 diopter of residual flattening was noted in the 8-incision radial keratotomy group. When extensive corneal neovascularisation was noted, no corneal flattening was observed and, surprisingly, 3.75–6.50 diopters of corneal steepening were observed. No corticosteroids were utilised in these monkey eyes, and, therefore, the morphological appearance of the incisions indicated normal wound healing following radial incisions in the owl monkey. Polymorphonuclear leukocytes and macrophages invaded the incisions at 48 hours, and this inflammatory infiltrate was replaced by epithelial cells at days 7–14. This epithelial plug was replaced at 1–2 weeks with fibroblasts which contained extensive rough endoplasmic reticulum, indicating collagen production or fibrous tissue proliferation. By 6 months, marked fibroblast contraction had occurred and residual scar tissue with fibres of 550–650 angstrom diameter were observed, compared to the normal 200–300 angstrom diameter collagen. The authors also noted a 14–15% endothelial cell loss. This cell loss was felt to be associated with inflammation in the anterior segment and surgical trauma. This significant loss of corneal power in the owl monkey was greater than observed in the stumptail macaque by the same group (Steel et al, 1981). They reported a 16-incision radial keratotomy in stumptail monkeys that demonstrated corneal flattening of 2.75 diopters, stabilising at

2.50 diopters of keratometric flattening 6 months after surgery. The owl monkey demonstrated 10–20% decrease in endothelial cells, whereas the stumptail monkey demonstrated no loss of endothelial cells. The authors suggested that the stumptail monkey's endothelial cell regenerative capacity might account for the disparate clinical result. The authors also suggested that the degree of wound healing might be related to the reversal of the flattening effect and theorised that topical corticosteroids might alter this operative result.

Careful analysis of radial keratotomy data from eye bank eyes revealed significant variations in corneal depth incisions with similar blade length extension, as reported by Jester et al (1981a). A Katena handle and razor knife were set at 80% of the central corneal thickness. Histological study of incision depth varied from 30–100% of corneal thickness, demonstrating the wide variability when a similar knife setting is attempted. The average depth of the incisions has 66.6%, with a range of 41.50–77.2% of the preset depth. The authors made the significant observation that 'as the incision extends beyond the corneoscleral limbus, there is a reduction in the flattening effect of the procedure.' (Jester et al, 1981a). The authors noted that a peculiarity in eye bank eye with increased apparent incision depths in the peripheral cornea. This clinical observation is disparate from the observed clinical result in human eyes in which a similar blade setting produces deep corneal incisions centrally and relatively shallow incisions peripherally. The preoperative eye bank eye radius of curvature was 42.6 diopters, with a range of 35.75–45.50 diopters. A change in corneal curvature of 8.5 diopters was noted, with a range of 5.75–10.75 diopters. In addition, the authors demonstrated marked corneal flattening, occurring with only 4 radial incisions. Four incisions produced 1.50–8.75 diopters of refractive change, or 62% of the total effect of the procedure; eight incisions produced 3.50–10.25 diopters of refractive change, or 85% of the total flattening seen with 16 incisions. Sixteen-incision radial keratotomy produced 5.75–10.75 diopters of refractive change.

In an additional study, Salz et al (1981) noted that 'the most striking finding (in eye bank eyes) was the variability between depth of incisions in a given eye, even though the blade setting and surgeon were constant.' They noted adjacent incisions with depths of 30% and 65% of the cornea, even though the blade setting was 80% of corneal depth. Occasional anterior chamber perforations occurred, obviously, over 100% of the prescribed depth.

An attempt at precision standardisation of radial keratotomy has been provided by several authors, including Salz et al (1981) and Jester et al (1981a). It is widely perceived that variations in incision depth may contribute to the biological variables both in wound healing and corneal flattening. Kramer et al (1981) designed a unique corneal template. Utilising a suction template in 36 eye bank eyes, eight radial corneal incisions, 3 mm in length and 0.5 mm in depth, were placed in a radial pattern. The overall depth of the 288 incisions was 0.49 mm, with standard deviation of 0.04 mm. The range of incision depth was 0.32–0.61 mm. Recognising the variability in incision depth with razor blades, Rowsey et al (1982c) designed a diamond knife with the blade anterior to the guard to allow for maximum corneal depth of cut. We felt that if the steel guard of the blade advanced in front of the diamond, corneal tissue would be pressed away from the cutting edge, decreasing the corneal incision depth. We, therefore, allowed the blade to proceed anterior to the guard for maximum corneal incisions with minimum incidence of perforation (Fig.

4.1). The 45 degree angle of the guard on the Micra diamond knife has been adapted to the KOI diamond knife with a similar 45 degree angle blade and guard design. Thin diamond knives are currently utilised in all radial keratotomy procedures at the University of Oklahoma and have been adopted in the Prospective Evaluation of Radial Keratotomy (PERK) Study sponsored by the National Eye Institute. We have outlined the methods by which the diamond should traverse the cornea, tangent to the corneal surface and parallel to the radius of curvature of the cornea, to maintain maximum incision depth.

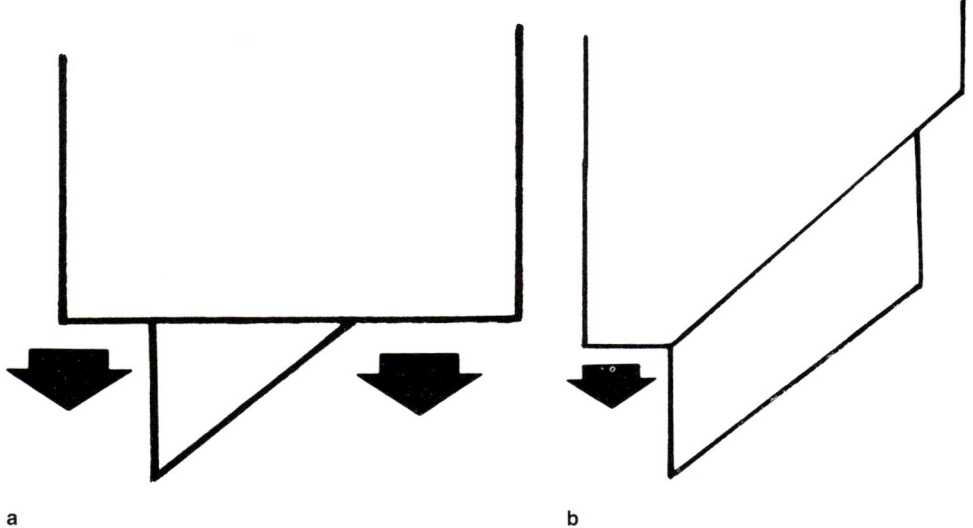

a   b

Fig. 4.1   **a** Schematic of diamond knife. The tissue pressure (arrows) of a blade guard tend to push corneal stroma away from the blade. **b** Rotating the blade away from a perpendicular to the cornea accentuates shallowing of the incision. The diamond blade design sets the blade anterior to the guard, minimising tissue distortion.

Maintenance of intraocular pressure during this procedure is important to counteract the diminished intraocular pressure which occurs with each incision. Eye bank eye studies reported by Unterman & Rowsey (1984) with the diamond knives currently available on the market demonstrate a better approximation of the incision depth to that prescribed. Salz et al (1983) presented a unique comparison of diamond and metal knives, and demonstrated similar incision depths, with the diamond reaching 84% and the metal 86% of the ultrasonically measured corneal thickness. Four incisions with a diamond knife produced 6.8 ± 1.6 diopters of corneal flattening, while a metal blade produced 7.9 ± 1.2 diopters of corneal flattening. The same blades produced 9.5 ± 1.0 diopters of flattening after eight incisions with a diamond, and 9.6 ± 0.8 diopters with a metal blade. The authors noted the range of cutting depth was from 61–98% of that desired. After comparison of scanning electron microscopy of diamond and razor blade tips, we conclude that maintenance of the sharp diamond tip might allow for vertical cuts in the optical zone and less variation (standard deviation and range) in the operative results. We have not, however, investigated a series of human eyes with razor blade fragments, superblade fragments, and the diamond knife to determine if this impression can be verified. We compared 3 mm optical zone radial keratotomies with superblades, and 25 patients demonstrated 5.50 ± 2.05 diopters of refractive change. The diamond knife design presented by Rowsey et al (1982c) produced 5.06 ± 1.32 diopters of refractive change at 3 months with an 8-incision, 3 mm optical zone radial keratotomy.

More recent studies have documented the results and complications of radial keratotomy. Nirankari et al (1982) reported a series of 33 eyes in 19 patients with an average decrease in myopia of 2.5 diopters with 8 or 16 incisions. The myopia decrease did not correlate with the preoperative keratometry readings or the number of corneal incisions. The main complications noted were corneal scarring, vascularisation and glare. Although the blade was placed at 100% of central corneal thickness, the postoperative examination confirmed that the cuts were approximately 50% of the corneal thickness. This small postoperative result of 2.50 diopters may be related to the rather shallow cuts routinely produced with razor blade fragments.

In a follow-up of this prospective clinical study by Nirankari et al (1983), an average of 2.7 diopters of myopia was corrected with keratometric flattening of 1.51 diopters. The second study by the same authors included 58 eyes in 33 patients who had been followed for a minimum of 6 months, with an average of 19 months. Refractive change was similar in patients with myopia under or over 5.00 diopters. Lower levels of myopia could therefore be approached with a reasonable expectation of improved visual acuity.

Fyodorov & Agranovsky (1982) updated their surgical results with radial keratotomy. Two different blade holders were utilised in the two separate groups reported. The authors stated that 4.75 diopters of refractive change were accomplished in an early group of 242 patients, and 6.25 diopters of refractive change were accomplished in a later group of 258 patients. Scarring diminished in the postoperative period of 1–2 years. Two to 5 years postoperatively, 52 patient eyes were reported, and 16 patients (57.1%) were emmetropic in the later group, whereas no patients were emmetropic in the early group.

Careful documentation of preoperative and postoperative ocular variables have been provided by Arrowsmith et al (1983). One hundred and fifty-six radial keratotomy procedures were carried out in 101 patients with a mean preoperative myopia, spherical equivalent of −5.00 diopters. An average change in spherical equivalent of +4.8 diopters was accomplished, and 51% of the patients were within 1 diopter of emmetropia postoperatively. The authors recommend that patients with under 6.00 diopters of myopia might be reasonable candidates for the procedure. The authors stated that 'while we did not expect full correction of myopia in many eyes, especially those with extremely high levels of preoperative myopia, we achieved at least 50% correction in 92% of all eyes 6 months after surgery.' Maximum corneal incision depth was attempted, and microperforations were seen in 35% of the patients, or 55 eyes. The operation was staged in an attempt to correct four levels of myopia, from −1.50 to −16.00 diopters. In 38 patients with −1.50 to 2.9 diopters, the spherical equivalent change was +2.6 diopters, with a range of 1.3–5.5 diopters. In the population of 70 patients, from −3.00 to 5.90 diopters, the mean spherical change was +4.7 diopters, with a range of +0.4 to +8.4 diopters. In the group of 36 patients with −6.00 to −9.90 diopters preoperatively, an average of +6.0 diopters of refractive change was observed, with a range of +1.5 to +15.8 diopters. In a smaller group of 12 patients with −10.00 to −16.00 diopters, an average of +8.6 diopters of refractive change was observed, with a range of +5.3 to +13.8 diopters.

Hoffer et al (1983) have provided a methodical analysis of the comparative results of three surgeons performing similar radial keratotomy procedures at the University of California, Los Angeles. An 8- and 16-incision protocol were reported. In 36 eyes, preoperative myopia of −3.80 diopters (±1.13) was reduced 2.80 (±1.00) diopters, utilising a 3.0 mm optical zone. This result was also accomplished by a second surgeon with −3.80 (±0.83) diopters of myopia preoperatively, with 3.00 (±0.80) diopters of correction seen. No progressive endothelial cell loss was observed, with 9% loss at 3 months and 2% net increase at 2 years.

MATERIALS AND METHODS: UNIVERSITY OF OKLAHOMA

Operative results and complications

We obtained Investigational Review Board approval at the University of Oklahoma Health Sciences Center to perform radial keratotomy as an experimental procedure in March, 1980. Rowsey & Balyeat (1982a) initially reported radial keratotomy results of 126 eyes in 102 patients, who continue in their follow-up at this time. The restrictive preoperative criteria excluded patients with external ocular infections or ocular diseases which might compromise visual acuity postoperatively. Patients eligible for the procedure had stable myopia of −2.00 to −14.00 diopters, with no sign of myopic degeneration in the posterior pole. Cycloplegic refractions were performed 30–45 minutes after 1% cyclopentolate drops were instilled. The patients with less than 4.00 diopters of regular astigmatism were considered acceptable for surgery as long as the corneascope topography revealed symmetry in the periphery and no keratoconus was present, as reported by Rowsey et al (1981) (Fig. 4.2). Endothelial cell counts exceeding 2000 sq mm were required, with corneal pachymetry readings of 0.45– 0.60 mm. The operation was, as it continues to be, performed as follows.

Under topical anaesthesia in the operating room, the eye is draped in a sterile manner after alcohol and iodine preparation of the periocular skin. The visual axis is marked by asking the patient to observe the operating light microscope on the Zeiss Omni-6 under decreased illumination. A 26-gauge needle is utilised to mark a small area of epithelium on the light reflex approximately 0.3 mm beneath the light reflex as observed from the corneal reflection. If the surgeon monocularly visualises the cornea with his own right eye, the left end of the corneal reflex is marked; conversely, if the surgeon views the light reflex with the left eye, the right end of the corneal reflex is marked, thereby compensating for movement of the light across the convex mirror of the cornea toward the eye being utilised by the surgeon, as described by Rowsey & Balyeat (1982b). A trephine mark with diameter of 3.0, 3.5, 4.0, or 5.0 mm is then circumscribed around the visual axis. Sixteen incisions were placed from the central optical zone toward the limbus in the first 50 patients, and eight in all subsequent patients. In March, 1981, diamond knife incisions were initiated to replace the 45 degree superblade previously used, allowing greater refractive results (Rowsey et al 1982c). No re-deepening is attempted on any patient. At the conclusion of the procedure, the incisions are carefully irrigated with balanced salt solution to eliminate the possibility of subsequent epithelial inclusion cysts, haemorrhage, and particulate

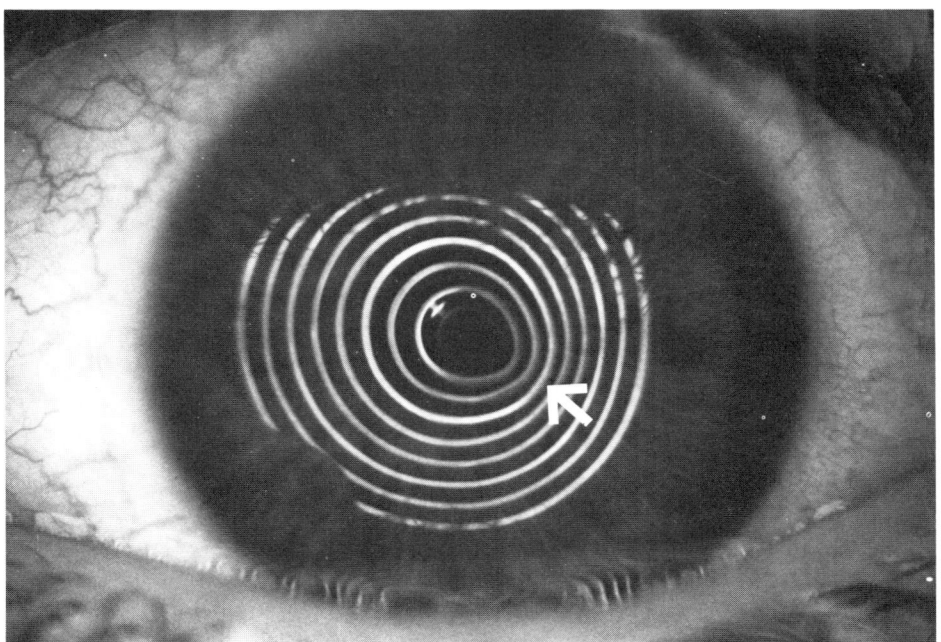

Fig. 4.2 Keratoconus. Corneascope photograph demonstrates diagnostic inferior temporal steepening (arrow) of the cornea. Early keratoconus patients may have sufficient contact lens fitting problems to request radial keratotomy. The diagnosis of keratoconus may be confirmed by Placido disc or corneoscopy imagery, and should preclude radial keratotomy surgery.

debris. We inject 0.5 ml betamethasone and 20 mg gentamicin sulphate subconjunctivally, and pressure patch the eye for 24 hours. Maxitrol eyedrops are utilised for 4 weeks postoperatively, one drop to the eye undergoing surgery 4 times a day. Maxitrol is a mixture of polymyxin-B sulphate, neomycin sulphate and dexamethasone. With a 3 mm optical zone, a refractive change of 5.16 diopters 1 year after surgery was reported by Rowsey & Balyeat (1982a).

In the first group of 13 patients undergoing radial keratotomy at the University of Oklahoma, the 16 incisions were deliberately carried 2 mm past the limbus, and in this patient population only 4.17 diopters of refractive change were observed. We recommended in Rowsey & Balyeat (1982a) that 'extending the incisions across the corneoscleral limbus may decrease the overall optical effect.' A 3 mm trephine has been utilised routinely for myopia of −4.00 diopters or greater, 3.5 mm for −3.00 to −3.75 diopters, and 4 mm for −2.00 to −2.75 diopters. The main predictive factors allowing us to estimate the operative results have recently been reviewed at the University of Oklahoma and reported in Rowsey et al (1983). The main preoperative variables which were significantly related to the operative result were the patient's age and the size of the optical zone utilised in the procedure. A 3 mm optical zone and 16-incision radial keratotomy in 39 eyes produced 5.18 diopters of refractive change at 1 year, with a range of 1.5 to 9.75 diopters. With 3 mm optical zone, an 8-incision procedure in 37 eyes produced 5.38 (±2.33) diopters of refractive change at 1 year, with a range of 1.25–14.00 diopters. A 3.5 mm optical zone and 8-incision procedure in 6 eyes produced 3.66 ($\pm$0.88) diopters of refractive change, with a range of 2.50–5.0 diopters, at 1 year. With a 4.0 mm optical zone, a 16-incision radial keratotomy in eight eyes produced 2.67 ($\pm$0.76) diopters of refractive change at 1 year, with a range of 1.50–3.50 diopters. Utilising simple bivariant linear regression analysis, we determined that the expected result from an 8-incision radial keratotomy with 3 mm optical zone was 2.53 diopters plus 0.087 multiplied by the patient's age. In other words, a patient 50 years of age with 10 diopters of myopia would obtain 3.05 diopters greater refractive change than a 20-year-old patient with the same level of myopia, or a total of 6.88 diopters of refractive change.

We report herein the longer follow-up of 2 years on the early surgical procedures and include the surgical accuracy, or lack thereof, which has constrained our enthusiasm for this procedure. We have defined the 'objective surgical accuracy' (OSA) as: delta diopters obtained divided by delta diopters desired. The accuracy and error from radial keratotomy are outlined in Table 4.1. A procedure that gives perfect

Table 4.1   Surgical accuracy formula

$$\text{Accuracy} = \frac{\Delta\text{Diopters obtained}}{\Delta\text{Diopters desired}} = \frac{\Delta\text{C.R.}}{\text{Pre-op C.R.}}$$

	Correction	Accuracy	Error
−5.00	10.00 Diopters	1.0	+1.0
	0.00 Diopters	0.0	−1.0
Average =	5.00 Diopters	1.0	1.00 = 100%

accuracy would have a result equivalent to the patient's preoperative myopia or the dioptric power of the eye, and would produce an accuracy of 1.00. The deviation from this degree of accuracy is termed the 'surgical error'. The surgical error is 1.00 minus the accuracy. For example, a patient with 10.00 diopters of myopia may obtain 8.00 diopters of refractive change and retain 2.00 diopters of residual myopia. $8.00 - 10.00 = 2.00$. Therefore, the error is 0.2 or 20%. When average refractive change alone following radial keratotomy is reported, the large standard deviation of the results is overlooked, but the prescient surgeon remains circumspect if there is a wide scatter of operative results around the desired mean. A patient (Table 4.1) who has 5.00 diopters of myopia and obtains 10.00 diopters of correction is 5.00 diopters overcorrected. If he obtains no diopters of correction, he remains 5.00 diopters undercorrected. If these two eyes are considered (0 and 10.00 diopters of refractive change), an average of 5.00 diopters of refractive change is observed, giving a spurious estimation of the true operative result. The error, however, may be averaged; the first patient obtaining 100% overcorrection and the second patient 100% undercorrection, thus the average error is 100%. This surgical error is subsequently reported, for it allows us to determine the accuracy of the procedure. Patients undergoing a 16-incision radial keratotomy with a 3 mm optical zone and all incisions traversing the limbus are summarised in Table 4.2. The preoperative myopia was −7.00 diopters, and these patients obtained a cycloplegic refractive change of 4.75 diopters at 1 year and 4.65 diopters at 2 years. The refraction is, therefore, reasonably stable. However,

Table 4.2 Radial keratotomy objective surgical accuracy 16 incisions 3 mm thru limbus

	Diopters Pre-op CR	Diopters 1 yr Δ CR	1 yr OSA	Error-1 yr	Diopters 2 yr Δ CR	2 yr OSA	Error-2 yr
	−5.50	4.25	0.77	−0.23	3.50	0.64	−0.36
	−4.75	5.50	1.16	+0.16	5.25	1.11	+0.11
	−7.25	7.25	1.00	0.00	6.50	0.90	−0.10
	−10.50	5.75	0.55	−0.45	5.75	0.55	−0.45
	−4.50	1.00	0.22	−0.78	0.50	0.11	−0.89
	−9.50	3.25	0.34	−0.66	3.25	0.34	−0.66
	−6.75	4.00	0.59	−0.41	4.25	0.63	−0.37
	−7.25	6.25	0.86	−0.14	6.25	0.86	−0.14
	−7.50	6.25	0.83	−0.17	7.25	0.97	−0.03
	−6.50	4.00	0.62	−0.38	4.00	0.62	−0.38
$\bar{x}$	−7.00	4.75	0.69	0.34	4.65	0.67	0.35
S.D.	+−1.91	+−1.83	+−0.29	+−0.25	+−1.98	+−0.31	+−0.27
Range	−4.25− −10.50	1.00− 7.25	0.22− 1.16	0− 0.78	0.50− 7.25	0.11− 1.11	0.03− 0.89

$n = 10$. CR = Cycloplegic refraction; OSA = Objective surgical accuracy.

the patients are largely undercorrected with an error of 34% at 1 year and 35% at 2 years. None of these patients has undergone any additional surgery, for we felt that 16 was the maximum number of incisions that we would routinely recommend if no astigmatism prevailed.

As previously discussed, we initiated a 16-incision radial keratotomy protocol, leaving all incisions in clear cornea after the first patients entered our study. The 16-incision, clear cornea radial keratotomy data is presented in Table 4.3. The mean preoperative myopia was −7.21 diopters, and the cycloplegic refractive change of this population at 1 year was 5.26 diopters and 5.03 diopters at 2 years. The error of the procedure, however, remains significant at 26% off of the desired visual refractive change at 1 year and 32% at 2 years. Although the cycloplegic refractive changes of over 5.00 diopters are greater than those frequently reported in radial keratotomy, the accuracy which we introduce and emphasise in this study is not sufficiently satisfactory to recommend that the procedure is predictable.

After the first 50 patients had entered the University of Oklahoma study, an 8-incision radial keratotomy was attempted to increase the surgical accurracy. We could, therefore, anticipate adding 8 incisions to the undercorrected population and defer further surgery on patients who became emmetropic or were overcorrected. Table 4.4 outlines the summary of data from this population of patients who were successfully corrected. The preoperative myopia of this population was −6.62 diopters, with a range of −3.50 to −11.25 diopters. The change in cycloplegic refraction was +5.91 diopters at 1 year postoperatively and +5.86 diopters at 2 years, indicating reasonable refractive stability in these patients. The error of the procedure was 23% at 1 year and 23% at 2 years. The standard deviation of the error of the successfully treated patients has diminished, however, from 26 to 14%, compared to the 16-incision radial keratotomy group. The remaining 8-incision population, which was more highly myopic and undercorrected with 8 incisions, underwent an additional 8-incision diamond knife radial keratotomy, utilising a similar 3.0 mm optical zone. We have not reopened any of the previous corneal incisions, fearing excessive scarring and fibrosis, but have placed additional incisions symmetrically between the previous

Table 4.3   Radial keratotomy objective surgical accuracy 16 incisions 3–11 mm OZ

	Diopters Pre-op CR	Diopters 1 yr Δ CR	1 yr OSA	Error-1 yr	Diopters 2 yr Δ CR	2 yr OSA	Error-2 yr
	−6.75	6.00	0.96	−0.04	6.25	1.00	0.00
	−5.50	5.25	0.95	−0.05	5.50	1.00	0.00
	−7.75	6.75	0.87	−0.13	5.75	0.74	−0.26
	−9.25	9.00	0.97	−0.03	7.50	0.81	−0.19
	−8.50	5.00	0.59	−0.41	3.75	0.44	−0.56
	−9.00	6.00	0.67	−0.33	6.00	0.67	−0.33
	−7.00	1.50	0.21	−0.79	1.75	0.25	−0.75
	−5.75	4.75	0.83	−0.17	5.75	1.00	0.00
	−8.75	5.50	0.63	−0.37	5.50	0.63	−0.37
	−4.50	4.00	0.89	−0.11	2.75	0.61	−0.39
	−4.25	3.00	0.71	−0.29	3.00	0.71	−0.29
	−3.50	3.50	1.00	−0.00	3.75	1.07	+0.07
	−4.50	5.50	1.22	+0.22	7.25	1.61	+0.61
	−6.00	4.50	0.75	−0.25	2.50	0.42	+0.58
	−9.50	5.50	0.58	−0.42	3.75	0.39	−0.61
	−4.50	3.50	0.78	−0.22	3.75	0.83	−0.17
	−8.25	6.25	0.76	−0.24	6.25	0.76	−0.24
	−8.25	5.75	0.70	−0.30	6.00	0.73	−0.27
	−15.75	4.00	0.25	−0.75	0.75	0.05	−0.95
	−9.50	9.25	0.97	−0.03	10.00	1.05	+0.05
	−9.75	8.50	0.87	−0.13	10.00	1.03	+0.03
	−9.00	4.50	0.50	−0.50	4.00	0.44	−0.56
	−8.50	4.75	0.56	−0.44	3.75	0.44	−0.56
	−4.00	3.25	0.81	−0.19	3.50	0.88	−0.12
	−5.50	6.25	1.14	+0.14	6.75	1.23	+0.23
	−4.50	5.25	1.17	+0.17	5.25	1.17	+0.17
x̄	7.21	Δ5.26	0.78	0.26	5.03	0.77	0.32
S.D.	+−2.69	+−1.79	+−0.25	+−0.20	+−2.25	+−0.34	+−0.26
Range	−3.50– −15.75	1.50– 9.25	0.21– 1.22	0.00– 0.44	0.75– 7.25	0.05– 1.61	0.00– 0.95

$n = 26$. CR = Cycloplegic refraction; OSA = objective surgical accuracy.

radial keratotomy gossamer scars. Table 4.5 reviews the data from the preoperative myopia of this population of patients, which was −7.72 diopters with a range of −4.50 to −10.75 diopters. The cycloplegic refractive change of this population was 4.30 diopeters from 3 to 15 months postoperatively, when a second 8-incision procedure was undertaken to correct remaining myopia. An additional refractive change of 2.24 diopters was obtained in these patients, with a range of 0.25–5.50 diopters. The follow-up time has been between 3 and 24 months in this population, with a total cycloplegic refractive change of 6.54 diopters and a range of 2.75–10.75 diopters. The final error of this population is 15%, with a range of 33–44%. This decreasing surgical error suggested to us that the staged radial keratotomy procedure for moderately high myopic individuals would be auspicious. In addition, two 8-incision procedures produced 12% greater effect than a single 8-incision operation. At this time, we have initiated a final graded radial keratotomy protocol that utilises 4 incisions and a 3.0 mm optical zone in an attempt to further decrease overcorrections, anticipating additional incisions in those patients who remain undercorrected. The preliminary data of this series of patients are reported in Table 4.6. The preoperative refractive error of this population was −7.41 diopters, and the 3-month change in cycloplegic refraction is 4.44 diopters. The 3-month error is therefore 38%. Those

Table 4.4 Radial keratotomy objective surgical accuracy 8 incisions 3–11 mm OZ

	Diopters Pre-op CR	Diopters 1 yr Δ CR	1 yr OSA	Error-1 yr	Diopters 2 yr Δ CR	2 yr OSA	Error-2 yr
	−5.75	7.00	1.22	+0.22	8.00	1.39	+0.39
	−6.75	6.75	1.00	0.00	7.50	1.11	+0.11
	−7.50	3.25	0.65	−0.35	3.75	0.75	−0.25
	−3.50	5.75	1.64	−0.36	5.00	1.43	+0.43
	−5.25	6.00	1.14	+0.14	5.25	1.00	0.00
	−6.25	3.25	0.52	−0.48	3.50	0.56	−0.44
	−5.25	3.25	0.62	−0.38	3.50	0.67	−0.33
	−11.25	9.75	0.87	−0.13	9.00	0.80	−0.20
	−4.50	3.75	0.83	−0.17	4.75	1.06	+0.06
	−6.00	5.50	0.92	−0.08	5.00	0.83	−0.17
	−6.50	7.25	1.12	+0.12	5.75	0.88	−0.12
	−4.75	6.25	1.32	+0.32	6.75	1.42	+0.42
	−4.75	6.50	1.37	+0.37	5.50	1.16	+0.16
	−5.00	6.50	1.30	+0.30	5.75	1.15	+0.15
	−9.25	8.25	0.89	−0.11	6.50	0.70	−0.30
	−9.25	7.25	0.78	−0.22	8.00	0.86	−0.14
	−5.00	4.25	0.85	−0.15	6.25	1.25	−0.25
x̄	−6.26	5.91	1.00	0.23	5.86	1.00	0.23
S.D.	+−2.02	+−1.86	+−0.30	+−0.13	+−1.62	+−0.27	+−0.14
Range	−3.50– 11.25	3.25– 9.75	−0.52– 1.64	0.00– 0.48	3.50– 9.00	0.56– 1.43	0.00– −0.44

$n = 17$. CR = cycloplegic refraction; OSA = objective surgical accuracy.

individuals who remain significantly undercorrected are candidates for four additional radial keratotomy incisions in an attempt to produce emmetropia, or up to 0.75 diopters of overcorrection. The number of corneal incisions and the optical zone size are therefore correlated to the potential operative result in radial keratotomy.

We have been intrigued by the additional response to the topical steroids utilised routinely in all patients in our study. With a 3.0 mm optical zone, an 8-incision radial keratotomy with topical steroids administered 4 times a day for 1 month revealed significantly greater response to the surgery in patients who were steroid responders. Steroid responders were identified as those patients with elevated intraocular pressure of 10 mmHg or greater (Table 4.7). Although the preoperative intraocular pressure was similar in the two populations, the non-steroid responders had an elevation of pressure of 17 to 19 mmHg at the end of 1 month preoperatively, whereas the steroid responders demonstrated an average intraocular tension of 16 to 27 mmHg. The population was similar in age at 33 years, and the myopia was statistically the same at −6.19 diopters in the non-steroid responders and −7.64 diopters in the steroid responders. The decrease in myopia of +5.10 diopters in the 52 patients who did not respond to the steroids was significantly less than the +7.04 diopters of refractive change demonstrated in the steroid responders. This difference of 1.94 diopters was statistically significant (p = 0.03). Table 4.7 demonstrates the preoperative horizontal (H) and vertical (V) keratometric readings of the steroid versus non-steroid responding group. We noted that the 7 steroid responders had an average preoperative horizontal K reading of 44.61 diopters, which was significantly steeper than the remainder of the population at 43.21 diopters (p = 0.02). In addition, the preoperative vertical radius of curvature was significantly steeper in the steroid responders, 45.96 compared to 43.97 diopters (p = 0.003). The change in keratometric reading between

Table 4.5 Radial keratotomy objective surgical accuracy 8 incisions 3.0 mm optical zone + 8 additional incisions

Diopters Pre-op CR	Diopters Δ CR01	OSA-1	Error-1	INT MO	ΔCR-2	FU MO	Diopters Final CR	Diopters CR 1–2	OSA 1–2	Error final
−5.75	3.00	−0.52	−0.48	9	0.75	3	−2.00	3.75	−0.65	−0.35
−9.50	5.25	−0.55	−0.45	5	0.25	3	−4.00	5.50	−0.58	−0.42
−8.25	4.00	−0.48	−0.52	8	3.50	3	−0.75	7.50	−0.91	−0.09
−4.50	1.50	−0.33	−0.677	5	1.25	6	−1.75	2.75	−0.61	−0.39
−7.00	1.25	−0.18	−0.82	4	5.50	6	−0.25	6.75	−0.96	−0.04
−6.75	3.00	−0.44	−0.56	5	1.75	6	−2.00	4.75	−0.70	−0.30
−7.75	4.50	−0.58	−0.42	3	2.50	12	−0.75	7.00	−0.90	−0.10
−8.00	3.25	−0.41	−0.59	15	1.25	3	−3.50	4.50	−0.56	−0.44
−7.50	3.50	−0.47	−0.53	6	2.25	6	−1.75	5.75	−0.77	−0.23
−9.75	8.50	−0.87	−0.13	6	2.00	12	0.75	10.50	−1.08	+0.08
−4.75	4.00	−0.84	−0.16	13	1.50	3	0.75	5.50	−1.17	+0.16
−9.00	7.00	−0.78	−0.22	7	1.25	3	−0.75	8.25	−0.92	−0.08
−8.25	3.75	−0.45	−0.55	7	2.75	6	−1.75	6.50	−0.79	−0.21
−8.75	4.00	−0.46	−0.54	9	3.00	6	−1.75	7.00	−0.80	−0.20
−10.25	7.75	−0.76	−0.24	4	3.00	3	0.50	10.75	−1.05	+0.05
−10.75	4.75	−0.44	−0.56	5	1.75	6	−4.25	6.50	−0.60	−0.40
−8.25	4.25	−0.51	−0.48	7	3.00	6	−1.00	7.25	−0.88	−0.12
−7.50	5.25	−0.70	−0.30	6	4.75	12	2.50	10.00	−1.33	+0.33
−4.50	3.25	−0.72	−0.28	3	0.50	24	−0.75	3.75	−0.83	−0.17
x̄ −7.72	4.30	−0.55	−0.45	6.68	2.24	6.79	−1.18	6.54	−0.85	−0.15
S.D. ±1.84	±1.87	±0.18	±0.18	±3.13	±1.37	±5.18	±1.68	±2.24	±0.21	±0.21
Range −10.75–	1.25–	−0.87–	−0.13–	3.00–	0.25–	3.00–	4.25–	2.75–	−1.33–	−0.33–
−4.50	8.50	−0.18	−0.82	15.00	5.50	24.00	2.50	10.75	−0.56	−0.44

n = 19. CR = cycloplegic refraction; OSA = objective surgical accuracy. Error = surgical error: 1 − OSA. INT MO = Time from original surgery to second operation. 1 − OSA. INT MO = Time from original surgery to second operation. Δ = charge.

Table 4.6 The University of Oklahoma Health Sciences Center Department of Ophthalmology 4 incisions: radial keratotomy results

Name	Eye	Zone	Sphere pre CR	Cyl pre CR	1 MO MR sphere	1 MO MR cyl	1 MO MR sphere Δ	1 MO MR CR Δ	3 MO CR sphere	3 MO CR cyl	3 MO CR sphere Δ	3 MO CR cyl Δ	1 MO% error	3 MO% error
L.M.	OS	3 mm	−6.25	2.00	−3.25	2.50	3.00	+0.50	−2.25	2.00	4.00	0.00	52%	36%
C.P.	OS	3 mm	−4.50	0.75	+1.50	1.25	6.00	+0.50	+0.75	1.00	5.25	+0.25	33%	17%
R.M.	OD	3 mm	−9.00	0.50	−5.75	0.00	3.25	−0.50	−7.00	0.50	2.00	0.00	64%	78%
D.P.	OD	3 mm	−7.25	0.00	−2.75	0.00	4.50	0.00	−2.50	1.25	4.75	+1.25	38%	34%
C.T.	OS	3 mm	−11.25	0.50	−3.50	1.25	7.75	+0.75	−5.75	0.50	5.50	0.00	31%	51%
M.R.	OD	3 mm	−6.00	1.50	+0.25	0.50	6.25	−1.00	−0.50	0.75	5.50	−0.75	4%	8%
R.M.	OS	3 mm	−10.00	0.00	−4.00	0.00	6.00	0.00	−6.50	0.50	3.50	+0.50	40%	65%
P.M.	OD	3 mm	−6.25	0.50	−1.50	0.00	4.75	−0.50	+0.50	0.00	6.75	−0.50	24%	8%
K.M.	OS	3 mm	−4.50	0.50	−2.00	1.25	2.50	+0.75	−1.25	1.75	3.25	+1.25	44%	28%
C.G.	OS	3 mm	−7.50	1.00	−2.75	0.50	4.75	−0.50	−4.00	1.25	3.50	+0.25	37%	53%
J.R.	OS	3 mm	−8.50	1.00	−2.00	1.00	6.50	0.00	−1.25	0.15	7.25	−0.85	24%	15%
C.T.	OD	3 mm	−9.25	1.25	−5.75	1.00	3.50	−0.25	−4.75	0.00	4.50	−1.25	62%	51%
S.B.	OS	3 mm	−10.00	0.50	−6.00	0.00	4.00	−0.50	−8.25	3.00	1.75	+1.25	60%	82%
D.T.	OD	3 mm	−6.50	0.50	−1.75	0.00	4.75	−0.50	−2.00	0.50	4.50	0.00	27%	31%
L.B.	OS	3 mm	−5.50	0.50	−2.25	0.00	3.25	−0.50	−2.00	0.00	3.50	−0.50	41%	36%
V.G.	OD	3 mm	−6.25	1.25	−3.00	0.75	3.25	−0.50	−0.75	0.00	5.50	−1.25	48%	12%
Mean			−7.41	0.77	−2.78/3.00	0.63	4.63	±0.14/0.45	−2.97/3.13	0.82	4.44	±0.02/0.62	39%	38%
S.D.			2.05	0.55	1.67	0.72	1.51	0.28	2.57	0.85	1.09	0.51	16%	24%

n = 19. Algebraic/absolute means.

Table 4.7

3 mm O.Z. RK + Non-steroid responders (52)	Mean	3 mm O.Z. RK + Steroid responders (7)	Mean
IOP pre-op =	17	IOP pre-op =	16
IOP 1 month =	19	IOP 1 month =	27
Age	33	Age	33
Myopia	−6.19	Myopia	−7.64
6 MO CR	−1.09	6 MO CR	−0.61
Decrease in myopia	+5.10	Decrease in myopia	+7.04

RK + Non-steroid responders (52)	H	V	RK + Steroid responders (7)	H	V
Pre-op K	43.21	43.97	Pre-op K	44.61	45.96
Post-op K	39.78	39.87	Post-op K	41.32	42.09
Decrease	4.43	4.10	Decrease	3.29	3.87

Steroid response accentuates radial keratotomy results.

the two populations, however, was not significant, nor was the postoperative K reading in the horizontal meridian. We had not been aware previously that steroid responders had significantly steeper keratometric readings than non-steroid responders. Since our operative results are greater than those reported in most populations by any combination of surgical manoeuvres in radial keratotomy, we feel that the topical steroids are useful in decreasing immediate wound healing and allowing the central and peripheral cornea to flatten, decreasing the myopia. However, topical steroids carry their own risks, including infection, glaucoma, and cataract, and cannot be recommended, except for the short postoperative period for which we have demonstrated their efficacy.

We have been pleased with the corneascope topography analysis following radial keratotomy which allows us to demonstrate the detailed shape of the cornea pre- and postoperatively with lighted Placido disc imagery as projected onto the cornea. The use of corneal topography in radial keratotomy has been reported in Rowsey et al (1981), Henslee & Rowsey (1983), and Isaac & Rowsey (1984). The cornea flattens asymmetrically following radial keratotomy procedures with the greatest corneal flattening occurring in the centre of the cornea, and diminished corneal flattening in the midperiphery and periphery of the cornea (Henslee & Rowsey, 1983). This is well demonstrated in Figures 4.3 and 4.4. The corneascope presents detailed map topography which we have analysed at the PERK Corneascope Reading Center at the University of Oklahoma. A curve fit algorithm, measuring the radius of curvature from the centre of the visual axis inside the central ring to the inside edge of any designated ring, is utilised by Rowsey & Isaac (1984). Flattening of the central cornea is associated with wide separation of the central rings. Steepening of the midperiphery of the cornea, or the corneal 'knee', demonstrates reversal of the aplanatic surface of the cornea following radial keratotomy (Henslee & Rowsey, 1983). We have been pleased that the Humphrey keratometer can measure this peripheral knee, or shorter radius of curvature, more rapidly than the corneascope, although the total of corneal topography is appreciated more easily with the photograph (Rowsey, 1983).

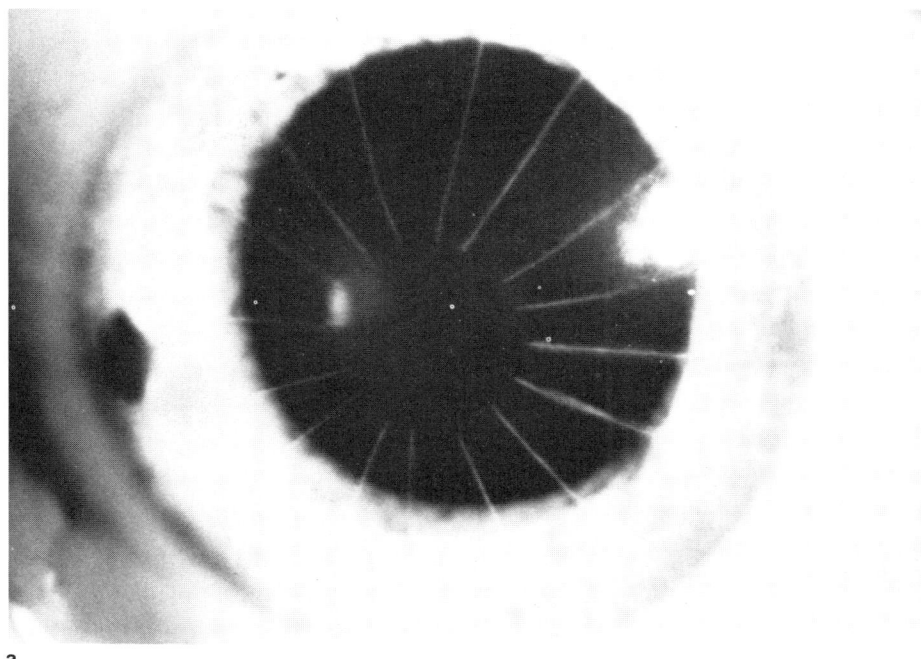

a

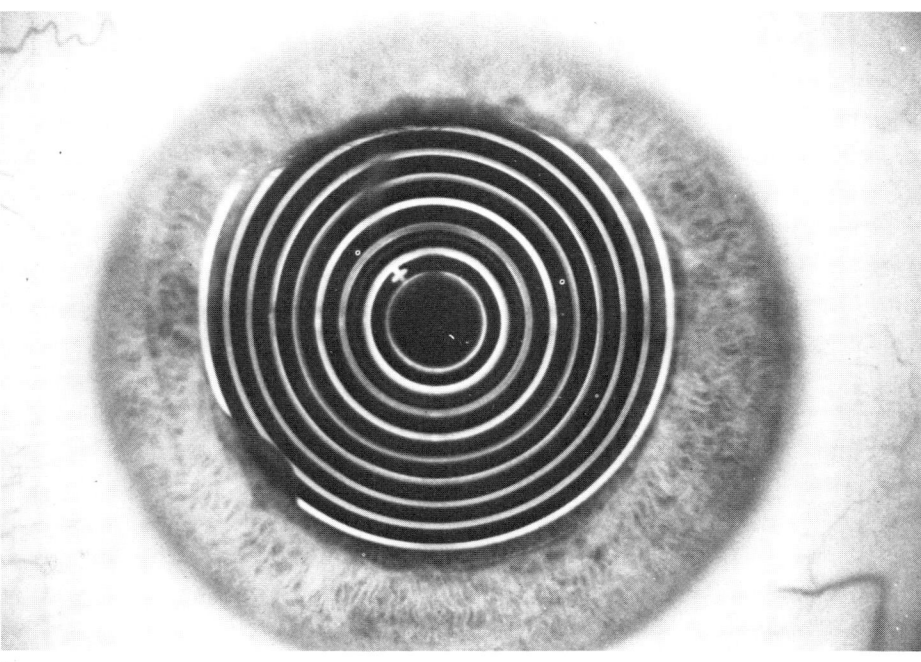

b

Fig. 4.3   a Slit lamp photograph of 16 incision radial keratotomy performed in June 1980. 5.75 diopters of myopia corrected. **b** Preoperative corneascope photograph of patient seen in 4a.

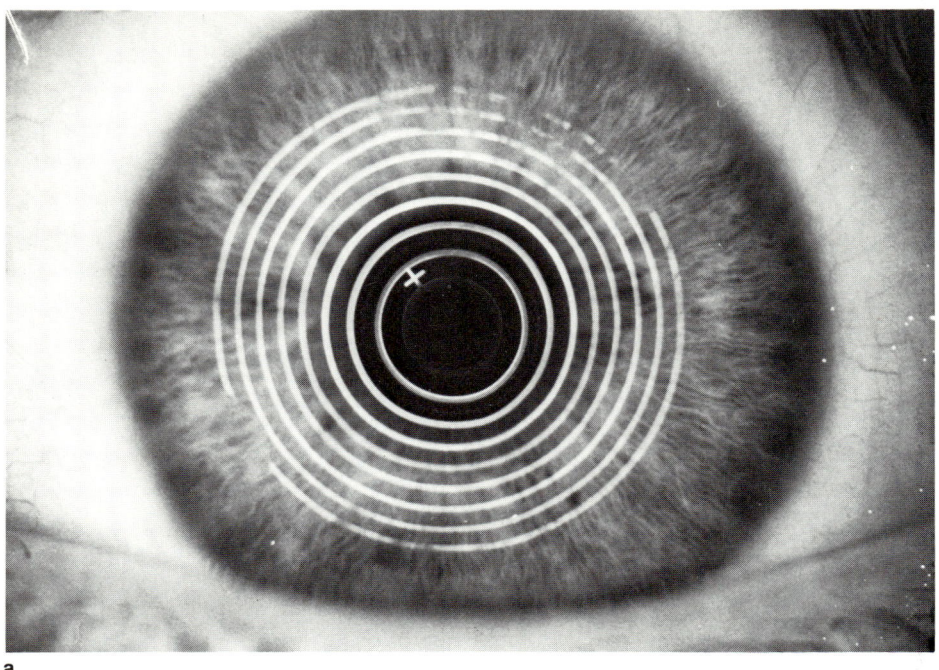

a

Fig. 4.4   a Postoperative corneascope photograph of patient seen in 4a. Note wide spacing (flattening) of central rings demonstrating reduction of corneal power from the operation. **b** Computer graphics comparator faceplate of corneascope photo seen in 5a. The dioptric power of the cornea is adjacent to the respective rings. The 'mean' corneal power of rings three to nine are presented adjacent to the 12:00 chord vertically. Note the central corneal flattening to 35.93 diopters with steepening toward the periphery (9th ring) to 39.45 diopters. This central corneal flattening remains stable over three years after surgery in our current follow-up of radial keratotomy patients.

COMPLICATIONS

The complications of radial keratotomy range from benign to disastrous, and patients should be aware of these complications before undergoing this experimental procedure. The lack of predictability of the operation and the range of surgical error have been discussed. Originally, the preliminary complications of the procedure were presented in Rowsey & Balyeat (1982a,b). The main complications that we have observed are the following: regression of myopic flattening, epithelial defects, recurrent erosions, stromal overgrowth, Cogan's map-dot-fingerprint corneal dystrophy, Moncreiff iron lines, blood in the incisions, vascular ingrowth with contact lens use, perforation of the anterior chamber, induction of astigmatic errors, incisional epithelial ingrowth, glare, decreased night vision, initial pain, persistently fluctuating vision, and overcorrection (Rowsey & Balyeat, 1982b). The data reviewed in Rowsey & Balyeat (1982a) demonstrated that perforations at the time of surgery contributed to induced astigmatism. These perforations have diminished with the use of ultrasonic pachymetry and diamond knife surgery (Rowsey et al, 1982c).

Patients are carefully questioned about the glare they experience in the evening. They are still able to observe scars when their pupils dilate, even 2 years after surgery.

CORNEASCOPE READING CENTER

UNIVERSITY OF OKLAHOMA
DEPARTMENT OF OPHTHALMOLOGY

DEAN McGEE EYE INSTITUTE
RESEARCH DIVISION

PATIENT NAME: EYE: O.S.   FILE: LCS26G1.1YR

TX HX: 14 MONTHS POST-OP 16 INCISION RADIAL KERATOTOMY 3-11 MM O.Z. (2TREP)
      DELTA CR: SPH=+5.75

CYCLOPLEGIC REF: PLANO   PHOTO DATE: 8/26/81   PRINTED: 10/21/83

CONTROL VALUE: 7.96   PHOTO MAG: 4.81 I.R.:1.3375 PERK #: N35448   MED REC#:035448

M.D./LOCATION: ROWSEY / MEI

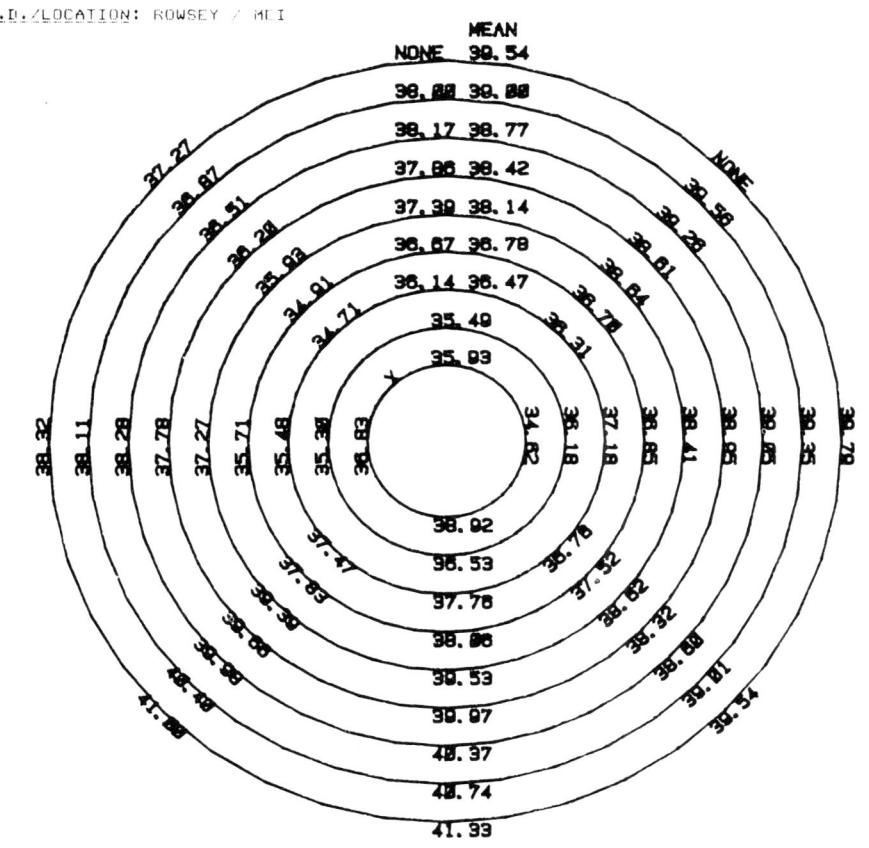

b

The Miller–Nadler glare tester has allowed us to document the gradual decrease in glare sensitivity to under 20% between 1 and 2 years. However, this glare does not appear to be incapacitating to the patient, and many who have undergone successful surgery will accept the glare in exchange for the myopic reduction accomplished.

The initial endothelial cell loss which we have documented in Rowsey & Balyeat (1982a) may not be progressive. Endothelial cell loss observed at both 1 and 3 months does not appear to be a progressive phenomenon at the 1 and 2 year gates, as demonstrated in Rowsey et al (1984). Steele et al (1982) demonstrated endothelial blebbing after radial keratotomy, with reversal of these blebs between 13 and 92 days postoperatively when wide field specular microscopy was accomplished. Cell loss of 5.8% was noted 3 months later in seven patients. The authors felt that the soft eye associated with additional incisions may contribute to undue flexing of the posterior cornea and endothelial cell loss. Hoffer et al (1981) noted a 10% endothelial cell loss at 3 months. These data are important, for Yamaguchi et al (1982) reported that of Sato's 281 eyes, 80 patients could be examined 10–20 years postoperatively, and 60 of these 80 eyes had bullous keratopathy. His data suggested that the older patients were more susceptible to this operative damage, and that it occurred approximately 20 years following the original operation. We re-emphasise that Sato's (1953) procedure frequently involved internal incisions through Descemet's membrane endothelium and superficial incisions through the anterior stroma. Yamaguchi et al (1982) reported 'patients who had many incisions developed bullous keratopathy more quickly'.

The careful work of Hull et al (1983) partially assuages our anxiety concerning eventual bullous keratopathy in patients undergoing radial keratotomy with the statement that 'fluorophotometry . . . showed no probable physiologically important change in endothelial fluorescein permeability' in rabbits. Similar studies in humans would be an important contribution.

Stainer et al (1982) examined a corneal transplant specimen that became cloudy following radial keratotomy and demonstrated persistent wound healing defects in the radial incisions, epithelial breakdown with irregular basement membrane changes, and persistent ingrowth into the incisions. The authors concluded 'we believe that radial keratotomy carries a potential risk of persistent optical and visual aberrations as well as the potential to endanger vision through delayed wound healing and widespread epithelial alterations.'

Similar epithelial inclusion cysts have been noted when circumferential and radial corneal incisions cross (Jester et al, 1983), suggesting that wound healing may be diminished because of inhibition of the centripetal spread of epithelial cells from the periphery of the cornea in a normal recruitment pattern. Jester reported a patient who had undergone both radial and concentric trephination to flatten the cornea, and his electron microscopic evaluation demonstrated extensive epithelial downgrowth into the incision sites and keratocyte degeneration with chromatin clumping and nuclear infolding consistent with an injury phenomenon. Abnormal anchoring fibrils and basal laminar material were noted between the surface epithelium and Bowman's membrane. The authors concluded that 'the integrity of the cornea has been altered, particularly with regard to the cornea's ability to withstand normal stress.'

The ability of the cornea to withstand subsequent trauma has been analysed by Luttrull et al (1982), Larson et al (1983) and Katz et al (1982). Luttrull demonstrated that following radial keratotomy in porcine eyes, incisions traversing the limbus were associated with ruptures of the globe at the limbus when incisions were at 70% of corneal thickness. Eyes which were incised to 95–100% of corneal thickness ruptured at the incision site. These data further contraindicate extension of the incisions through the limbus.

Ninety days after radial keratotomy in 33 rabbits, a controlled ocular trauma model was utilised by Larson et al (1983). The authors noted that at 90 days postoperatively, only 50% of the force of the normal eye could be tolerated before rupture occurred in the healed radial keratotomy eyes. Wound gape was noted, in which the wound margin separated for the length of the incision, along with a progressive pattern of lamellar dehiscence of the posterior corneal stromal collagen from the base of the incision sites. These areas were noted prior to frank perforation. The abnormality of wound healing may be associated with the peripheral corneal vascularisation that has been noted in Rowsey & Balyeat (1982b). The wound healing characteristics may also account for the complications of contact lens wear in a rabbit model following radial keratotomy (Katz et al, 1982). Corneal vascularisation was noted in rabbits following contact lens fitting after radial keratotomy. Under the lens contact point, the association of corneal scar formation near the limbus and contact lens anoxia may be associated with wound healing abnormalities and peripheral corneal neovascularisation. We have observed a patient referred to us who has undergone radial keratotomy on three occasions with minuscule effects on his myopia, but with significant corneal vascularisation 360 degrees underneath a continuous wear contact lens. Discontinuation of the contact lens was recommended, but corneal vascularisation persisted.

Gelender et al (1982) reported endophthalmitis following a corneal perforation in a patient referred to them after radial keratotomy. Gelender has also reported cataract formation in a 31-year-old patient referred to him after radial keratotomy (Gelender & Gelber, 1983). Corneal perforations had been noted at the time of surgery in both patients. The surgeon should note the peripheral shallowing of the anterior chamber as the intraocular pressure decreases after each incision, and the increased potential for engaging the iris and lens capsule with the diamond tip as Descemet's is inverted posteriorly into the anterior chamber. Even if a perforation does not occur, maintenance of high intraocular pressure during the operative procedure maintains an open angle and protects the lens. The corneal endothelium should never be allowed to touch the iris during the procedure.

SUMMARY

Radial keratotomy reduces myopia in the −2.00 to −6.00 diopter range. Advances in ophthalmic instrumentation, including diamond knives, corneoscopy, ultrasonic pachymetry, fixation devices, and control of wound healing, may allow greater predictability of this procedure's results in the future. Many surgical and postoperative nuances of the procedure are increasing the operative predictability and reducing the surgical error. The long-term complications of this technique on consecutive patients are not yet available. The most significant common complications, to date, appear to be the lack of predictability of results, glare, and fluctuating vision. Multivariant analysis of the preoperative and operative factors in the future may allow sufficient precision to recommend the procedure in selected myopic patients.

REFERENCES

Arrowsmith P N, Sanders D R, Marks R G 1983 Visual, refractive, and keratometric results of radial keratotomy. Archives of Ophthalmology 101: 873–881
Bores L D, Myers W, Cowden J 1981 Radial keratotomy: an analysis of the American experience. Annals of Ophthalmology 13: 941–951
Cowden J W 1982 Radial keratotomy: a retrospective study of cases observed at the Kresge Eye Institute for six months. Archives of Ophthalmology 100: 578–580
Cowden J W, Bores L D 1981 A clinical investigation of the surgical correction of myopia by the method of Fyodorov. Ophthalmology 88: 737–741

Fyodorov S N, Agranovsky A A 1982 Long-term results of anterior radial keratotomy. Journal of Ocular Therapy and Surgery 1: 217–223

Fyodorov S N, Durnev V V 1979 Operation of dosaged dissection of corneal circular ligament in cases of myopia of mild degree. Annals of Ophthalmology 11: 1885–1890

Gelender H, Gelber E C 1983 Cataract following radial keratotomy. Archives of Ophthalmology 101: 1229–1231

Gelender H, Flynn H W, Mandelbaum S H 1982 Bacterial endophthalmitis resulting from radial keratotomy. American Journal of Ophthalmology 93: 323–326

Henslee S L, Rowsey J J 1983 New corneal shapes in keratorefractive surgery. Ophthalmology 90: 245–250

Hoffer K J, Darin J J, Pettit T H, Hofbauer J D, Elander R, Levenson J E 1981 UCLA clinical trial of radial keratotomy: preliminary report. Ophthalmology 88: 729–736

Hoffer K J, Darin J J, Pettit T H, Hofbauer J D, Elander R, Levenson J E 1983 Three years experience with radial keratotomy: the UCLA study. Ophthalmology 90: 627–636

Hull D S, Farkas S, Green K, Laughter L, Elijah R D, Bowman K 1983 Radial keratotomy: effect on cornea and aqueous humor physiology in the rabbit. Archives of Ophthalmology 101: 479–481

Issac, Rowsey J J 1984 Corneoscopy in Keratorefractive surgery. Cornea (in press)

Jester J V, Villasenor R A, Miyashiro J 1983 Epithelial inclusion cysts following radial keratotomy. Archives of Ophthalmology 101: 611–615

Jester J V, Venet T, Lee J, Schanzlin D J, Smith R E 1981a A statistical analysis of radial keratotomy in human cadaver eyes. American Journal of Ophthalmology 92: 172–177

Jester J V, Steel D, Salz J, Miyashiro J, Rife L, Schanzlin D J, Smith R E 1981b Radial keratotomy in non-human primate eyes. American Journal of Ophthalmology 92: 153–171

Katz H R, Duffin R M, Glasser D B, Pettit T H 1982 Complications of contact lens wear after radial keratotomy in an animal model. American Journal of Ophthalmology 94: 377–382

Kramer S G, Yavitz E Q, Sulonen J 1981 Precision standardisation of radial keratotomy. Ophthalmic Surgery 12: 561–566

Larson B C, Kremer F B, Eller A W, Bernardino V B 1983 Quantitated trauma following radial keratotomy in rabbits. Ophthalmology 90: 660–667

Luttrull J K, Jester J V, Smith R E 1982 The effect of radial keratotomy on ocular integrity in an animal model. Archives of Ophthalmology 100: 319–320

Nirankari V S, Katzen L E, Karesh J W, Richards R D, Lakhanpal V 1983 Ongoing prospective clinical study of radial keratotomy. Ophthalmology 90: 637–642

Nirankari V S, Katzen L E, Richards R D, Karesh J W, Lakhanpal V, Billings E 1982 Prospective clinical study of radial keratotomy. Ophthalmology 89: 677–686

Rowsey J J 1983 Ten caveats in keratorefractive surgery. Ophthalmology 90: 148–155

Rowsey J J, Balyeat H D 1982a Preliminary results and complications of radial keratotomy. American Journal of Ophthalmology 93: 437–455

Rowsey J J, Balyeat H D 1982b Radial keratotomy: preliminary report of complications. Ophthalmic Surgery 13: 27–35

Rowsey J J, Balyeat H D, Yeisley K P 1982c Diamond knife. Ophthalmic Surgery 13: 279–282

Rowsey J J, Reynolds A E, Brown R 1981 Corneal topography: corneascope. Archives of Ophthalmology 99: 1093–1100

Rowsey J J, Balyeat H D, Rabinovitch B, Burris T E, Hays J C 1983 Predicting the results of radial keratotomy. Ophthalmology 90: 642–654

Rowsey J J et al 1984 Complications of radial Keratotomy. Ophthalmology (To be published)

Salz J, Lee J S, Jester J V, Steel D, Villasenor R A, Nesburn A B, Smith R E 1981 Radial keratotomy in fresh human cadaver eyes. Ophthalmology 88: 742–746

Salz J, Lee T, Jester J V, Villasenor R A, Steel D, Bernstein J, Smith R E 1983 Analysis of incision depth following experimental radial keratotomy. Ophthalmology 90: 655–659

Sato T 1950 Posterior incision of cornea: surgical treatment for conical cornea and astigmatism. American Journal of Ophthalmology 33: 943–948

Sato T, Akiyama K, Shibata H 1953 A new surgical approach to myopia. American Journal of Ophthalmology 36:823–829

Stainer G A, Shaw E L, Binder P S, Zavala E Y, Akers P 1982 Histopathology of a case of radial keratotomy. Archives of Ophthalmology 100: 1473–1477

Steel D, Jester J V, Salz J, Villasenor R A, Lee J S, Schanzlin D J, Smith R E 1981 Modification of corneal curvature following radial keratotomy in primates. Ophthalmology 88: 747–754

Steele A D McG, Buckley R J, Sherrard E S 1982 Early experiences with radial keratotomy. Transactions of the Ophthalmological Society of the UK 102: 35–41

Unterman, Rowsey J J 1984 Diamond knife cornea incisions. Ophthalmic Surgery (in press)

Yamaguchi T, Kanai A, Tanak M, Ishii R, Nakajima A 1982 Bullous keratopathy after anterior-posterior radial keratotomy for myopia and myopic astigmatism. American Journal of Ophthalmology 93: 600–606

5. Intraocular lenses

M. J. Roper-Hall   W. J. C. C. Rich

Optically, the best position for correction of the refraction after cataract surgery is as close as possible to that of the normal crystalline lens. The level of safety and the visual results with intraocular lenses now justify their implantation immediately after most cataract extractions, but a high degree of skill and careful choice of lens and method are essential. Problems such as temporary loss of the anterior chamber, or a small peripheral iris adhesion would probably not threaten the end result in orthodox cataract surgery, but when an intraocular lens has been inserted, these complications assume greater importance and may lead to irreversible damage to the corneal endothelium. Despite such potential problems, if patients are suitably selected and proper precautions are observed, the incidence of complications with intraocular lens surgery should, in the same hands, differ little from that of simple cataract surgery. Rehabilitation after surgery is much easier and quicker than with other methods, the postoperative vision and orientation seem natural and the patient can often see well without glasses. The scope of cataract surgery has been extended to those unilateral lens opacities which used to be left untreated when the fellow eye remained unaffected. Blindness from bilateral cataract has become less common.

Intraocular lenses have gained great popularity and there may often be considerable pressure upon surgeons to carry out this type of surgery. Whether they are implanting lenses themselves or not, ophthalmologists are aware of the very good and some very bad results: often these are attributed to the use of a particular lens, which is being promoted or criticised. With around 200 different lens designs to choose from and so many changes and new introductions taking place all the time, choice is extremely difficult. We intend in this chapter to set out the present position in relation to the use of intraocular lenses and important matters which are emerging. Many different techniques are being used; we would like to point out the important principles and indicate the best management.

STATISTICS

In 1982, 496 000 lenses were implanted in the United States of America (US) and approximately 37 500 in the United Kingdom (UK). This represents 78% of cases of cataract extraction in the US and approaching one half of those in the UK. The types of intraocular lenses being used show interesting changes (Stark et al, 1983). A trend is now becoming apparent away from iris fixated lenses. In 1978 in the US 52% of intraocular lenses were iris supported, while in 1982 57% were capsule supported, 40% anterior chamber angle supported and only 3% iris supported. In the UK in 1982 the proportions were almost evenly shared between the three main groups.

In association with the widespread adoption of intraocular lens surgery, an absolute increase is occurring in the number of cataract operations being performed (Taylor, 1981).

RESULTS

It is very difficult to make a clear comparison of results of cataract surgery because there are so many variables in selection and assessment. The age of the patient, the level of visual acuity at the time of surgery, whether to operate on unilateral cataract all have a bearing on surgical method and the potential for a good result. In published reports the duration of follow-up can vary from a few weeks to several years. The case study may also be over a short period or several years. If the latter, there are other variables which are not immediately apparent: a lens of nominally the same design is not always made by the same manufacturer, there are subtle differences in dimension, material and handling. Some of the changes are planned for a purpose, but others are unplanned and forced by variation in supply of materials or fluctuations of demand.

None of us are satisfied unless our results show continuing improvement over succeeding decades. During a period of time many subtle changes of surgical method have a bearing on safety of the operation and the quality of results. We are now doing different operations, with different standards of evaluation, and it is difficult to compare our own results using different lenses; it is certainly not possible to take two lenses used by different surgeons at different times and make a valid comparison of results. As a general standard, in the 1980s none of us should be satisfied with a corrected vision of less than 6/12 in the long term after an uncomplicated cataract is removed from an otherwise healthy eye.

CLASSIFICATION

Lenses can be classified by the position of their refractive element and their method of support.
1. Anterior chamber — Angle supported
2. Pre-pupillary — Iris supported
3. Posterior chamber — Iris supported
        — Capsule supported
        — Ciliary body supported

Lens materials
Polymethylmethacrylate (PMMA) was first produced at the beginning of the century, but until it was needed during the 1939–45 war its development was slow. The success of intraocular lens surgery owes much to the availability of the material, which in chemical, physical, biocompatible and optical qualities is still the most satisfactory. PMMA was not exposed to the laboratory tests which would now be demanded before such a material could be applied to clinical use. Nevertheless, PMMA has stood the test of time outstandingly well and its characteristics are so far unmatched; it has high tensile strength, it is not affected by hydrolysis, optically it has a very low scattering coefficient and very high direct transmission of light. In the eye, the fact that it is brittle is not important and it is not exposed to the physical forces which degrade it,

especially heat and ionising radiation, but this susceptibility introduces problems in sterilisation of the lens before surgery. Heat methods cannot be used, gamma irradiation turns it brown and may cause cracking. The intrinsic problems of PMMA within the eye are its hydrophobic property which makes it a danger to corneal epithelium and the fact that it cannot withstand sterilisation by heat. Major problems have been encountered in the past and could occur again due to contamination of PMMA by chemicals introduced during manufacture or handling and particularly during sterilisation and storage. Glass intraocular lenses have been produced with claimed optical benefits and biocompatibility, but they have problems caused by the necessity for complicated supporting systems made from other materials.

Materials used for supporting loops of intraocular lenses do not have the same satisfactory record as PMMA; nylon has been show to degrade (Drews et al, 1978) so much so that complete loops could disappear; polypropylene is now used for the loops of many lenses and by some surgeons for suturing the lens to the iris. Degradation of polypropylene does occur in vivo with superficial cracking and flaking, but the equivalent of a lifetime of ultraviolet light in vitro has been shown to produce only slight reduction in the tensile strength of polypropylene (Mobray et al, 1983). A greater degree of degradation has been noted in actively metabolising tissues so that permanency of loops in the anterior chamber angle must be questioned, particularly if engulfed by peripheral anterior synechiae (Drews, 1983).

Many lenses, including the loops, are made entirely from PMMA and the report of an earlier Boberg Ans all-PMMA anterior chamber lens, showing no evidence of biodegradation after 23 years in an eye, must encourage this trend.

Sterilisation
Until 1956 the generally accepted method of sterilisation was immersion in 1% quaternary ammonium compounds for one hour. The use of this antiseptic was one undoubted cause of serious postoperative reactions. The caustic soda method of Frederick Ridley (1957) has been used for nearly 30 years. The lens is sterilised in 10% caustic soda (NaOH) and stored in 0.1% NaOH solution; used correctly this method has proved very safe and effective. Galin et al (1983) now recommend that 5% rather than 0.1% NaOH is used for storage and the lens thoroughly washed three times in sterile water or balanced salt solution before use. Caustic soda has been criticised on theoretical grounds particularly because of the difficulty in proving that an individual lens has been completely sterilised. Gas sterilisation is used exclusively in some countries as a replacement method, but has been associated with an increased incidence of intraocular inflammation.

CONCEPTS OF LENS DESIGN

Lens designs may attempt to copy nature, but it usually proves impractical to simulate the natural construction. Simpler substitutes are often found to have perfectly adequate function. The development of intraocular lenses has shown that dimensions can be much reduced. To be effective implants need to be surgically convenient, simple, safe and quick to insert, so that their advantage can be applied by the average surgeon, not only those with special skill. The implant must maintain its purpose efficiently after implantation.

The scientific basis is important, but in addition the value of the whole procedure depends on selection of materials and designs appropriate to the particular need, and technical skill in avoiding complications in what is, at first, a relatively unknown field.

There is a tendency for the success rate of implants to deteriorate noticeably when they are made available for general use. There are a number of reasons for this: the pioneering surgeon may select his cases very carefully and pay great attention to detail. During development, experience will be accrued and problems solved, but such details may not be published. The initial implants are prototypes made in a laboratory with great care. Once released for general use there may be a demand greater than the supply and commercial manufacture introduces mass production and cost-cutting competition. Materials thought to be the same may prove to be quite different in their biocompatibility. If, in addition, such an implant is used by someone inexperienced, disasters can follow, which bring the implant and everyone involved into disrepute.

Quality control

There have been steady improvements in the quality of most intraocular lenses, but, with many new lens designs and manufacturers, it is more important than ever to keep this aspect under close scrutiny. Optical performance of some products has been vigorously tested and found to be very close to specification (Olson, 1980). The surface of some lenses has been shown to be excellent, others have been less satisfactory with rough edges and inconsistent angulation or length of loops or feet (Dersch, 1981). The practice of engraving or embossing information on the lens is questionable, because it produces an unnecessary surface defect and deposits of grinding polish have been noted in crevices.

Current trends in lens design

While there is general agreement that PMMA of clinical quality is the best material to use for optical implants, there is no agreement on the best design. A lens design needs to be capable of commercial production, surgically convenient and safe with regard to intra- and post-operative complications. There is at present a general trend towards lenses which require a less critical fit and which are made of one lens material. Angle supported lenses of the rigid or semi-rigid type require very accurate measurement of the diameter of the anterior chamber and hence lenses have been designed to have a tolerance in this respect and some are claimed to fit all diameters. It is very obvious that lenses must not be flexible antero-posteriorly or they will reintroduce the dangers of corneal touch demonstrated in mobile iris supported lenses (Jagger & Jacobi, 1979); anterior flexion of the lenses might well occur when, for example, the patient rubs the eye. The safety of such lenses is certainly not yet proved. Indeed, serious complications have occurred with the Azar 91–Z flexible loop anterior chamber lens which necessitated withdrawal of the lens from further use. Erosion of such loops into the angle has been followed in a significant number of cases by glaucoma, uveitis and hyphaema; this is an example of how a lens design can become widely adopted, while complications only become apparant all too late. In the relatively short history of intraocular lenses there have been several examples of similar avoidable complications.

The manufacture of lenses and supporting loops entirely in PMMA would seem to be sensible, but it brings with it some problems. The angle of supporting loops can be very critical, for example, the Little-Arnott iris supported lens became much less stable when one manufacturer made a 5° change in the angulation of the anterior loops without informing all the surgeons who used this lens. Some posterior chamber lenses are being made with anterior angulation of the loops by 5–10° in order to move the lens posteriorly and produce a tight fit against the posterior capsule. A plano-convex lens with the convex surface facing posteriorly may help to delay opacification of the posterior capsule by tight contact. This gives the optical advantages of reduced magnification and less spherical and chromatic abberration (Wang & Pomerantzeff, 1982). The effectivity of the lens in this form is reduced because the principal plane is more posteriorly situated in the eye (Downing & Sayano, 1983).

The use of the YAG laser for postoperative capsulotomy has encouraged the introduction of posterior chamber lenses such as the Hoffer ridge lens which deliberately produce a gap between the lens and the posterior capsule, so that the laser energy focused on the capsule will not damage the lens itself.

It can be observed that currently there is a turmoil of activity in lens design, but it must be emphasised that changes need to be made with great care to ensure that they result in *improvement* in design, material or technique. Often during the past 30 years well-intentioned changes have had unexpected and undesirable results.

Withdrawal of lenses

Some examples have already been given of lenses which have had to be withdrawn because of unacceptable complications; many were quite small modifications of existing lenses, sometimes without changing the description of the lens, but sometimes attaching the name of another surgeon. At the time the alteration might seem a small detail, but have important effects, which are not immediately apparent. Twenty-five modifications were made by one manufacturer during the development of a widely used lens; most of the modifications were not obvious, but some led to a high incidence of endothelial corneal dystrophy. When such complications occur there is a risk of widespread public criticism of intraocular lenses in general.

Europe has had previous experience of serious intraocular lens disasters which led a majority of surgeons to discontinue implant surgery, so it is disturbing that recent indiscriminate attempts were made to sell lenses in Europe which had already been withdrawn in the US. The competing lenses made by different manufacturers should be carefully inspected for obvious faults as well as any other variations from those of proved reliability. Differences may be revealed between them, some of which may be the cause of a higher incidence of complications.

Refractive considerations

It should now be possible to predict the intraocular lens power to be inserted for a given patient to achieve the best possible optical correction, and it is no longer acceptable to insert a 'standard' power lens in all cases. Hillman (1983) reports that it should be possible to attain 80% within one diopter spherical equivalent of the predicted postoperative refraction. To achieve this, very accurate measurement of the axial length by A-scan ultrasonography and corneal radius by keratometry are required. The position of the intraocular lens within the eye must be carefully considered (Shammas, 1980) and formulae devised by Binkhorst (1975), Colenbrander (1973) or others can be used to predict the required intraocular lens power. If ultrasound and keratometry are not available and predictions are based on the patient's refractive history, there will be a number of unexpectedly high errors.

The quality of vision with intraocular lenses can be quite outstanding. Many patients see much better than they had expected and achieve a quite extraordinary depth of focus which enables them to obtain satisfactory distance and near vision without spectacle correction (Nakazawa & Ohtsuki, 1983). To make this desirable achievement most likely, it is necessary to aim for a postoperative degree of ametropia of −1.5 diopters spherical equivalent power. Huber (1981) has pointed out that the depth of focus can be enhanced by simple myopic astigmatism between −0.75 and −3.00 diopters at an axis of 180 degrees. With such a result many patients can see 6/6 and read N5 without glasses.

LENS IMPLANTATION AND GLAUCOMA

Chronic simple glaucoma, whether or not medically controlled, is now a relative rather than an absolute contraindication to lens implantation if cataract surgery is required. Considerations such as the depth of the anterior chamber and the supportive ability of the iris and pupil may make a posterior chamber lens after extracapsular surgery a preferred choice if a trabeculectomy or other drainage operation has already been carried out. If trabeculectomy is to be combined with cataract removal, then an extracapsular extraction offers the advantage of keeping the vitreous away from the drainage site. A posterior chamber lens is unlikely to be able to touch the cornea if there is any shallow anterior chamber after surgery. The thinned atrophic iris of many patients with glaucoma has been reported as making pupil capture a rather common (28%), but not serious, complication with posterior chamber implants (Rock & Rylander, 1983).

The postoperative pressure elevation, which normally follows cataract surgery if wound closure has been secure, is transient and rarely lasts more than 24 hours (Rich et al, 1974), but the degree and duration can be significantly greater if alpha chymotrypsin or sodium hyaluronate has been used (Hoopes, 1982).

Pupil block glaucoma occurs most frequently with angle supported lenses when the lens itself blocks badly placed iridectomies; iris supported lenses also can be associated with blockage of the pupil if there is no functioning iridectomy. Adequate iridectomies are obviously necessary with these lenses, but seem unnecessary with posterior chamber lenses, as pupil block glaucoma is very rare. Treatment by pupillary dilatation may be successful, but, if not, an iridectomy will have to be performed either by open surgery or more elegantly by neodymium YAG or Argon laser.

LENS IMPLANTATION AND DIABETES

Most patients with diabetes seem to be suitable for lens implantation (Clayman et al, 1979) and indeed an intraocular lens could be argued to minimise the optical effect of a scotoma or distortion caused by macular problems of background retinopathy. Known proliferative retinopathy or rubeosis iridis should be considered as contraindications. The intraocular lens must not make treatment for diabetic retinopathy more difficult, and adequate pupillary dilatation must be possible for laser treatment.

LENS IMPLANTATION AND SENILE MACULAR DEGENERATION

The normal optical relationships which can be regained by implantation surgery mean that patients who might not previously have been considered suitable for cataract surgery, because of known senile macular degeneration and the doubtful improvement to central vision which cataract surgery would bring, can now receive real benefit in overall vision. As the possibility of treatment of macular disease becomes better established, the criteria for surgical management of the cataract may need further modification.

MYOPIA

Patients who have a significant degree of axial myopia are often not happy to be rendered aphakic, both because of aniseikonia and because the resultant hypermetropia is less useful than a mild degree of myopia. Livernois & Sinskey (1983) reported good results in a series of myopic patients who received implant lenses ranging between an equivalent power of +10.00 and +6.00 diopters giving them a final refractive error between −3.00 and +1.25 diopters.

The greater risks of retinal detachment in myopic patients must be borne in mind and a lens design chosen which will allow very adequate examination of the peripheral retina. The presence of an intraocular lens does not seem to predispose to the development of retinal detachment (Clayman et al, 1981). The extracapsular technique has been shown to carry a lower risk of postoperative retinal detachment and is, therefore, to be preferred in cases at risk.

SURGICAL CONSIDERATIONS

Anaesthesia

Good anaesthesia is essential for a satisfactory outcome of the operation, but bad anaesthesia can be disastrous.

The choice of general or local anaesthesia for intraocular lens surgery needs to be made after considering all the relevant facts about the patient's general condition and mental state, the surgical environment and the quality of supporting staff. In Europe, unlike the United States (Jaffe, 1981), there is a growing preference for general anaesthesia. The administration of general anaesthesia is now so skilled that many of the dangers and disadvantages of the past no longer exist. The introduction of non-depolarising muscle relaxants has been an important factor in securing satisfactory akinesia and in reducing intraocular pressure during implant surgery. The patient's recovery is usually quick and quiet. Good, safe general anaesthesia needs special skill and monitoring, thus making extra demands on medical resources. There are greater risks unless general anaesthesia is given in these ideal conditions.

Akinesia

A local anaesthetic agent will block sensory and motor nerve conduction and thus produce akinesia of the orbital muscles as well as anaesthesia.

Muscle relaxants under general anaesthesia will produce akinesia of all muscles, not only those of the orbit. This has an unarguable advantage in that the fully anaesthetised patient cannot make any unexpected movement. Respiratory movements continue, but under regular and controlled mechanical ventilation.

Vasoconstriction
Local anaesthetic solutions containing adrenaline (epinephrine) will constrict vessels. Under general anaesthesia vasoconstriction is obtained by using controlled positive pressure ventilation, which reduces the carbon dioxide level in the blood.

Ocular hypotension
Reduction of intraocular pressure is obtained by abolition of the tone of the extraocular muscles so that the eye is not compressed. Reduction of volume in the vitreous can also effect reduction of intraocular pressure. Agents such as oral glycerol, intravenous urea, or mannitol have been used, but they have disadvantages such as nausea, vomiting and urinary retention.

Under local anaesthesia ocular hypotension is obtained by digital or balloon pressure exerted in such a way that volume is reduced without embarrassing flow through the central retinal artery. It should be noted that the effect of digital pressure is maximal at the end of its application, but as soon as it is discontinued, the effect on vitreous volume will be reversing and this will be during surgery (Obstbaum et al, 1971).

Under general anaesthesia ocular hypotension is obtained by controlled positive pressure ventilation alone, and the effect will continue to be exerted throughout the operation. This is, therefore, an advantage over the preoperative compression techniques.

Volume reduction
Reduction of vitreous volume has additional advantages for intraocular lens surgery in increasing the depth of the anterior chamber so that there is more room for insertion of the lens and work on the lens or iris without endangering the corneal endothelium. In addition, the concave vitreous face is much less vulnerable to damage. Successful volume reduction may induce a danger, in the intracapsular technique, of trapping air behind the implant unless the anterior chamber is reformed with fluid.

NEW MATERIALS AND INSTRUMENTS

Fluids
Attention has recently been drawn to the vulnerability of the corneal endothelium to damage during implant surgery. Surgeons are now very aware of this and while some have chosen a different lens design, others have modified their surgical technique in order to minimise the problem. Damage is caused directly; the endothelium is vulnerable not only to contact by the implant but also to other mechanical contact and to irrigating fluids. Saline solutions need to be physiologically balanced in all their constituents, in buffering, in tonicity, in sterility and in temperature. Some of these factors are more important than others, but none can be ignored. Surgeons must

ensure that high quality is maintained, keep alert to the possibility of contamination and observe closely that no particles are present in solutions used within the eye.

In the performance of cataract surgery, a percentage of endothelial cells is lost; the major cause is direct trauma. If the endothelial cell count has already become reduced to a critical level below $1000/mm^2$, there is a risk that surgery will precipitate bullous keratopathy.

Roper-Hall & Wilson (1982) showed an overall drop in endothelial cell density of 23.2% in patients who underwent cataract extraction with intraocular lens; a very similar result to the prospective studies reviewed by Bourne et al (1981) which gave an overall figure of 23.8%. However, those cases where there was no evidence at operation of endothelial damage during the intraocular lens insertion, showed no greater reduction in cell density than with cataract extraction alone. Although the reduction of endothelial cell density was greater when there was endothelial contact with the implant this still remained within safe levels when no abrasive force was applied. It was when endothelial contact was prolonged and the lens was rubbed against the endothelium, that an unacceptably large cell loss occurred. Great damage is caused by PMMA because it is hydrophobic and sticks firmly to the endothelium. When it is moved, it will tear cells off. This damage will be minimised if the PMMA is irrigated away from the endothelium and rubbing is carefully avoided. The reduction of endothelial cell density related to endothelial trauma is comparable with the retrospective results of Sugar et al (1978). All possible steps must, therefore, be taken to avoid damage to the endothelium.

Sodium hyaluronate

Sodium hyaluronate has recently been introduced for use during cataract surgery. It appears to have even greater advantage if an intraocular lens is to be inserted (Percival, 1981) when it can protect the endothelium from touch by the implant. Other products with similar properties such as methylcellulose are being studied for use in anterior segment surgery and these may be less expensive (Fechner, 1979).

The proprietary preparation of sodium hyaluronate (Healon, Healonid) is manufactured within physiological limits. It can be injected into the anterior or posterior chamber through a fine cannula keeping tissues separated so that damage can be avoided during manipulation. It is claimed that endothelial cell loss is greatly reduced (Pape & Balazs, 1980; Percival, 1981). However, Lazenby & Brooker (1981) showed no significant difference in endothelial cell density or corneal thickness when comparing cases in which sodium hyaluronate preparation was used and those which received balanced salt solution or air. There are reports of a significant protective function of sodium hyaluronate to the corneal endothelium (Grane, 1980) and it would seem desirable to coat the intraocular lens and all instrument tips which will enter the anterior chamber with this material before insertion. The preparation has certainly been used enthusiastically as a means of avoiding endothelial problems in implant surgery, but is is important that it is not used as an alternative to improved surgical technique, or an excuse for continuing a technique which should have been modified in some other way in order to make it safer.

Instruments

Individual instruments have been designed to hold, insert and manipulate intraocular lenses. A wide range is available, but each surgeon will have his own preferences and a set of instruments should be selected by experience and observation.

Needles

Special needles for ophthalmic surgery are now so sharp that they can be passed through tissues almost without fixation. This means that a corneal wound can be closed without losing the anterior chamber during suturing giving greater safety during implant techniques. These very good needles need to be handled with care, misdirection may bend them and a momentary touch against the needle holder or forceps will blunt them so that subsequent passages are difficult and not accomplished without distortion and potential inaccuracy of wound closure.

There is disagreement on the ideal shape and size of the needle. Most eye surgeons prefer a needle of 3/8ths of a circle, the 'eye curved needle', but some ask for a half circle needle and recently there have been designs which have a variable curvature i.e. a shorter radius near the tip to enable a more vertical deeper bite to be taken, followed by a shaft which is easier to control during the subsequent passage of the needle.

Neodymium YAG laser

The introduction of the YAG laser has brought a new tool with particular applications in the field of implant surgery. Aron-Rosa (1981) has carried out anterior capsulotomy prior to extracapsular surgery and claims that capsular flaps well suited to intraocular lens retention can be fashioned by this technique. It is doubtful whether this offers a real advantage over surgical capsulotomy and it seems to constrict the pupil and increase viscosity of cortical lens material, which can cause problems during extraction.

Much more useful is the ability of the YAG laser to achieve posterior capsulotomy painlessly and rapidly through the slit lamp. The laser energy must be the minimum necessary for the task and accurate focusing is essential, otherwise it is easy to produce small areas of damage to the implant; there have been reports of lens fracture. Unless there are very many of these spots of damage there is no noticeable visual deficit and liberation of free monomer is stated to be minimal. Vitreous bands and adhesions from intraocular lenses can be divided with ease. Claims have been made that some cases of cystoid macular oedema may be relieved by division of bands of vitreous between lens and wound by the YAG laser (Katzen et al, 1983). Complications such as pupil block glaucoma can be treated very effectively by making an iridotomy or a hole in the vitreous face with this new instrument. There can be no doubt that the availability of a Neodymium YAG laser will alter the extracapsular surgeon's approach, so that primary capsulotomy should no longer be needed and excessive capsular cleaning at the time of surgery is now unwarranted. The influence this has on lens design has already been mentioned (see p. 87 [Ridge]).

COMPLICATIONS

The incidence of complications was reported in the very valuable interim FDA report on intraocular lenses (Worthen et al, 1979). This studied data on 117 503 lenses of different classes. Over 80 million bytes of information were recorded. Two sets of data resulted, a core study and an adjunct study. The core study had more detailed and frequent reporting and included 27 914 cases of lens implantation and 3132 controls (these were patients referred for lens implantation and who were considered suitable, but refused to have it and so had an orthodox cataract extraction without lens).

The complications recorded for all lenses and controls included lens dislocation, retinal detachment, iritis, endophthalmitis, vitritis, cyclitic membrane, pupillary block, secondary glaucoma, hyphaema, macular oedema, and corneal oedema. The incidence of retinal detachment was highest in the control group. The incidence of macular oedema was highest with anterior chamber fixated lenses (6650 cases studied), next highest with posterior chamber lenses (1182 cases studied), and then with the control group of 3132 cases. The incidence with iris fixation and irido-capsular lenses (20 082 cases studied) was less than with the controls or any of the other groups!

There is, therefore, conflicting evidence on the frequency of various complications. Most of the complications which are cited in arguments for and against various methods, do, in fact, occur with all methods. The total effect of all the complications which occur needs to be taken into account and, in the last analysis, the best way of deciding on success is the quality of long term corrected vision in our patients.

Dislocation problems
Anterior chamber angle supported lenses may be unstable and the feet of the implant may rotate in the angle because of too small a lens diameter. A foot of such a lens may protrude backwards through an iridectomy or forwards into the lips of the limbal incision. These situations sometimes stabilise and can then safely be left alone.

Iris supported lenses vary greatly in their propensity to discloation according to design characteristics such as number, position and angulation of supporting loops and also to surgical method including whether an iris suture is used or not. When the haptic of such lenses is in the anterior chamber, dislocation forwards endangers the corneal endothelium. When iris supported posterior chamber lenses dislocate they usually do so backwards. One loop dislocations may be a simple matter to retrieve using gravity and a mydriatic followed by a miotic, but if all loops dislocate then a serious retrieval problem may exist. The McCannel suture (McCannel, 1976) is very useful in securing a replaced lens.

Cystoid macular oedema
Wide variations in diagnostic criteria, onset and duration of this non-specific condition has made it possible for different investigators to come to conflicting conclusions. Fluorescein leakage at the macula is very commonly evident (47%) in patients after cataract extraction (Hitchings et al, 1975) and it seems that this angiographic leakage is more common with intracapsular surgery and iris supported lenses than with extracapsular and posterior chamber lenses (Miami study group, 1979). Clinically significant cystoid macular oedema is accompanied by a reduction in central vision which is often transient and occasionally permanent. Many series have been published and there is great variation in the reported frequency of clinical cystoid macular oedema. It is abundantly clear that the individual surgeon's technique is of the greatest importance. The difference between an incidence of 8% following intracapsular surgery and an iris supported lens and 1.4% following extracapsular surgery and angle supported lens (Moses, 1979) and similarly 4.5% after intracapsular

surgery and iris supported lens falling to 1.8% after extracapsular surgery and posterior chamber lens (Miami study group 1979) does seem impressive. However, important factors such as progressive learning and surgical technique do have to be taken into account and equally low incidence after intracapsular surgery and iris supported lenses is reported (Roper-Hall, 1981, 1983).

COMMERCIAL ASPECTS

The number of lens implantations being carried out and the cost of lenses make it obvious that very large finances and presumably profits are involved. The industry advertises widely and considerable pressures are exerted upon surgeons to favour different lenses, often with attractive introductory offers or other inducements to deviate the surgeon from making his own choice upon his own and other surgeons' experience and the authentic reported results of a particular lens and manufacturer.

The cost of lenses means that there is very little prospect of them being used in developing countries and strenuous efforts should be made to make this possible. It seems likely that such a step forward will depend upon the satisfactory performance of a lens material which can be mass produced cheaply.

As demand for intraocular lenses increases with patient awareness of the method and its advantages, there is a danger that new manufacturers will try to enter the field and expand their share of the market. This they may do without the essential background knowledge. This has already happened with serious consequences. Quality control and experience is most important and some manufacturers have established their reliability in this respect.

THE FUTURE

As time goes on we shall have authentic long term reports of visual results and complications. In the meantime it will be most important for us to be wary of jumping to the conclusion that any lens with less than two years follow up is going to be better than one with a longer record.

The great interest which has been given to the quality and protection of the corneal endothelium means that it will be studied carefully in all cases before operation and a decision made on the most appropriate management. The calculation of intraocular lens power should be made in all cases by applying a standard formula to measurements of corneal curvature and axial length of the eye.

As experience and confidence increases there will be a reduction of the lower age limit applied for intraocular lens insertion. Traumatic cataract is particularly suitable for consideration, since the majority are unilateral and occur in the most active age group with a requirement for good binocular vision to do precision work. There is difficulty in the case of traumatic cataract in young children and at present no lens design seems really satisfactory.

Polymethylmethacrylate has been a most fortunate first choice for the modern intraocular lens. Despite the later introduction of other materials PMMA lives on as the most suitable material at present available. It is not ideal, and we must hope that at a future time a better substitute will be found. In the meantime, attempts to convert the hydrophobic surface to a less damaging hydrophilic one may be successful. Failing that it can be coated with a suitable viscoelastic material.

The proof of the aetiological mechanism of cystoid macular oedema is still needed, and since it is receiving much attention, we can hope that this will come, with the prospect of prevention or effective therapy.

Bullous dystrophy from endothelial cell loss and decompensation is at present managed by keratoplasty. It is tantalising that endothelial cells can be grown quite easily in tissue culture, but not in the anterior chamber. If the inhibiting factors can be identified and controlled, it may be possible to encourage regeneration in cases of threatened dystrophy with dangerously low cell counts.

If these predictions are fulfilled, many of the problems will be solved, but others will certainly remain.

The training of junior surgeons in implant techniques can be difficult and time consuming, not to mention a source of considerable anxiety. Techniques such as closed circuit colour television and step-by-step play back analysis can be very helpful. It has been shown that results are better when the operation is performed by an experienced surgeon (Sutton, 1980). In the final analysis, for the individual patient, the choice of surgeon will probably continue to be more important than the choice of lens implant.

REFERENCES

Aron-Rosa D 1981 Use of a pulsed neodymium-YAG laser for anterior capsulotomy before extracapsular cataract extraction. American Intraocular Implant Society Journal 7: 332–333

Binkhorst R D 1975 The optical design of intraocular lens implants. Ophthalmic Surgery 6: 17–31

Bourne W M, Waller R R, Liesegang T J, Brubaker R F 1981 Corneal trauma in intracapsular and extracapsular cataract extraction with lens implantation. Archives of Ophthalmology 99: 1375–1376

Clayman H M, Jaffe N S, Light D S 1979 Lens implantation and diabetes mellitus. American Journal of Ophthalmology 88: 990–996

Clayman H M, Jaffe N S, Light D S, Jaffe M S, Cassidy J C 1981 Intraocular lenses axial length and retinal detachment. American Journal of Ophthalmology 92: 778–780

Colenbrander M C 1973 Calculateion of an iris-clip lens for distance vision. British Journal of Ophthalmology 57: 735–740

Dersch M F 1981 Comparative surface analysis of intraocular lenses. American Intraocular Implant Society Journal 7: 226–232

Drews R C 1983 Polypropylene in the human eye. American Intraocular Implant Society Journal 9: 137–142

Drews R C, Smith M E, Okun N 1978 Scanning electron microscopy of intraocular lenses. Ophthalmology 85(4): 415–424

Downing J E, Sayano J J 1983 Change in effective power of posterior chamber lenses placed with the plano surface anterior. American Intraocular Implant Society Journal 9: 297–300

Fechner P U 1979 Methylcellulose als gleitsubstanz für die implantation künstlicher augenlinsen. Klin. Monats. Augenheilkünde 174: 136–139

Galin M A, Sawan S P, Asano Y, Salamone J C, Maghraby A, Tassone D 1983 Studies of residual alkali on intraocular lenses sterilised with NaOH. American Intraocular Implant Society Journal 9: 290–292

Grane E L, Polack F M, Balazs E A 1980 The protective effect of Na-hyaluronate to corneal endothelium. Experimental Eye Research 33: 119–127

Hillman J S 1983 Intraocular lens power calculation for planned ametropia: a clinical study. British Journal of Ophthalmology 67: 255–258

Hitchings R A, Chisholm M, Bird A C 1975 Aphakic macular oedema incidence and pathogenesis. Investigative Ophthalmology Visual Science 14: 68

Hoopes P C 1982 Sodium hyaluronate in anterior segment surgery: a review and a new use in extracapsular surgery. American Intraocular Implant Society Journal 8: 148–154

Huber C 1981 Planned myopic astigmatism as a substitute for accommodation in pseudophakia. American Intraocular Implant Society Journal 7: 244–249

Jaffe N S 1981 Cataract Surgery and its Complications. 3rd Edition. Mosby, St Louis

Jagger J S, Jacobi K W 1979 An analysis of pseudophakodonesis and iridodonesis. American Intraocular Implant Society Journal 3: 203–206

Katzen L E, Fleischman J A, Trokel S 1983 YAG laser treatment of cystoid macular oedema. American Journal of Ophthalmology 95: 589–592

Lazenby G W, Brooker G 1981 The use of sodium hyaluronate (Healon) in intracapsular cataract extraction with insertion of anterior chamber intraocular lenses. Ophthalmic Surgery 12: 646–649

Livernois R, Sinskey R M 1983 Lowpower intraocular lenses. American Intraocular Implant Society Journal 9: 321–323

McCannel M A 1976 A retrievable suture idea for anterior uveal problems. Ophthalmic Surgery 7(2): 98–103

Miami Study Group 1979 Cystoid macular edema in aphakic and pseudophakic eyes. American Journal of Ophthalmology 88: 45–48

Moses L 1979 Cystoid macular edema and retinal detachment following cataract surgery. American Intraocular Implant Society Journal 5: 326–329

Mowbray S L, Chang S M, Casella J F 1983 Estimation of the useful lifetime of polypropylene fiber in the anterior chamber. American Intraocular Implant Society Journal 9: 143–147

Nakazawa M, Ohtsuki K 1983 Apparent accommodation in pseudophakic eyes after implantation of posterior chamber intraocular lenses. American Journal of Ophthalmology 96: 435–438

Olson R J 1980 Intraocular lens optical quality: update 1979. American Intraocular Implant Society Journal 6: 16–17

Obstbaum S A, Robbins R, Best M, Galin M A 1971 Recovery of intraocular pressure and vitreous weight after ocular compression. American Journal of Ophthalmology 71: 1059–1063

Pape L G, Balazs E A 1980 The use of sodium hyaluronate (Healon) in human anterior segment surgery. Ophthalmology 87: 699–705

Percival P 1981 Protective role of Healon during lens implantation. Transactions of the Ophthalmological Societies of the United Kingdom 101: 77–78

Rich W J, Radtke N D, Cohan B E 1974 Early ocular hypertension following cataract extraction. British Journal of Ophthalmology 58: 725–731

Ridley F 1957 Safety requirements for acrylic implants. British Journal of Ophthalmology 41: 359–367

Rock R L, Rylander H G 1983 Spontaneous iris retraction occurring after extracapsular extraction and posterior lens implantation in patients with glaucoma. American Intraocular Implant Society Journal 9: 45–47

Roper-Hall M J 1981 Intraocular lenses with intracapsular cataract extraction. Transactions of the Ophthalmological Societies of the United Kingdom 101: 56–57

Roper-Hall M J 1983 The long term reliability of intracapsular extraction with Binkhorst 4-loop implant. Transactions of the Ophthalmological Societies of the United Kingdom 103: 195–196

Roper-Hall M J, Wilson R S 1982 Reduction in endothelial cell density following cataract extraction and intraocular lens implantation. British Journal of Ophthalmology 66: 516–517

Shammas H J F 1980 Postoperative anterior chamber depth for anterior chamber lenses. American Intraocular Implant Society Journal 6: 153–155

Stark W J, Leske M C, Worthen D M 1983 Trends in cataract surgery and intraocular lenses in the United States. American Journal of Ophthalmology 96: 304–310

Sugar J, Mitchelson J, Kraff M 1979 Endothelial trauma and cell loss from intraocular lens insertion. Archives of ophthalmology 96: 449–450

Sutton G A 1980 Intraocular lens implantation by surgeons in training. British Journal of Ophthalmology 64: 687–688

Tagger W S, Jacobi U W 1979 An analysis of pseudophakodonesis and iridodonesis. American Intraocular Implant Society Journal 3: 203–206

Taylor J M 1981 Medicare payments and charges in the rate of cataract extraction. Ophthalmology 88: 41A

Wang J, Pomerantzeff O 1982 Obtaining a high quality retinal image with biconvex intraocular lens. American Journal of Ophthalmology 98: 87–90

Worthen D M, Boucher J A, Buxton J N, Hayreh S S, Lowther G, Reinecke R D, Spencer W H, Talbott M, Weeks D F 1979 Interim FDA report of intraocular lenses.

6. Treatment of congenital cataracts

C. S. Hoyt

INTRODUCTION

Most ophthalmologists have considered the monocular congenital cataract a nearly hopeless clinical problem in which successful visual rehabilitation is virtually unknown (Frey et al, 1973; François, 1979). The failure to obtain good visual acuity in these eyes has been ascribed to the high incidence of associated ocular anomalies including microphthalmos, nystagmus, foveal dysplasia, and strabismus. Such anomalies have been said to occur in 30–70% of eyes with monocular congenital cataracts (Bagley, 1949). Surgical technique, timing, and complications have also been considered significant factors in determining the final visual outcome. However, until recently no consistent relationship between the type of surgery performed, the associated ocular abnormality or the final visual result had been demonstrated.

Several clinical and laboratory investigators have suggested that ideally surgery should be performed in the first few days of life, followed by immediate optical correction and amblyopic therapy in order to produce the most favourable visual outcome in these patients (von Noorden et al, 1970a,b).

Although the long term visual outcome of bilateral congenital cataracts has usually been more encouraging than those obtained in monocular congenital cataracts, a significant portion of these patients have persisted with major visual handicaps. Although immunisation programmes for rubella have significantly reduced the incidence of this embryopathy and its associated ocular anomalies, binocular congenital cataracts remain a major cause of visually handicapped infants in developed countries.

Recent advances in our understanding of the importance of visual deprivation syndromes and their application to the clinical problems of congenital cataracts have prompted renewed vigour and enthusiasm among those treating congenital cataracts. Moreover, the advances in surgical technology, especially those of the closed eye vitrectomy techniques, have offered ophthalmologists new approaches to surgical removal of congenital cataracts. The aphakic correction of these children remains difficult. Improvements in paediatric aphakic contact lenses, as well as promising new experimental techniques to correct the aphakic condition, also have been responsible for the excitement surrounding the changing concepts in the management of congenital cataracts.

THE CONCEPT OF A SENSITIVE PERIOD AND VISUAL DEPRIVATION SYNDROMES

The notion of a sensitive or critical period in visual development has been one of the central concepts to emerge over the last 15 years from the many studies on the effects of various manipulations of early visual input on the development of the visual pathways. Although there are obvious clinical antecedents, the conviction that visual experience exerts a greater influence on the development of the visual pathways at certain stages of life than at others has arisen primarily from the observations of the effect of periods of monocular and binocular occlusion imposed on experimental animals of different ages (Wiesel & Hubel, 1963a,b; Hubel & Wiesel, 1970). These monocular and binocular deprivation syndromes have been characterised by anatomical, physiological, and behavioural characteristics.

Wiesel & Hubel (1963b) reported atrophy of the lateral geniculate cells receiving input from eye of the kitten, visually deprived shortly after birth, together with almost complete inability to drive striate cortical cells observed by the deprived eye. They later established that there was a critical or sensitive period beyond which deprivation of this type had no comparable measurable effect (Wiesel & Hubel, 1970). They showed that binocular deprivation produced similar but less pronounced changes in the lateral geniculate nucleus and significantly decreased the usually large number of binocularly driven cells in the striate cortex (Wiesel & Hubel, 1965).

von Noorden and co-workers (1970a,b, 1973) documented similar results in experiments with monkeys whose visual systems are closer to those of humans. They deduced from eyelid closure experiments that the sensitive period in these animals extended through the first 12 weeks of life. Moreover, they demonstrated that short periods of deprivation during this sensitive period could result in severe and irreversible amblyopia.

More recent detailed physiological studies have shown that only a few days of constant monocular deprivation within the sensitive period of visual development can have a striking effect on the ocular dominant histogram of the visual cortex (Olson & Freeman, 1978). A definite bias occurs in favour of the non-deprived eye at the expense of the deprived eye. In addition, physiologically determined visual acuities of single cells in that part of the lateral geniculate nucleus subserving the deprived eye are found to be decreased after monocular deprivation (Lehmkuhle et al, 1980). Morphological studies of the cortical ocular dominant columns have demonstrated that columns from the non-deprived eye expand at the expense of the shrunken columns representing the deprived eye (Hubel & Wiesel, 1977). Geniculate neurons from the deprived eye are smaller than comparable neurons in the non-deprived pathway (Crawford, 1978). The potential for recovery from this monocular deprivation has also recently been documented. Recovery by part-time reverse deprivation (occlusion) has been studied in kittens and the physiological basis of this effect has been demonstrated (Crewther et al, 1981).

These experiences with monocular deprivation syndromes are not entirely applicable to binocular deprivation, because experiments have shown that the neurophysiological substrates of unilateral and bilateral amblyopia are different (Wiesel & Hubel, 1963a; Wiesel & Hubel, 1965; Crawford et al, 1975). However, the temporal characteristics of the vulnerability of the visual system to amblyopia are probably comparable in binocular and monocular deprivation.

Data from experiments in cats and monkeys have shown that long term binocular deprivation commencing at birth results in a large number of cortical cells becoming unresponsive to stimuli from either eye (Wiesel & Hubel, 1965; Crawford et al, 1975). It is not clear what the minimum period of deprivation needed to produce these changes is. However, bilateral occlusion for as little as 8 weeks has led to seemingly irreversible behavioural and physiological effects in monkeys (Crawford et al, 1975). Even after prolonged bilateral eyelid closure, a partial behavioural recovery can be produced in cats by extensive visual training of the re-opened eye (Chow & Stewart, 1972). Further demonstrations of binocular visual recovery following bilateral visual deprivation has been demonstrated in other experimental animals as well (Olson & Freeman, 1978; Giffin & Mitchell, 1978).

I would like to caution the reader, however, from drawing direct parallels from the experimental animal models of binocular deprivation and the human infant with bilateral congenital cataracts. It should be noted that none of the experimental animal models with binocular visual deprivation ever develop significant abnormalities of ocular movements. That is, none of them demonstrate nystagmus as the result of binocular deprivation. This is clearly not the case in children with significant bilateral congenital cataracts, where nystagmus heralds a poor visual outcome. Complete understanding of the motor consequences of bilateral visual deprivation in children will be necessary before it is possible to draw direct comparisons from the experimental animal models that are applicable to this clinical situation.

The best evidence for loss of visual acuity or amblyopia elicited by visual deprivation in infants and children has come from retrospective studies of the consequences of abnormal visual experience on lateral visual functions (for binocular functions — Banks et al, 1975; Hohmann & Creutzfeldt, 1975; for meridional deprivation — Mitchell et al, 1973; and for unilateral patching — Awaya et al, 1973; Hartwig et al, 1976). Awaya et al (1973) noted that eyes patched for as little as one week in children aged less than one year were subsequently found to experience the development of a deep and intractable amblyopia. In contrast Hartwig et al (1976) indicated that 7–9 days of patching had no lasting effect on infants who were aged 4, 5, and 8 months old.

Unfortunately, even analysing the recent results in those studies in which good visual acuities have been obtained in monocular congenital cataracts does not provide sufficient data to define precisely the timing and duration of the critical period in humans. However, Taylor (1981) and Vaegan & Taylor (1979) have argued that the critical period may be deduced by studying children with amblyopia occurring after uncomplicated unilateral cataract and the subsequent aphakic blur. These authors have argued that in unilateral congenital cataracts, surgery and optical correction if indicated should be completed within the first 4 months of life. Although occasional results of good visual function have been obtained in children between 6 and 12 months of age (Morgan et al, 1983; Pratt-Johnson & Tilson, 1981; Ben-Ezra & Paez, 1983), extensive data from previously published series clearly document that good visual results are rare in children 6 months of age or older (von Noorden et al, 1970b; François, 1979).

Although some have criticised the specificity with which the animal models of monocular visual deprivation reproduce the clinical situation of infantile cataracts, I agree with von Noorden (1981) that the treatment of form deprivation amblyopia during infancy must be initiated very early in order to avoid the deleterious effects on the developing neural visual system. Moreover, the recent study of the lateral geniculate nucleus in a human anisometropic amblyope has clearly established that similar anatomical changes occurred as those produced in monocularly deprived experimental animals (von Noorden et al, 1983). Although there may be species specific variations in terms of the duration of the sensitive period and in particular the ocular motor consequences of sensory deprivation, the clinical importance of the experimental models of monocular and binocular visual deprivation can no longer be denied. The single most important factor in our study of congenital cataracts that has resulted in improved visual rehabilitation has been the early detection and initiation of treatment of these cataracts, even at the time of birth.

SURGICAL TECHNIQUES

Neonatal and infantile cataracts are considered complete when no fundus details are ophthalmoscopically visible, even with full dilatation of the pupil. Effective visual stimulation in this setting is obviously impossible. There can be no question of the necessity for surgical removal of these cataracts if they are detected at such a time as to allow for visual rehabilitation. The more difficult and, unfortunately more common, clinical problem is the assessment of the infant with incomplete cataracts. No absolute rules or objective techniques are available for identifying those partial cataracts that will invariably produce severe visual deprivation and those that will spare the developing visual system. Certain clinical guidelines have been offered by Parks (1982) including the suggestion that if more than 30% of the visual axis is occluded by a congenital cataract it should be removed. The development of an objective technique to assess the effects of partial congenital cataracts on the developing visual system would be a significant advancement in our management of infants with congenital cataract.

The history of the surgical techniques for removal of congenital cataracts is replete with one new technique after the other. Simple discussions gave way to linear extractions and then to a variety of aspirating techniques through small incisions, once the soft consistency of these cataracts became generally recognised. The high incidence of operative and postoperative complications in the earlier techniques of congenital cataract removal were certainly a driving force behind the technical innovation in this area. On the other hand, the uncritical adoption of new instrumentation by some ophthalmologists have resulted in ridiculous proposals for congenital cataract surgical removal, for example, the suggestion that these lenses should be removed using phakoemulsification equipment. Obviously the soft lens of the congenital cataract does not require this type of instrumentation with its increased risk of corneal damage.

At the present time, the two primary techniques utilised for removal of congenital cataracts are various adaptations of the basic aspiration technique and the lensectomy–vitrectomy approach utilising closed eye vitrectomy procedures. No long term clinical study is available at the present time to compare directly and contrast these two techniques and their long term visual results and complications. However, Taylor (1981) reported a study in which 28 eyes with congenital cataracts were treated using a lens aspiration technique, leaving the posterior capsule intact. Nineteen of these eyes required re-operation a total of 32 times to keep the pupillary axis clear for refraction and accurate contact lens prescription within the first 18 months of life. In contrast, a similar group of eyes operated on during the same period utilising the lensectomy–vitrectomy approach through a limbal incision resulted in no secondary operations. It is noteworthy that 5 of the 23 eyes treated by lensectomy and vitrectomy were seen to have strands of vitreous across the iris to the corneal–scleral wound on postoperative slit lamp examination.

Those who advocate the routine use of the standard lens aspiration technique for the removal of congenital cataracts cite its simplicity, well documented low incidence of intraoperative complications, and its preservation of the posterior capsule and maintenance of the integrity of the vitreous body. Most authorities utilising this technique are concerned that the routine violation of the vitreous cavity may predispose the developing eye to later complications. Those experts utilising the lensectomy–vitrectomy approach suggest that the clear visual axis created by this technique prevents any subsequent visual deprivation as the result of opacifications of the posterior capsule. Moreover, it permits rapid and precise retinoscopy at frequent intervals in the first several months of life, even in the unsedated patient. Whether macular oedema occurs with this technique as the result of the vitreous strands pulled across the iris, remains controversial (Hoyt & Nickel, 1982; Gilbard et al, 1983). At the 1983 American Academy of Ophthalmology meeting, Parks and co-workers presented a study comparing the lens aspiration technique with the lensectomy approach and analysed the incidence of chronic glaucoma, retinal detachment and secondary membrane formation. Although this is a short-term study, the findings of this group of investigators suggest that secondary glaucoma is certainly no more common in a lensectomy–vitrectomy approach, and perhaps less frequently seen. Moreover, as was the case in the study of Taylor (1981), the incidence of secondary procedures following the lensectomy–vitrectomy technique was greatly reduced, indeed entirely eliminated. The one remaining question, however, that will take a study of much longer duration to answer, is whether these patients are more prone for retinal detachment. The pathogenesis of retinal detachment in aphakic congenital cataracts remains incompletely understood but secondary changes at the vitreous retinal interface may be important (Jagger et al, 1983).

We have adopted the lensectomy–vitrectomy approach for all of our monocular congenital cataracts and those binocular cataracts in children under 18 months of age. We concur with Parks (1982) that the necessity for repeated retinoscopy examinations and attended changes in contact lens (or glasses) are so imperative that the greater facility for these examinations provided by the lensectomy–vitrectomy approach seems to warrant any potential risk of this procedure at the present time. We do, however, prefer to utilise the lens aspiration approach in those children older than 18 months of age in whom the consequences of visual deprivation are much less likely to be severe. If long term studies, however, document that the risk of retinal detachment in the lensectomy–vitrectomy approach is no greater than those with lens aspiration, it seems almost certain that the lensectomy–vitrectomy approach will be accepted by most authorities dealing with these problems. This technique may be utilised using either an anterior chamber incision or a pars plicata approach. The pars plicata approach has been advocated in order to reduce the incidence of vitreous adhesions to the iris and cornea. I believe one can also minimise the risk of this complication by injecting filtered air through the infusion needle prior to the removal of the vitrectomy machine from the eye. The injected air tamponades the remaining vitreous and prevents the vitreous from being pulled forward during the time of removal of the vitrectomy instrument through the limbal wound. This technique has significantly reduced the incidence of vitreous strands to the corneal scleral wound in our patients and the subsequent development of macular oedema.

Although there has been a tendency in the past several years to omit the iridectomy from the routine congenital cataract procedure, I cannot endorse this. Several studies have documented the incidence of aphakic glaucoma in congenital cataracts (François, 1979; Chandler, 1968). Although it is certain that the incidence of glaucoma is much less in non-rubella cataract eyes, the management of aphakic glaucoma in infants is difficult and usually visually devastating. The best treatment is prevention of the predisposing conditions responsible. Most authorities agree that the primary cause of aphakic glaucoma in congenital cataracts is synechia formation with subsequent iris bombé (Chandler, 1968; François, 1979). A peripheral iridectomy or iridotomy to prevent this devastating complication still seems warranted. Care should be taken, however, not to damage the iris sphincter so that a small round pupil can be maintained. The greater depth of focus resulting from the small pupil may be important in providing a greater tolerance to minor defocusing problems with the aphakic correction especially during the early sensitive period.

Postoperative management of patients with congenital cataracts should pay special attention to continuing pupillary dilatation, anti-inflammatory therapy (sub-Tenon's and topical steroid treatment), and routine antimicrobial therapy. Termination of pupillary dilatation and anti-inflammatory therapy should not be precipitated by early contact lens fitting. Although the external appearance of the infantile aphakic eye appears to be uninflamed, the potential for serious synechia formation has repeatedly been demonstrated (Chandler, 1968; François, 1979). In contrast, the single suture required to close the corneal scleral wound, either following a lens aspiration or a lensectomy–vitrectomy approach, does not prevent successful fitting of a contact lens within 2–7 days following surgery. The need for immediate aphakic correction of these children is apparent from the previous discussion of visual deprivation syndromes.

APHAKIC CORRECTION AND AMBLYOPIA THERAPY

The need to place the infant aphakic eye in precise optical focus is implicit from the discussion in the first section concerning the visual deprivation syndromes in infancy. However, several pragmatic difficulties face the clinician attempting to perform this task. First and foremost is the difficulty of obtaining reliable retinoscopy data from the tiny, unco-operative infant. I choose to perform all retinoscopy in the outpatient setting with the infant unsedated. I have chosen to do this since the rapid change in refractive power that occurs in the first year of life requires retinoscopy to be performed frequently (in our clinical research protocol every 2 weeks for the first year of life) and thus precludes the use of sedation or general anaesthesia for this task. I am aware of the difficulties of performing retinoscopy in infants and the anomalous reflexes that may occur as the result of both the short axial eye length of the infant eye, and the problem of off-axis retinoscopy (Howland, 1978). I usually have two different examiners retinoscope each infant on every visit so as to be certain of the accuracy of our measurements.

Even once an estimate of the refractive error of the aphakic infant has been accomplished, the fitting of contact lenses in this situation is hardly simple. The aphakic neonatal eye is smaller than the adult eye, its cornea has a lower vault above the scleral wall, central corneal radius of curvature is generally only slightly steeper than that found in the adult cornea, but the required hyperopic correction is very high with lenses of +35 to 40 sometimes required in the first few weeks of life (Enoch, 1972). The conjunctiva pulls away from the globe closer to the limbus in the infant than the adult. Obviously, therefore, to support the very high power plus aphakic correction, the contact lens fit has to be good. Contact lens fit is basically a problem of capillary attraction distributed over an adequate lens bearing area versus the gravitational pull caused by the weight of the lens. Clearly, the thinner the contact lens and the smaller the lenticular zone, the less the weight. In those cases which require particularly high refractive power, too thin a scleral flange and/or corneal carrier for the inevitably thicker and less flexible lenticular component may result in splitting of the contact lens (Enoch, 1972).

I prefer to use soft contact lenses in this population because they are readily accepted by the infant, as a corrective device and easily inserted and removed by the parent. I have not been able to achieve the same parental compliance with hard contact lenses. Although I am aware of the controversy surrounding the incidence of astigmatic errors in the normal human infant (Howland et al, 1978), I have not found that our aphakic children have a significant incidence of major astigmatic errors. Astigmatism can be created, however, by pulling the suture too tight in closing the corneal wound.

In the first few weeks of life, a soft contact lens diameter is usually limited to no more than 13.5 mm, because of the relative shallowness of the conjunctival fornix. As a basic principle, however, I try to fit the widest contact lens possible at all times in order to minimise contact lens losses. Later in the first year of life, lenses of 14.5–15.5 mm in diameter may be utilised.

The availability of high plus aphakic contact lenses for the paediatric population has been woefully inadequate in the United States until recently. Although several additional lenses are now available, we are still a long way away from the ideal paediatric aphakic contact lens. In general, we have experienced a contact lens loss or replacement rate of approximately 7–8 lenses per eye per year. Both the rapid change in refractive error as well as the frequency of lost lenses had been responsible for this high contact lens turnover. The cost of these lenses is not insignificant and in some circumstances has actually been responsible for the termination of visual rehabilitation.

I can fully understand the frustration of those who have worked with contact lenses in the aphakic infant and understand the search for alternative forms of aphakic correction. I do not hesitate to use aphakic spectacles in the management of bilateral congenital cataracts, even in the first few months of life. I have no experience either with intraocular lenses (BenEzra & Paez, 1983) or epikeratophakic grafts (Morgan et al, 1983). Preliminary results utilising both of these techniques, however, have been promising, and further clinical trials are warranted in order to establish their efficacy. Both techniques will probably require overcorrection with contact lenses in order to provide a means of changing the refractive power in the first several months of life as axial eye elongation reduces the hyperopic correction of the aphakic infant. Although I am aware of the clinical research data suggesting that sharp optical focus may not be essential for the development of normal visual function in the first few weeks of infancy (Powers & Dobson, 1982), I believe at the present time clinicians would be best advised to continue in their attempts to correct the aphakic prescription in these infants as precisely as possible.

In the experimental animal models in which monocular visual deprivation is created, spontaneous recovery of visual acuity in the deprived eye may occur if the lid occlusion is terminated early in the sensitive period without cross occluding the previously non-deprived eye (Movshon, 1976; Mitchell et al, 1977). In clinical practice, however, it seems unwise to assume that even in the child of a few days old with a monocular congenital cataract that no patching of the contralateral eye is indicated. Knowing the problems of contact lens fitting cited above, it is unlikely that the correction of the aphakic eye is ever precisely matched to the phakic eye. I advocate institution of patching therapy of the phakic eye in the treatment of monocular congenital cataracts as soon as the contact lens has been fitted. This usually is within 72 hours of surgery. Strategies for patching therapy in tiny infants are still being developed. Schedules including total occlusion of the phakic eye for several days have been advocated. I prefer to utilise a patching scheme of 4–6 hours a day in the first several months of life. This is based upon our observations with visual evoked potential measurements (Odom et al, 1981; Jastrzebski et al, 1984) that have documented visual function in the aphakic eye returns rapidly with only a few hours of patching a day. Moreover, it has been our observation that if total occlusion is used in the first several weeks or months of life a secondary esotropia invariably occurs. A number of our children who have been treated with patching of no more than a few hours a day have recovered reasonable vision in their monocular aphakic eye and appear to have retained some binocular function. Further long term studies, however, are required before we will be certain whether the image size disparity created by the optical correction (Enoch, 1978) or the total occlusion of the phakic eye has been responsible for the secondary strabismus observed in most monocular congenital cataract patients. Full-time occlusion is recommended if visual function of the aphakic eye appears to be very poor and strabismus is already present.

It should be emphasised that amblyopia occurs commonly in patients with bilateral congenital cataracts. I believe the incidence and severity of this amblyopia can be minimised if the interoperative period for correction of the right and left eyes is kept to a maximum of 72 hours and bilateral occlusion therapy be utilised upon completion of the lens removal in the first eye and the initial contact lens or spectacle fitting. A careful search for evidence of amblyopia should be part of the routine follow-up of all of these patients. Patching therapy when necessary should utilise the same principles as outlined in the discussion of monocular congenital cataracts.

VISUAL RESULTS AND CONCLUSIONS

That improved visual acuity results have been accomplished in the treatment of monocular and binocular congenital cataracts in the last decade cannot be denied (Enoch & Rabinowicz, 1976; Pratt-Johnson & Tilson, 1981; Beller et al, 1981; Rogers et al, 1981; Jacobsen et al, 1981; Gelbart et al, 1982; Parks, 1982; Morgan et al, 1983; BenEzra & Paez, 1983; Mohindra et al, 1983). All workers in the field would, I believe, agree that the important work of von Noorden in bringing to the clinician's attention the significant aspects of form deprivation amblyopia and its early irreversible changes in infancy is an essential part of this evolving story (von Noorden, 1981). There is, however, no agreement among the many authorities working in the area as to when the amblyopia in monocular congenital cataracts might be no longer reversible. Pratt-Johnson & Tilson (1981), BenEzra & Paez (1983), and Morgan et al (1983) have reported good visual acuity results in some patients with monocular congenital cataracts operated on between 6 and 12 months of age. I, however, have not had this experience. My best results have been achieved in those patients operated on in the first 6 weeks of life, and none of my patients treated after 4 months of age have achieved better than 20/200 vision in the aphakic eye. In the case of bilateral congenital cataracts, the importance of early detection and surgery is also well established. However, the high frequency of incomplete cataracts in the bilateral circumstance as well as the frequent progression of some forms of cataracts make a precise analysis of the timing of visual deprivation more difficult. Nevertheless, the clear association of nystagmus with a poor prognosis in these patients and the documentation that the nystagmus, if it is to occur, usually has its onset within the first 8–12 weeks (Rogers et al, 1981; Gelbart et al, 1982; Parks, 1982) seem to be irrefutable evidence to suggest that there is again no justification for delay either in detection or treatment of visually significant bilateral congenital cataracts.

Although the understanding of visual deprivation in early infancy is continuing to evolve, and the surgical and postoperative techniques of treatment of infants with congenital cataracts continues to change rapidly, I suggest that the following conclusions are warranted at the present time in regards to management of congenital cataracts:

1. Visually significant monocular or binocular congenital cataracts require early detection (ideally in the neonatal period), prompt referral for definitive surgical therapy and immediate visual rehabilitation if the irreversible neural consequences of visual deprivation are to be avoided.

2. Although there is no long term prospective study to document the incidence of complications, as well as, the visual results obtained with the 2 primary surgical procedures used in the treatment of congenital cataracts, (lens aspiration and lensectomy–virectomy) the following seems clear. If one chooses to use lens aspiration as the primary form of therapy in the management of congenital cataracts, a high percentage of patients will require a secondary procedure within the first few months following surgery. Any delay in the removal of secondary membrane or lens remnants may be responsible for further visual deprivation and irreversible amblyopia. On the other hand, the incidence of secondary procedures in the lensectomy–vitrectomy approach is minimal, and retinoscopy in the awake alert child can be accomplished much more readily than following the lens aspiration, either with or without a posterior capsulotomy. However, the long-term risks of routinely violating the vitreous cavity in patients with congenital cataracts have yet to be determined. Although the incidence of glaucoma certainly seems to be no more frequent and perhaps less common utilising this approach, the potential risk of macular oedema and retinal detachment utilising this technique has not yet been defined.

3. The aphakic correction of congenital cataracts remains the major obstacle in the successful rehabilitation of these children. Contact lens fitting requires a patient, meticulous fitter, willing to pay specific attention to the unique qualities of the infant eye. The frequent replacement and loss of contact lenses in the management of these

patients is costly and, in the case of monocular congenital cataracts, may not be thought to be cost effective at the present time. Improvements in contact lenses or other forms of aphakic therapy will be necessary in order that more universally good results may be obtained in the management of congenital cataracts.

4. Patching therapy for the treatment of amblyopia in patients with congenital cataracts should be instituted whenever required, immediately following surgery and visual rehabilitation. I believe there is strong evidence to suggest that, at least in the first year of life, part-time daily occlusion therapy is efficacious and may perhaps preserve some forms of binocular interactions in some patients.

5. The importance of a team approach to the problem of congenital cataracts cannot be overemphasised. The need for careful meticulous postoperative follow-up and repeated contact lens fitting requires more than one medical professional to accomplish this.

6. Finally, it is the general practitioner and paediatrician who hold the key to good visual outcome in the management of congenital cataracts. Ophthalmologists should continue to be diligent in their efforts to educate these non-ophthalmic physicians in the absolute necessity for a specific search for cataracts at the time of the newborn examination or, at the very latest, the first well-baby checkup.

REFERENCES

Awaya S, Miyake Y, Imaizumi Y 1973 Amblyopia in man suggestive of stimulus deprivation amblyopia. Japanese Journal of Opthalmology 17: 69–82

Bagley C H 1949 Congenital cataract. American Journal of Ophthalmology 32: 411–419

Banks M S, Aslin R N, Letson R D 1975 Sensitive period for the development of human binocular vision. Science 196: 675–677

Beller R, Hoyt C S, Marg E, Odom J V 1981 Good visual function after neonatal surgery for congenital monocular cataracts. American Journal of Ophthalmology 91: 559–565

BenEzra D, Paez J H 1983 Congenital cataracts and intraocular lenses. American Journal of Ophthalmology 96: 311–314

Chandler P A 1968 Surgery of the congenital cataract. American Journal of Ophthalmology 65: 663–673

Chow K L, Stewart D L 1972 Reversal of structural and functional effects of long-term visual deprivation in the cat. Experimental Neurology 34: 409–420

Crawford M J 1978 Visual deprivation syndrome. Ophthalmology 85: 465–477

Crawford M J, Blake R, Cool S J 1975 Physiological consequences of unilateral and bilateral eye closure in Macaque monkeys: Some further observations. Brain Research 84: 150–154

Crewther D P, Crewther S G, Mitchell D E 1981 The efficacy of brief periods of reverse occlusion in promoting recovery from the physiological effects of monocular deprivation in kittens. Investigative Ophthalmology and Visual Science 21: 357–362

Enoch J M 1972 The fitting of hydrophilic (soft) contact lenses to infants and young children. I. Mensuration data on aphakic eyes of children born with congenital cataracts. Contact Lens Bulletin 5: 3–4

Enoch J M 1978 Restoration of binocularity in unilateral aphakia by non-surgical means. International Ophthalmology Clinics 18: 273–282

Enoch J M, Rabinowicz I M 1976 Early surgery and visual correction of an infant born with unilateral eye lens opacity. Documenta Ophthalmologica 41: 371–382

François J 1979 Late results of congenital cataract surgery. Transactions of the American Academy of Ophthalmology Otolaryngology 86: 1586–1598

Frey T, Friendly P, Wyatt D 1973 Reevaluation of monocular cataracts in children. American Journal of Ophthalmology 76: 381–388

Gelbart S S, Hoyt C S, Jastrebski G, Marg E 1982 Long-term visual results in bilateral congenital cataracts. American Journal of Ophthalmology 93: 615–621

Giffin F, Mitchell V E 1978 The rate of recovery after early monocular deprivation in kittens. Journal of Physiology 274: 511–537

Gilbard S M, Peyman G A, Goldberg M F 1983 Evaluation for cystoid maculopathy after pars plicata lensectomy–vitrectomy for congenital cataracts. Ophthalmology 90: 1201–1206

Hartwig H, Haver U, Kanther A 1976 Zur frage der deprivations-amblyopie. Klinische Monatsblatter für Augenheilkunde 168: 414–418

Hohmann A, Creutzfeldt O D 1975 Squint and the development of binocularity in humans. Nature 254: 613–614

Howland H C 1978 Retinoscopy of infants at a distance: Limits normal and anomalous reflexes. Vision Research 18: 597–599

Howland H C, Atkinson J, Braddock O et al 1978 Infant astigmatism measured by photo-refraction. Science 202: 331–333

Hoyt C S, Nickel N 1982 Aphakic cystoid macular edema: Occurrence in infants and children after transpupillary lensectomy and anterior vitrectomy. Archives of Ophthalmology 100: 746–749

Hubel D H, Wiesel T N 1970 The period of susceptibility to the physiologic effects of unilateral eye closure in kittens. Journal of Physiolology 206: 419–436

Hubel D H, Wiesel T N 1977 Functional architecture of the Macaque monkey visual cortex. Proceedings of the Royal Society London 199: 1–59

Jacobsen S G, Mohindra I, Held R 1981 Development of visual acuity in infants with congenital cataracts. British Journal of Ophthalmology 65: 727–781

Jacobsen S G, Mohindra I, Held R 1983 Monocular visual form deprivation in human infants. Documenta Ophthalmologica 55: 199–211

Jagger J D, Cooling R J, Fison L G 1983 Management of retinal detachment following congenital cataract surgery. Transactions of the Ophthalmological Societies of the UK 103: 103–107

Jastrzebski G, Marg E, Hoyt C S 1984 Amblyopia measurements with visually evoked potentials. Archives of Ophthalmology (in press)

Lehmkuhle S, Kratz K E, Nangel S C et al 1980 Effects of early monocular lid suture on spatial and temporal sensitivity of neurons and dorsolateral geniculate nucleus of the cat. Journal of Neurophysiology 41: 65–74

Mitchell D E, Cynader M, Movshon J A 1977 Recovery from the effect of monocular deprivation in kittens. Journal of Comparative Neurology 176: 53–64

Mitchell D E, Freeman R D, Millodot 1973 Meridional amblyopia: Evidenced for modification of the human visual system by early visual experience. Vision Research 13: 535–558

Mohindra I, Jacobsen S G, Held R 1983 Binocular visual form deprivation in human infants. Documenta Ophthalmologica 55: 237–249

Morgan K S, Asbel P A, MacDonald M B, Kaufman H 1983 Preliminary visual results of pediatric epikeratophakia. Archives of Ophthalmology 101: 1540–1544

Movshon J A 1976 Reversal of the physiological effects of monocular deprivation in the kitten's visual cortex. Journal of Physiology 261: 125–174

Odom J V, Hoyt C S, Marg E 1981 Effect of natural deprivation and unilateral eye patching on visual acuity of infants and children. Evoked potential measurements. Archives of Ophthalmology 99: 1412–1416

Olson C R, Freeman R D 1978 Monocular deprivation and recovery during sensitive period in kittens. Journal of Neurophysiology 41: 65–74

Olson C R, Freeman R D 1980 Cumulative effect of brief daily periods of monocular vision on kitten striate cortex. Experimental Brain Research 38: 53–56

Parks M M 1982 Visual results in aphakic children. American Journal of Ophthalmology 94: 441–449

Powers M K, Dobson V 1982 Effect of focus on visual acuity of human infants. Vision Research 22: 521–528

Pratt-Johnson J A, Tilson G 1981 Visual results after removal of congenital cataracts. Canadian Journal of Ophthalmology 16: 19–21

Rogers G L, Rishler C L, Tsou B H 1981 Visual acuities in infants with congenital cataracts operated on prior to six months of age. Archives of Ophthalmology 99: 999–1003

Taylor D I 1981 Choice of surgical technique in the management of congenital cataracts. Transactions of the Ophthalmological Societies of the UK 101: 114–117

Vaegan, Taylor D 1979 Critical period for deprivation amblyopia in children. Transactions of the Ophthalmological Societies of the UK 99: 432–439

von Noorden G K 1973 Experimental amblyopia in monkeys: Further behavioral observations and clinical correlations. Investigative Ophthalmology 12: 721–726

von Noorden G K 1981 New clinical aspects of stimulus deprivation amblyopia. American Journal of Ophthalmology 92: 416–421

von Noorden G K, Crawford M L J, Levacy R 1983 The lateral geniculate nucleus in human anisometropic amblyopia. Investigative Ophthalmology and Visual Science 24: 788–790

von Noorden G K, Dowling J E, Ferguson D C 1970a Experimental amblyopia in monkeys: Behavioral studies of stimulus deprivation amblyopia. Archives of Ophthalmology 84: 206–214 von Noorden G K, Ryan S J, Maumenee A E 1970b Management of congenital cataracts. Transactions of the American Academy of Ophthalmology and Otolaryngology 74: 352–358

Wiesel T N, Hubel D H 1963a Effects of visual deprivation on morphology and physiology in the cats lateral geniculate body. Journal of Neurophysiology 26: 978–993

Wiesel T N, Hubel D H 1963b Single cell responses in striate cortex of kittens deprived of vision in one eye. Journal of Neurophysiology 26: 1003–1017

Wiesel T N, Hubel D H 1965 Extent of recovery from the effect of visual deprivation in kittens. Journal of Neurophysiology 28: 1060–1072

7. Ocular phototoxicity

S. Lerman

BACKGROUND

The biological effects of electromagnetic radiation are wavelength dependent. The photon energies (expressed as electron volts [eV]) in the UV, visible, and IR portions range from approximately 12 to less than 1 eV. These energies, when absorbed, will induce specific molecular alterations depending on the radiation wavelength involved (Fig. 7.1). In order to understand photobiological mechanisms, it is important to remember that light must be absorbed by a molecule before photochemical effects can occur (Grotthus-Draper's first law of photochemistry). The second law of photochemistry (Stark-Einstein) postulates that the absorption of only one photon is required to affect one molecule; however, it should be noted that absorbed light does not always result in photochemical changes since there are a variety of nonchemical mechanisms available for the molecule to dissipate energy and return unaltered to its ground (resting) state (Lerman, 1980c).

EFFECTS OF NON-IONISING RADIATION ON BIOLOGICAL SYSTEMS

The effect of nonionising radiation on a cell depends on the specific chemical composition within the cell, that is, on the presence of absorbing molecules (or chromophores). This type of radiation must be absorbed in order to cause a change in the molecule since absorbed energy is required to promote a chemical change. Molecules in excited electronic states have different chemical and physical properties than their counterparts in the ground state (prior to absorption of energy). Thus cells that do not contain chemical compounds absorbing at certain wavelengths will transmit these wavelengths. For example, the nucleic acids and most proteins in a cell are essentially transparent to and completely transmit visible light but absorb certain wavelengths in the UV region (between 250 and 320 nm) and can be damaged by this form of radiation, while other macromolecules in a cell such as rhodopsin, which absorbs at 498 nm, and haemoglobin, which has absorption peaks in the UV and visible region (275, 400, and 540–576 nm) appear coloured since they absorb visible light. These latter macromolecules can be damaged by visible radiation at their specific absorption wavelengths. These principles have been utilised in the phototherapeutic approach for certain types of malignancy. Haematoporphyrin derivatives (HPD) are infused into the tumour and their absorption characteristics (in the red portion of visible radiation) can result in the destruction of the malignancy with red light (Dougherty et al, 1981). Attempts are currently under way to treat intraocular tumours in this fashion (Menon et al, 1982).

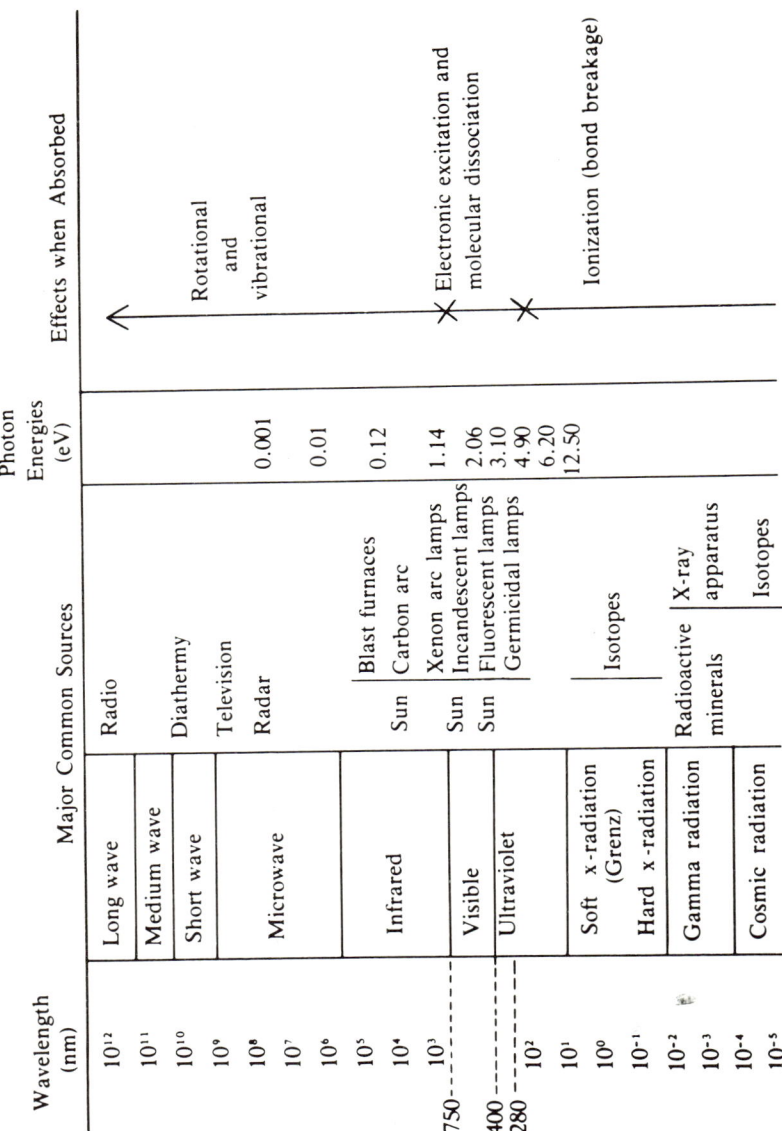

Fig. 7.1   The electromagnetic spectrum

The absorption on non-ionising radiation is determined by the chemical composition of the tissue being exposed; thus, the more radiation that the molecules absorb the greater the effect of the radiation. The term "action spectrum" is used as a measure of the relative effect of different wavelengths of radiation on a chemical compound, macromolecule, cell, or entire organism. That is, it is a plot of the relative effect versus the wavelength. For example, the maximum efficiency for experimental photokeratitis has been shown to occur at approximately 288–290 nm, with a smaller peak at 254–260 nm. This type of action spectrum is due to the presence of specific absorbing chromophores in the cornea (nucleic acids at 260 nm; tyrosine and tryptophan at 275–295 nm).

Aside from the skin, the eye is the only organ or tissue in the body that is particularly sensitive to the non-ionising wavelengths of optical radiation (280–1400 nm) normally present in our environment. In addition to infrared and visible radiation, we are constantly exposed to ultraviolet radiation (solar and man-made) throughout life. At sea level, we are exposed to 2–5 mW/cm^2 of UV radiation (280–400 nm) depending on geographical location and season (Lerman, 1980c). Man-made ultraviolet radiation can also play a role in ocular phototoxicity, albeit a relatively small one under normal circumstances. The spectral output of fluorescent lamps commonly utilised is relatively low at these wavelengths and should not pose a problem except in special circumstances, e.g. in patients who are being treated with photosensitising drugs and in aphakes and pseudophakes. However, exposure to photo flood lamps or the black light lamps frequently used in various laboratories might present a potential hazard since their output can approach approximately 5–10% of the average levels of solar radiation in our atmosphere (Lerman, 1980c). Furthermore, a much more significant hazard may exist in certain industries which utilise UV radiation in certain polymerisation reactions.

Since the normal cornea, aqueous, ocular lens and vitreous are almost completely transparent to all but the shorter wavelengths of visible light [although the aging eye does absorb increasing amounts of shortwave visible radiation (Lerman, 1980c)] one would not anticipate photic damage to these tissues from visible radiation. As will be discussed in a later section, only the retina is susceptible to photodamage from visible radiation. Furthermore, in order for non-ionising radiation to exert an effect, it must be absorbed. While the retina contains chromophores whose function it is to absorb visible radiation (the photoreceptor rods and cones and the macular pigment), the other ocular tissues anterior to the retina, have very few chromophores which can absorb such wavelengths. Nature has provided us with transparent ocular media which are essentially avascular and contain very few visible wavelength absorbing chromophores in order to transmit effectively (as well as refract) the specific wavelengths required to initiate the visual process by photochemical reactions. However, these tissues do have the ability to absorb varying amounts of ultraviolet radiation (particularly the ocular lens). The shorter the wavelengths of radiation absorbed the greater the potential for photic damage since there is an inverse relationship between a wavelength and the photon energy associated with it (Fig. 7.1). Thus, UV radiation is the non-ionising portion of the electromagnetic spectrum which could cause the most damage, provided that it is absorbed. As we shall see, this applies to all the ocular tissues including the retina in the very young eye (where the lens has not as yet become an effective UV filter), but in particular, the ocular lens sustains the greatest amount of photochemical change during a life of exposure to ambient UV radiation.

Infrared radiation (750 nm–1M) has a much lower photon energy than visible or UV radiation (Fig. 7.1) and exerts its action by increasing the motion of molecules; i.e., a heating effect. Under normal circumstances, ambient infrared radiation is by itself incapable of exerting damage to ocular tissues. Although it is absorbed by water (hence by most biological tissues) the amount of IR radiation we are normally exposed to is insufficient to cause any significant heating. Obviously very high exposure levels (e.g., CO_2 laser or Nd:YAG laser) can exert significant damage due to shockwaves (acoustic gradients) as well as intense heating (Lerman, 1983). Blast furnaces can also cause IR cataracts (Glass Blower's Cataract). However, normal daily life does not expose us to such levels of radiation, and the only effects of IR radiation at ambient levels, are those associated with small temperature elevations (1–5°C) in the absorbing tissues (mainly the lens and retina) which can exert their action by enhancing UV induced photochemical changes.

This discussion will therefore be devoted mainly to delineating the effects of UV and visible radiation on normal ocular tissues, their relationship with aging changes in these tissues, in particular, the lens and retina, and their role in the pathogenesis of cataracts and retinal degenerative diseases.

UV RADIATION (UV LIGHT)

Ultraviolet induced changes in human and animal ocular tissues can be attributed to two mechanisms: a direct or intrinsic process in which the radiation is absorbed by specific naturally occurring chromophores within these tissues (e.g., the nucleic acids or aromatic amino acid residues), and an indirect or photosensitised process in which the radiation is initially absorbed by photosensitising drugs or other extrinsic compounds.

Direct UV radiation

Corneal photodamage from ultraviolet radiation has long been appreciated, a typical example being snow blindness experienced by polar explorers. This type of photo-keratitis is due to the relatively high levels of ultraviolet radiation which can be reflected by snow compared with less than 5% from earth or grass. Aside from the well-known polar and industrial photokeratitis, ultraviolet radiation has also been implicated in a variety of conjunctival and corneal lesions. These include pingueculae and pterygiums, exposure keratosis (which involves epithelial changes related to actinic radiation and is analogous to actinic keratosis of the skin), nodular band shaped keratopathy, experimentally induced tumours in animals, and the relatively rare dysplasia and intra-epithelial carcinoma. Certain corneal diseases can also be triggered by exposure to ultraviolet radiation; for example, herpes simplex keratitis and recurrent erosions of the cornea. Experimental UV photokeratitis is generally associated with an action spectrum showing a major peak at 280 nm and a minor one at μ 260 nm (Lerman, 1980c).

The normal human cornea and aqueous humour transmit almost all of the UV radiation longer than 300 nm, although there is a small but progressive decrease in the percentage of UV radiation transmitted as the cornea ages (this may be due to an accumulation of UV induced chromophores in the cornea as it ages (Lerman, 1980c). Thus the human ocular lens is constantly exposed to ambient UV radiation (300–400 nm) throughout life.

UV radiation can markedly affect the intact lens by direct absorption both in vivo and in vitro. During the past decade a considerable amount of evidence has accumulated implicating UV radiation (between 300 and 400 nm) as a significant factor in the in vitro generation of fluorescent compounds and in protein cross linking associated with lens aging and cataractogenesis in the mouse, rat, and human lenses (Lerman, 1972, 1976, 1980b, 1980c; Lerman et al, 1970, 1976; Zigman, 1971; Pirie, 1972; Satoh et al, 1973; Augusteyn, 1974, 1975; Dilley & Pirie, 1974; Spector et al, 1975; Bando et al, 1975; Lerman & Borkman, 1976, 1978; Zigman et al, 1979; Castineiras et al, 1979; Yu et al, 1979; Garner & Spector, 1980; Borkman et al, 1977; Borkman & Lerman, 1977). In vivo studies have also demonstrated that UV radiation of wavelengths longer than 300 nm are capable of generating experimental cataracts in mouse, rat, rabbit and primate lenses, and human UV radiation cataracts have been reported (Zigman & Vaughn, 1974; Pitts et al, 1977; Lerman, 1980a). The consequences of chronic cumulative photochemical damage are an increasing absorption of UV radiation and some visible light due to the presence of photochemically generated chromophores which increase in concentration and in number as the lens ages. At least two such chromophores have been partially characterised. One absorbs at 360 nm and fluoresces at 440 nm and a second absorbs at 435 nm and fluoresces at 520 nm (Lerman, 1980; Lerman & Borkman, 1976). These fluorescent compounds increase in number and in concentration as the lens ages, the lens nucleus becomes yellower, and there is a progressive decrease in the transmission of visible light as well as UV radiation with age (Fig. 7.2). The discoloration is mainly confined to the lens nucleus since the cortex has much higher levels of glutathione and other compounds capable of aborting most of these photochemical reactions (Lerman, 1980). Extreme examples of this age-related photochemical generation of lens pigments are the brown and black cataracts.

Although only a small amount of UV radiation from the sun enters the eye under normal circumstances, the cumulative effect of many years exposure is significant, particularly when one considers man's ever increasing life span. Epidemiologic surveys provide some support for the thesis that sunlight plays a role in lenticular aging and senile cataracts. For example, cataracts, and the rate of cataract extraction, are much higher in India, Pakistan, and certain areas of Africa than in the temperate zones. A recent epidemiologic investigation into the relationship between sunlight and cataract in the United States reported that '. . . cataract to control ratios for persons aged 65 years or older were significantly larger in locations with large amounts of sunlight . . .' (Heller et al, 1977). A more detailed study in Nepal, involving a relatively homogeneous population demonstrated a striking relationship between the prevalence of cataracts and hours of solar exposure (Brilliant, 1983). Those regions with the highest exposure experiences a cataract incidence of >75% which decreased to 15–20% in the areas with the least solar exposure. Obviously other factors play a role in cataractogenesis including heredity, nutrition, metabolism, etc.

Thus, it is now generally accepted that chronic exposure to UV radiation (300–400 nm) over an individual's lifetime leads to the generation and increased accumulation of various chromophores in the lens which are, to some extent,

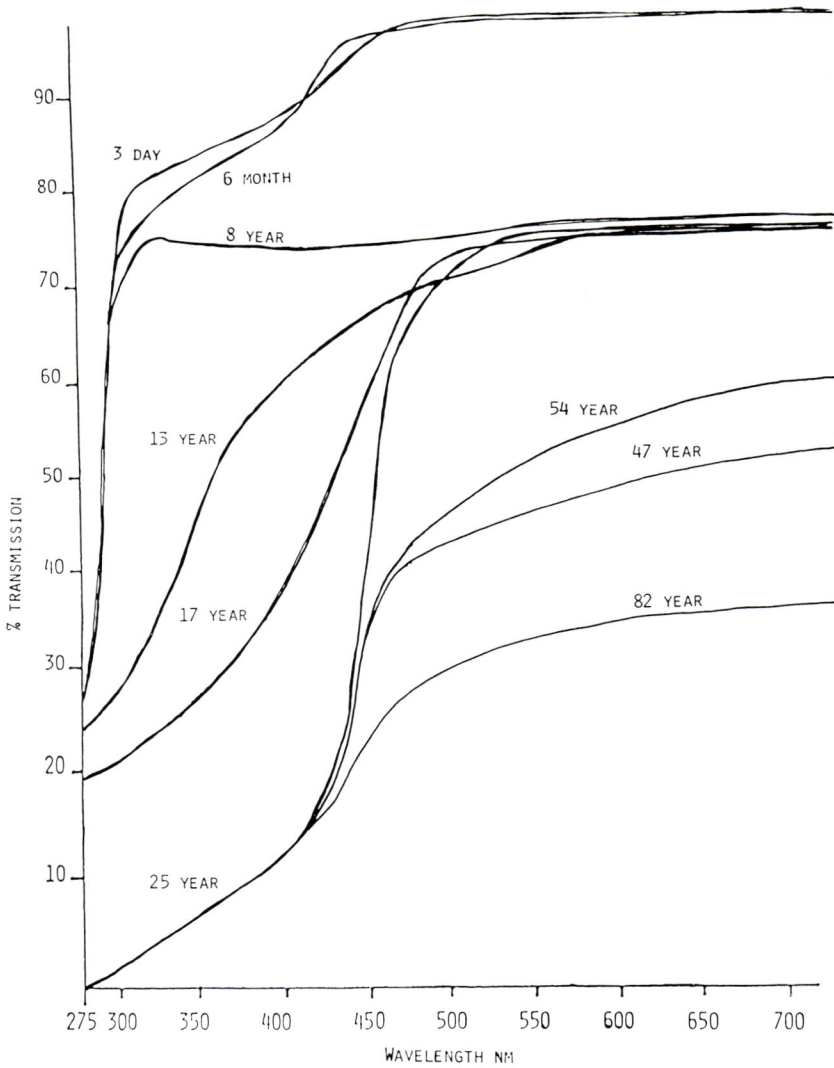

Fig. 7.2   Transmission of UV and visible radiation in the normal aging human lens

responsible for the increased yellow colour of the lens nucleus as it ages. In about 10% of our population this process progresses at a more rapid pace, resulting in the development of the brown (nuclear) cataract. This type of discoloration, in moderation, is actually beneficial since it enables the lens to become a very effective filter for UV and short wavelength visible radiation (by the second to third decade) thus protecting the retina from cumulative photochemical damage which could occur during a lifetime. Recent studies have shown that such radiation can cause irreversible retinal photodamage in the aphakic Rhesus monkey and even in man (Ham et al, 1982; Hochheimer, 1981; Berler & Peyser, 1983). It is interesting that nature has provided us with the ability to develop a lenticular UV filter to protect the retina from continuous radiation exposure which could be harmful, particularly in the older individual where the retinal metabolism and repair process are no longer as effective as in the young. We are now beginning to see confirmation of the hypothesis (Lerman, 1980b) that long wavelength UV radiation may play a role in certain retinal diseases (e.g., cystoid macular oedema) which tend to occur in older patients following removal of their cataractous lenses and even in degenerative processes such as macular degeneration and retinitis pigmentosa.

Aside from the effects of chronic exposure to ambient UV radiation, exposure to higher radiation levels can produce cortical opacities in human, rat and rabbit lenses in vitro and in vivo (Zigman & Vaughn, 1974; Pitts et al, 1977; Lerman, 1980a; Lerman et al, 1981b). Thus more intense UV radiation (300 nm and longer) can induce lens changes involving the cortex while chronic exposure mainly affects the lens nucleus. These effects appear to be dose and time related (Lerman, 1980c; Lerman et al, 1981b). It is postulated that UV radiation is capable of inducing severe photochemical damage to important enzyme systems (e.g., catalase, GSH dehydrogenase). There is also the possibility that more intense UV radiation may affect the protein/water order within the lens resulting in the formation of 'water lakes' associated with protein aggregates. This would give rise to localised areas of marked changes in refractive index in the injured site resulting in light scattering and opacification. Recent studies on rabbit lenses exposed to 337 nm laser irradiation demonstrate marked changes in their water component (Thomas & Schepler, 1980). These wavelengths have sufficient energies (c.a. 1–1.5 eV) to disrupt the protein/water order in the lens and give rise to sudden changes in refractive index resulting in localised opacities.

Vitreous
As previously noted, the vitreous is normally protected from UV radiation by the filtering action of the cornea (up to 295 nm) and by the lens as it ages (> 295 nm). However, patients who have had their cataracts removed (aphakes and pseudophakes) have lost a significant and protective intraocular filter. The normal vitreous is a gel-like material composed mainly of water, collagenous protein, and long-chain carbohydrates. These compounds do not contain any significant chromophores absorbing above 250–260 nm, although a small number of aromatic amino acids are present. In this respect the cornea plays a much more significant role as an UV filter (for the vitreous) since it prevents UV radiation below 295 nm from entering the eye. However, the vitreous does contain some tryptophan residues and several cell types; the hyalocytes and fibrocytes. Thus, some chromophores are present that are capable of absorbing UV radiation longer than 295 nm, provided that the filtering action of the ocular lens is removed. There is some experimental evidence that exposure of the vitreous to UV radiation up to 320 nm results in shrinkage of the vitreous gel and denaturation of the collagen network (Balazs et al, 1959). There is also a decrease in the viscosity of hyaluronic acid preparations derived from UV exposed vitreous which can be attributed mainly to a decrease in molecular weight and length. Ultraviolet irradiation causes an increase in the reducing power of the polysaccharide solution due to a breakdown of the glucosidic linkages, an increase of the reducing end groups, and the formation of smaller fragments (Balazs et al, 1959). The absorption spectra of hyaluronic acid subjected to UV irradiation shows significant alterations with the

development of new chromophores absorbing at approximately 267 nm. Other studies in which human vitreous gels were subjected to monochromatic UV radiation (280–300 nm) resulted in the generation of one or more fluorescent compounds. A 320–340 nm excitation and a 420-fluorescence emission peak could be demonstrated following 4–6 hours of irradiation, suggesting the possible photodegradation of certain amino acids.

It would thus appear that the cornea, which filters all UV radiation shorter than 295 nm, plays a major role in protecting the vitreous from UV damage. There is still insufficient experimental evidence to assess the effect of UV radiation longer than 295 nm, but there are indications that the vitreous is also sensitive to longer wavelength UV radiation (Lerman, 1980c). Thus the 295–400 nm filtering action of the ocular lens may also be of significance in protecting the vitreous.

RETINAL PHOTODAMAGE

The fact that visible light is required in the cyclic process of shedding and renewal of the outer membrane discs that contain visual pigments might explain the finding that even moderate but prolonged exposure to visible light, at thresholds of illumination well below those capable of causing thermal damage to the retina, can result in retinal pathology in a variety of experimental animals (Lerman, 1980c; Lanum, 1978; Marshall, 1982; Tso, 1973, 1982). Aging is known to be characterised by a loss of rod and cone cells (Lerman, 1980c; Marshall, 1982). The recent observation that photic trauma can damage the receptors, suggests a potential cumulative action of light resulting in an enhanced loss of visual cells over a period of years. That is, phototoxic effects may be cumulative in the normal aging process of the retina. Photon energies in the electromagnetic spectrum increase as the wavelength decreases, from 1.6 eV at 750 nm to 3.3 eV at 400 nm and higher energies in the UV wavelengths capable of penetrating to the retina in the aphakic or psuedophakic eyes. One would anticipate that photic damage would be greatest for UV radiation (320–400 nm) and short wave visible light in the blue region (400–475 nm) and decrease with increasing wavelengths of light, with the least photic damage occurring with red light. Recent studies strongly implicate longwave UV and short wave visible radiation (320–450 nm) as a significant factor in retinal photodamage in primates as well as other experimental animals, and even in man (Lerman, 1980c; Ham et al, 1982; Hochheimer, 1981; Berler & Peyser, 1983; Lanum, 1978; Marshall, 1982; Tso, 1973, 1982). These data are of particular concern in young patients as well as aphakes and pseudophakes who are on photosensitising drugs and to all patients exposed to prolonged or above ambient levels of UV radiation (e.g. occupational exposure in industries where UV polymerisation is employed, sailors, etc.).

The spectral sensitivity of the human retina plays a role with respect to the efficiency of a specific wavelength in producing retinal damage. The ocular lens also protects the retina from visible as well as UV radiation since it filters more of the shorter wavelengths of visible light (blue) as compared with the longer wavelengths. Thus, the aging retina, which metabolically should be more susceptible to photic damage caused by visible light (as well as ultraviolet radiation), is in fact protected by the ocular lens which increasingly filters out the ultraviolet and shorter wavelengths of the visible spectrum as the person ages. This might explain why human retinas are normally capable of withstanding much higher thresholds of radiation intensity as compared with other animals such as the rat, rabbit and pigeon. The retinas of these animals can be damaged by levels of environmental light that are not damaging to the normal human eye.

PHOTOCHEMICAL DAMAGE TO THE RETINA

Although it has long been recognised that visible as well as infrared radiation is capable of causing thermal damage to the retina when the eye is exposed to sufficiently intense sources at these wavelengths (solar retinopathy, xenon arc, and laser photocoagulation), the potential for non-thermal light injury has only recently become apparent. During the past two decades a growing body of literature has accumulated that attests to the deleterious effects of long term exposures to low levels of visible light as well as UV radiation (Lerman, 1980c; Ham et al, 1982; Hochheimer, 1981; Berler & Peyser, 1983; Lanum, 1978; Marshall, 1982; Tso, 1973, 1982). These investigations demonstrate that visible light at intensities well below levels that would cause thermal photocoagulation can damage retinal tissue in a variety of animals including man. This damage is manifested by electroretinographic and/or histopathological changes.

Deleterious effects of long term exposure of the growing chick eye to light was reported in 1961 (Lauber et al, 1961). The effects of the photoreceptor cells could not be explained in terms of thermal injury alone. The following year it was demonstrated that light exposure accelerated the degeneration of the photoreceptor cells in rats afflicted with hereditary retinal degeneration (Dowling & Sidman, 1962). In 1965, Noell first demonstrated that the retinas of rats could be damaged by light of moderate intensity (Noell, 1965). This report was followed by a series of papers (Noell et al, 1971; Noell & Albrecht, 1971; Organisciak & Noell, 1977; Noell, 1974) which established that long term exposure of normal albino rats to visible light at levels well below possible thermal damage, resulted in the degeneration and loss of rod photoreceptors. The wavelength that produced maximum damage corresponded to the peak absorption of rat rhodopsin, and body temperature was noted to be an important factor in these photic effects. Photic damage to the retina after long term exposure to low levels of visible light has now been reported in pigeons, rats, mice, rabbits, piglets, monkeys and even humans (Lerman, 1980c; Lanum, 1978; Marshall, 1982; Tso, 1973, 1982, Lauber et al, 1961; Dowling & Sidman, 1962; Noell, 1965, 1974; Noell et al, 1971; Noell & Albrecht, 1971; Organisciak & Noell, 1977).

A schematic outline of a typical course of retinal damage following long term exposure to light is shown in Figure 7.3. The initial effects involve the outer segments of the photoreceptor cells, in which the outer tip of the photoreceptor shows vacuole formation. The damage proceeds until the outer segment loses its normal lamellar structure and breaks off from the inner segment of the visual cell. As the outer segments are phagocytosed by the pigment epithelium, the inner segments develop pyknotic nuclei and also disappear. The final result is a retina in which most of the photoreceptor cells have disappeared but the remaining layers appear to be intact.

There is still a considerable amount of controversy regarding the effect of light on the pigment epithelium. Some workers believe that damage to the pigment epithelium occurs prior to the destruction of the photoreceptors; other believe that it occurs at the

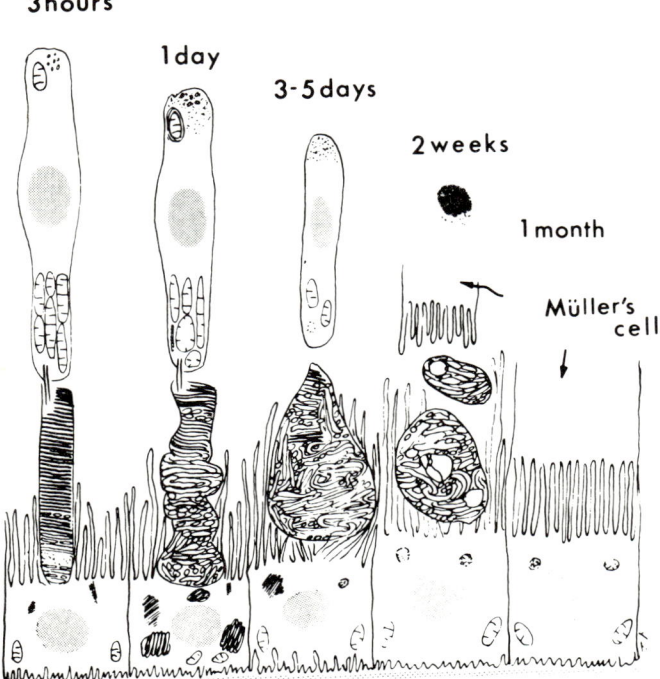

Fig. 7.3   Schematic representation of retinal damage following exposure of albino rats to visible light. At a three-hour exposure only outermost tip of photoreceptor shows vacuoles. At 24 hours photoreceptic outer segment is tortous and swollen. Myelin membranes separate from each other and form vesicular and tubular structures. The synaptic end of the photoreceptic cell shows pathologic changes. Pigment epithelium shows conspicuous increase in myeloid bodies. At 3–5 days damaged outer segment is isolated from inner segment and becomes large, round or pear-shaped body filled with tubular material, followed by cellular degeneration at 2–3 weeks and complete adhesion of pigment epithelium and Muller's cell in one month. (From Kuwabara T, Gorn R A 1968 Archives of Ophthalmol 79: 69–78, Copyright 1968 American Medical Association.)

same time as photoreceptor cell destruction, and it has also been proposed that damage to the pigment epithelium occurs subsequent to the destruction of the receptor cells. Some investigators believe that damage to the pigment epithelium plays a major and primary role, with outer segment degeneration being a secondary response to this damage and subsequent repair processes (inflammatory response). There is, however, considerable evidence of direct photic damage to the photo-receptor cells of the retina which occurs very soon after the animal has been exposed to light. It appears that the relative emphasis on photoreceptor cell damage versus pigment epithelial cell damage as the primary lesion, can be related to the use of pigmented versus albino strains of experimental animals. Thus, the role of melanin in retinal photopathology may be significant and awaits further elucidation. Recent studies on melanin haematoparphyrin photobinding suggest such a role for this pigment (Persad et al, 1983).

Although most of the work relating retinal damage to visible light comes from studies with experimental animals, there is increasing evidence indicating that the human retina can also be damaged by relatively low levels of visible light (Lerman, 1980c). The normal dark-adaptation reaction requires 30–40 minutes; an individual's sensitivity to light begins to increase immediately after being placed in the dark and reaches its normal level after 30–40 minutes, at which time there is no further increase in sensitivity. However, several investigators have demonstrated that exposure to strong sunlight for 3–4 hours results in dark adaptation thresholds that are elevated for 24 hours or more above normal levels and that there is a chronic effect on night vision that may persist for up to 10 days (Clark et al, 1946; Hecht et al, 1948). Another study involving patients suffering from solar retinopathy, reported that there was complete recovery in about half of the eyes 6 months after the injury (Penner & McNair, 1966). This would not be expected if the damage was due to retinal coagulation caused by thermal injury. It has been proposed that solar retinopathy in the rhesus monkey cannot be explained solely in terms of thermal injury; some type of thermally enhanced photochemical effect must also play a role. Some investigators believe that solar retinopathy can be accounted for almost entirely in terms of the photochemical effects of the shortwave visible components of the sun's spectrum (Ham et al, 1982).

A recent study has demonstrated that a simulated solar spectrum (400–1400 nm) with a predominant portion of the energy in the short visible wavelengths was more damaging to the retina than a long wavelength spectrum (700–1200 nm), by a factor of 5 (Ham et al, 1973). These workers inferred that for a continuous solar spectrum, as the retinal irradiance is reduced and exposure duration is prolonged, thermal insult becomes less pronounced while photochemical effects with thermal enhancement become more prominent. This reasoning is supported by theoretic considerations. Thermal damage to the retina would be expected for radiation in the near-infrared region since the energy absorption takes place predominantly in the melanin granules of the pigment epithelium and choroid while the photoreceptors are not involved (they do not absorb at these wavelengths). The absorption of the near infrared by the melanin involves wavelengths with photon energies ($< 1\,eV$) that would essentially induce vibrational changes in the molecule without adversely affecting its molecular structure, that is, a thermal effect. However, the shorter the wavelength the greater the photon energy; in the UV and shortwave visible spectra (320–475 nm) the photon energies approach levels in which electronic excitation becomes the dominant mode of energy absorption (2.0 eV at 475 nm to 3.5 eV at 320 nm). Molecular systems in electronically excited states above the ground state are subject to photochemical reactions. Thus, overbleaching of the photo pigments results in a new chain of metabolic events that appears to be capable of leading to irreversible as well as reversible damage to the visual cells depending on the duration and intensity of exposure to light.

Recovery from visible light damage

It has now been shown that visible light plays a normal physiological role in maintaining the health of the outer segments of the visual cells. In man and other diurnal animals, a certain amount of photic damage followed by repair and recovery of the receptor cells is a significant factor in the maintenance of the photoreceptor elements and normal visual acuity. One would also predict that diurnal animals should be less susceptible than nocturnal animals to the same intensity of visible light, since nature must have provided them with a more efficient recovery mechanism, because scotopic vision (daylight vision) plays such an important role in their daily lives.

The absorption characteristics of the ocular media (the cornea and lens) must be considered in determining the threshold level of visible light that is capable of causing retinal damage. We have shown that the human lens plays an increasingly important role with respect to its ability to filter UV radiation as it ages. The increasing yellow colour of the lens nucleus with age also functions as a partial filter for visible radiation, particularly in the shorter wavelengths (in the blue region). Thus, the human ocular lens may serve an additional function in the older individual by virtue of its ability to filter out a significant portion of the visible radiation, particularly the shorter wavelengths (with a higher photon energy), thereby protecting the aging and metabolically less efficient retina from photic damage due to visible light.

It should be noted that the irradiance levels of energy incident on the retina (intensity measured as watts per square centimeter) is determined by the imaging properties (focusing properties) of the ocular media (the cornea and lens), the absorbing properties of the ocular media, and the size of the pupil. Utilising these parameters, one can predict that the nocturnal animal should be more sensitive to the same threshold of light compared with the diurnal animal, and this appears to be borne out by experimental data (Lerman, 1980c; Lanum, 1978). Thus, the rat (particularly the albino rat) and rabbit appear to be the most sensitive animals to experimental retinal damage, with the diurnal animals (the monkey and human) displaying a decreasing order of sensitivity to the same intensity of visible light. There is as yet insufficient data available to determine the specific dose of photons absorbed, per receptor, for sustaining retinal damage. It is estimated that 1.5×10^3 to 1.5×10^4 photons/receptor/sec continued for a relatively long period of time are necessary to cause retinal damage by visible light (Lanum, 1978). Although the early studies indicated that visible light damage to the retina was irreversible, there is now evidence that the retina is capable of recovering from a moderate amount of photic damage, particularly if the pigment epithelium of the retina and the photoreceptor cell body are preserved (Kuwabara, 1970). These studies demonstrate that retinas from albino rats exposed to 750–1000 footcandles ($1.2–1.6 \times 10^{-3}$ watts/cm²) of light are capable of recovering within 3–6 weeks after such an exposure, as evidenced by a return of the electroretinogram to normal levels. The pathological damage includes loss of the outer segments of the photoreceptor cells and moderate damage to the pigment epithelium. These damaged areas recover slowly with the latter cells showing the first recovery response followed by regeneration of the membranes to form somewhat irregular outer segments.

BODY TEMPERATURE AND LIGHT DAMAGE

It is important to note that the body temperature of the animal plays an important role in determining whether the damage is reversible or irreversible. There is a direct relationship between an increase in body temperature and the degree of reversibility of photic damage to the retina; a rise in body temperature by 3–5°C above normal will significantly increase the photic damage to the retina at the same exposure threshold compared with an animal kept at normal body temperature (Noell et al, 1966).

Most of the studies on retinal pathology have utilised fluorescent and incandescent light sources. As previously noted, the spectral output of the fluorescent light source more closely approximates daylight, particularly in the UV region, while the incandescent illumination has a large infrared spectral output that serves as a heat source. Since even a relatively small increase in body temperature (1–3°C) can have a great influence on increasing the degree of light damage, it is important to differentiate experimental retinal photopathology from its purely photochemical versus its thermal mechanism.

OPHTHALMOSCOPY, THE OPERATING MICROSCOPE AND RETINAL DAMAGE

One should also consider the potential problem with respect to indirect ophthalmoscopy and retinal damage. Several workers have demonstrated that indirect ophthalmoscopy is capable of producing retinal damage in primate eyes (Dawson & Herron, 1970; Tso et al, 1972). It should be noted that the standard method employed in indirect ophthalmoscopy involves the use of a 20-diopter convex lens placed between the light source and the patient's eye, which in effect will serve to act as an additional focusing element, thereby concentrating the light and energy per unit area on to the patient's retina (in addition to the concentrating properties already inherent in the patient's eye). It has been estimated that the amount of focal energy applied to the retina and choroid by the indirect ophthalmoscope is about $0.1–0.2 \, \mathrm{w/cm^2}$, which approximates the amount of irradiance received at the retinal surface from the sun. However, it should also be noted that the indirect ophthalmoscope has 90% of its power in the infrared region (longer than 750 nm). The retinal irradiance levels with an indirect versus a direct ophthalmoscope have been measured and the data indicate a tenfold increase in retinal irradiance with the indirect ophthalmoscope (Pomerantzeff et al, 1961). It is estimated that at the patient's retina the total irradiance is composed of one-third visible light to two-thirds infrared radiation. Some workers have proposed that infrared filters should be incorporated into all ophthalmoscopes to prevent potential thermal damage from extensive indirect ophthalmoscopy. They also proposed that reasonably short exposures should be used when examining the posterior pole of the eye. Intense illumination and frequent re-examination at short intervals should be avoided. It should be pointed out that the energy delivered during indirect ophthalmoscopy is only 200 times less than the energy that is capable of producing a retinal burn.

Recent reports have described clinically demonstrable retinal lesions in patients undergoing intraocular surgery with the operating microscope (Hochheimer, 1981; Berler & Peyser, 1983; Henry & Henry, 1977). Lesions resembling central serous retinopathy have been demonstrated in primate eyes exposed to longwave UV radiation (Tso, 1982). One must therefore consider the potential for retinal damage with these clinical techniques, particularly in certain conditions, such as retinitis pigmentosa, which might be accelerated by light exposure. Photic damage has also been shown to result in pathologic changes in the pigment epithelium as well as the outer segments; this suggests the possibility that such damage would weaken the adhesions between the retina and pigment epithelium and potentiate retinal detachment (Lerman, 1980c).

Two recent reviews have considered the possibility of ocular hazards resulting from ambient light exposure (Lanum, 1978; Sliney, 1976). They indicate that ambient light levels are currently approaching the threshold level for permanent retinal damage (following chronic exposure). The levels of artificial illumination that we are exposed to at present vary between 20 and 50 footcandles $(3.2-8.1 \times 10^{-5} \text{watts}/\text{cm}^2)$. Although these levels of irradiance are well below the levels that are capable of producing retinal photopathology in primates and man, they have been shown to be of sufficient intensity to produce permanent as well as reversible retinal damage in certain experimental animals, particularly albino rats. The recent trend by lighting engineers toward higher levels of illumination (e.g., 100–1000 footcandles) should be approached with extreme caution in view of the potential photic damage that could be incurred at these levels of illumination. It sould also be noted that the lowest reported retinal damage threshold in primates occurs at wavelengths in the blue region of the spectrum, and the potential adverse effects of UV radiation on the retina must also be considered, particularly in the aphakic eye. Another point to bear in mind is the fact that the pigment epithelium is one of the major sites of primary photic damage; thus the melanosomes in the pigment epithelium may play a significant role as transducers of photic energy in the eye. These organelles seem to play a central role in both the thermal and chemical mechanisms or primary photic damage to the retina and may play a role in the pathogenesis of senile macular degeneration. One must also consider the role of photosensitising agents in retinal photobiology. The fact that the psoralens absorb mostly in the longer wavelength UV spectrum (between 320 and 360 nm) has allayed concern about the risk of this drug to the retina. However, the ocular hazard from such photosensitising drugs should be of concern in aphakic eyes that have lost their natural UV filter (the ocular lens), in pseudophakes, and in young children (whose own lens has yet to develop as an effective UV filter).

Photosensitised UV radiation
In addition to the demonstrated direct photochemical action of UV radiation on the ocular lens, there is the possibility of photobiologic damage by means of photosensitised reactions due to the accumulation of certain drugs within this organ. After the 13 mm stage of development the ocular lens is completely encapsulated and never sheds its cells throughout life. Thus, photobinding a drug to the lens proteins and nucleic acids ensures its lifelong retention within the lens with the potential for enhanced photodamage if the photoproducts are capable of acting as photosensitising agents.

The psoralen compounds are well-known photosensitising agents and have been used (under controlled conditions) in many dermatology clinics to treat psoriasis and vitiligo (Parrish et al, 1974, 1976). This form of phototherapy, commonly referred to as PUVA therapy, involves the ingestion of 8-methoxypsoralen (8-MOP) or related compounds followed by exposure to UVA radiation (320–400 nm) for short periods of time. 8-MOP can be found in a variety of ocular tissues within two hours after the animal (rat, dogfish and monkey) is given a single dose (equivalent to a human therapeutic level) and can become photobound to lens proteins and DNA if there is concurrent exposure to ambient levels of UVA radiation (Lerman & Borkman, 1977, 1978; Lerman et al, 1977, 1980a, 1980b, 1981c; Jose & Yielding, 1978; Megaw et al, 1980; Wulf & Andreasen, 1981, 1982; Lerman, 1982a). Since the mature ocular lens is a very effective filter to UVA radiation in most mammals (including man) there can be no photobinding of 8-MOP in the retina. However, UVA radiation can penetrate to the retina in aphakic and pseudophakic experimental animals and in young eyes (where the ocular lens still permits significant penetration of UVA radiation) and 8-MOP photobinding can also occur in these retinas.

Psoralen-UVA (PUVA) therapy and cataract formation have been documented in experimental animals and presumptive human cataracts have been reported (Cloud et al, 1960, 1961; Freeman & Troll, 1969; Crylin et al, 1980; Lerman, 1983a). Cataracts from patients on PUVA therapy were subjected to high resolution phosphorescence spectroscopy. The lens proteins from these patients showed phosphorescence peaks identical (in shape and lifetime) with the previously reported 8-MOP lens protein photoproduct seen in PUVA treated cataractous rat lenses (Lerman et al, 1981b, 1982b; Koch et al, 1982). These data provide proof that this drug can generate specific PUVA photoproducts in human lenses which have been shown to be associated with the formation of PUVA cataracts in experimental animals. These data are the first objective demonstration of an 8-MOP lens protein photoproduct in material derived from human PUVA patients and provide further evidence to substantiate the previous clinical reports of PUVA cataracts. However, this observation should not deter anyone from prescribing this form of therapy for psoriasis since simple and effective preventive measures are available. It should be noted that 8-MOP can be found in the lens *for only 24 hours, provided* that the eye is protected from UVA radiation. Thus, many dermatologists are now providing proper UV filtering glasses to all their PUVA patients with instructions to put them on as soon as they ingest the drug and continue to wear them for at least 24 hours. They must be worn indoors as well as out of doors, since there is sufficient UVA radiation in ordinary fluorescent lighting to photobind the 8-MOP (Lerman, 1980c; Lerman et al, 1977, 1981b). A 2-year follow-up study using UV slit lamp densitography has proven the efficacy of this approach. All the patients were provided with proper UV filtering glasses for at least 24 hours following drug ingestion, and none developed enhanced or abnormal lens fluorescence levels. In contrast, patients whose eyes had not been properly protected (those treated prior to 1978) had anomalous and enhanced lens fluorescence and three of them developed PUVA cataracts (Lerman, 1983a). It should be noted that PUVA therapy could pose a potential hazard not only to the ocular lens but to the retina in young people whose lenses are not effective UV absorbers and/or in aphakic and pseudophakic individuals, particularly if they are exposed to repeated PUVA therapy (Lerman et al, 1981c; Lerman 1982b, 1983a, Takei et al, 1983). The intraocular lenses currently in use are excellent transmitters of UV radiation and thus provide less protection from UVA radiation than the natural lens or even ordinary glass (which absorbs all UV radiation up to 320 nm). UV absorbing intraocular lenses are now being tested by several manufacturers and should provide a simple solution in preventing potential UVA photodamage to the pseudophakic retina.

Allopurinol is a commonly used antihyperuricaemic agent in treating gout. Scattered reports have appeared regarding the possible relationship between the development of lens opacities in relatively young patients (2nd–4th decade) and chronic ingestion of this drug (Fraunfelder et al, 1982; Lerman et al, 1982a). Cataracts obtained from 11 patients on chronic allopurinol therapy (> 2 years) were subjected to high resolution phosphorescence spectroscopy. The characteristic allopurinol triplet was demon-

AGE   VISIBLE   UV

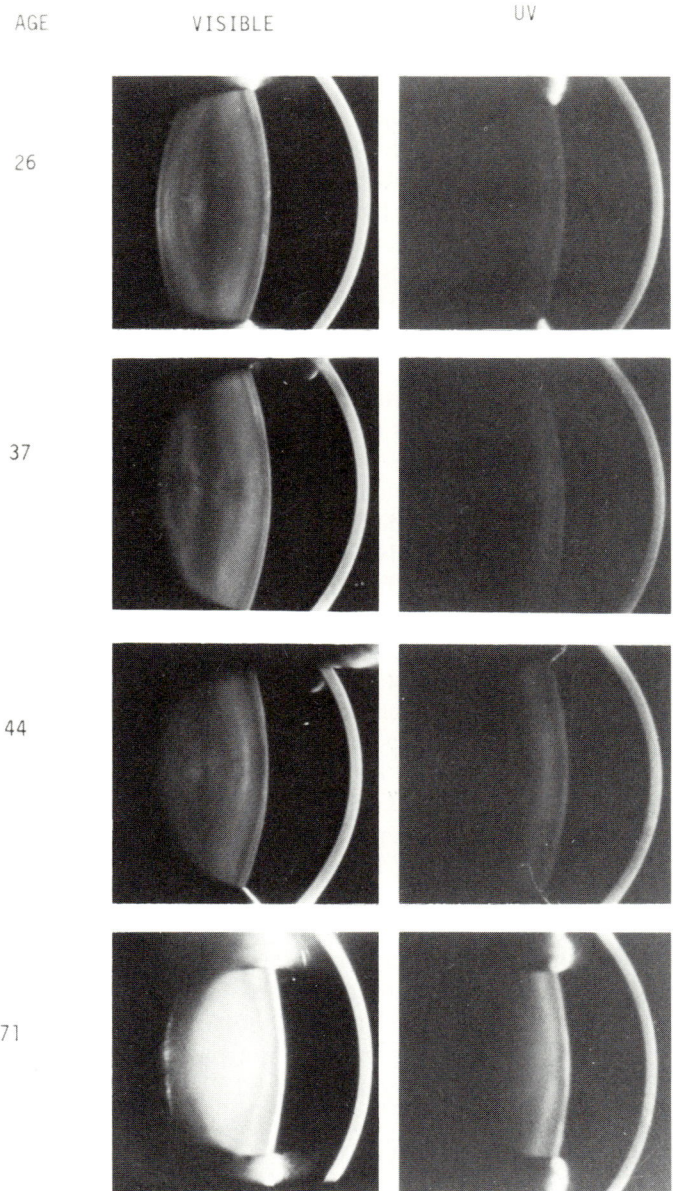

Fig. 7.4 Visible (left) and UV (right) slit lamp photography of normal lenses in patients aged 26, 37, 44 years, and nuclear sclerosis in a patient aged 71 years. The UV photos represent fluorescence from lens and cornea.

strated in all the cataracts. Indentical spectra were obtained on normal human lenses incubated in media containing 10^{-3}M allopurinol and exposed to $1.2 \, mW/cmn^2$ UV radiation for 16 hours; control lenses (irradiated without allopurinol) were negative. Similar data were obtained on lenses from rats given one dose of allopurinol and exposed to UV radiation overnight. However, the allopurinol triplet could not be

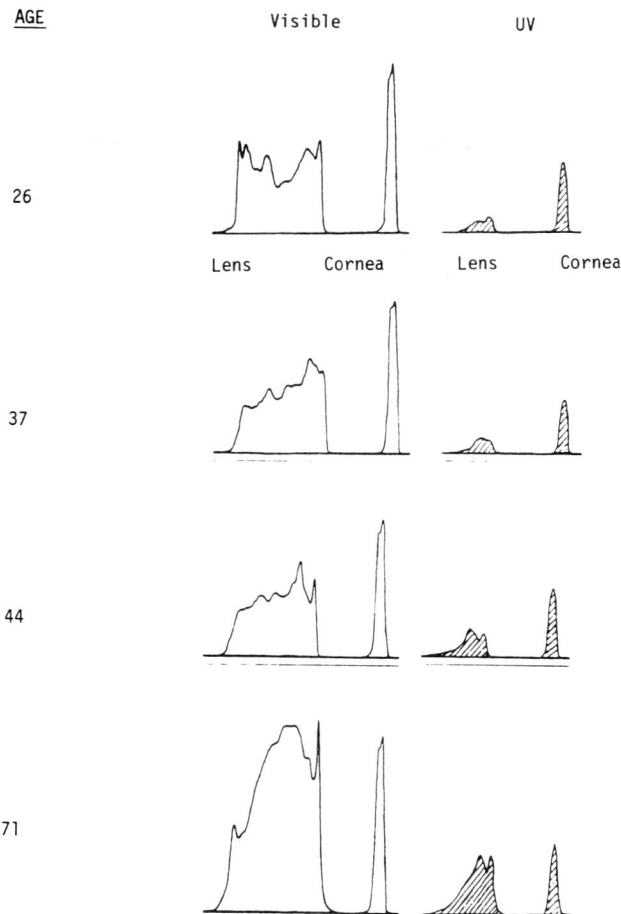

Fig. 7.5   Corresponding densitometric analysis of lenses in Fig. 7.4. Note increasing fluorescence levels with age and in nuclear sclerosis.

demonstrated in normal eye bank lenses derived from patients who had been on chronic allopurinol therapy for more than 2 years without developing ocular problems. These data suggest that allopurinol can act as a cataractogenic enhancing agent in some patients when it is permanently photobound within their lenses probably as an additional extrinsically derived photosensitiser (Lerman et al, 1982a; Fraunfelder et al, 1983). However, chronic allopurinol therapy (by itself) does not necessarily result in the retention of allopurinol if it is not photobound. The relationship between levels of UVA exposure, circulating allopurinol levels (and renal function) in the genesis of photosensitised allopurinol cataracts will require further studies.

CLINICAL STUDIES

Since laboratory studies have demonstrated enhanced fluorescence in the ocular lens associated with aging and drug therapy, and photosensitised cataracts have also been reported, a method to monitor lens fluorescence in vivo has been developed (Lerman, 1982b; Lerman et al, 1981a, 1983a; Lerman & Hockwin, 1981; Hockwin & Lerman, 1982). A new slit lamp densitographic apparatus (based on the Scheimpflug principle) capable of accurately and reproducibly recording visible changes in lens density as it ages was recently introduced (Dragomirescu et al, 1978, 1981; Hockwin et al, 1983). This apparatus has been modified to utilise UV radiation (300–400 nm) to measure and quantify the age related fluorescence levels in the normal lens in vivo and correlate them with in vitro data (Lerman, 1976, 1980b, 1980c; Lerman & Borkman, 1976;

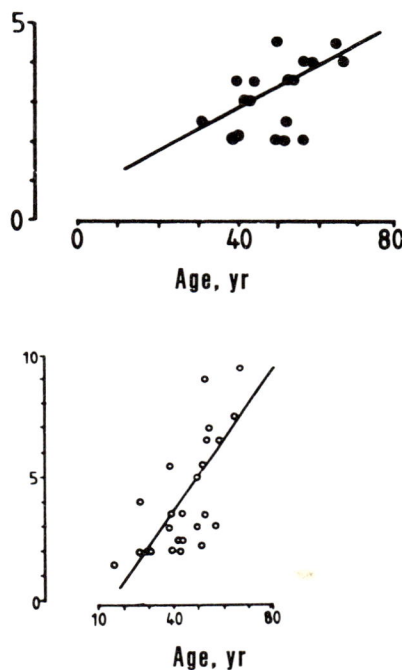

Fig. 7.6   Normal age-related increase in two densitographic regions derived from UV slit lamp photos in vivo) which correspond to the 440 nm (Fig. 7.1) and 520 nm (Fig. 7.2) fluorescence emission levels obtained in vitro.

Lerman et al, 1983a). Representative visible and UV slit lamp photographs taken with the Scheimpflug (Topcon) camera on normal eyes and corresponding densitograms show increased lens fluorescence with age (Figs. 7.4 and 7.5). A series of UV and visible slit lamp photographs of normal patients ranging in age from 5–82 years demonstrate a lack of fluorescence in the young lens and a progressive increase in fluorescence with age (Lerman et al, 1983a). These data can be expressed in graphic form (Fig. 7.6) showing the normal age related increase in lens fluorescence (in vivo) which corresponds well with the in vitro data (Figs. 7.7 and 7.8) previously reported (Lerman, 1976, 1980b; Lerman & Borkman, 1976). The in vitro studies were performed on lenses from normal eye bank eyes and represent two (non-tryptophan) fluorescence peaks obtained by fluorescence spectroscopy.

Aside from demonstrating the normal age related increase in lens fluorescence, abnormally enhanced fluorescence caused by occupational (or accidental) exposure to higher levels of UV radiation can also be detected. This is shown in Figure 7.9a which is a photograph of a 40-year-old patient who was exposed to excessive UV radiation in his workplace. The increased fluorescence can easily be appreciated by comparing this lens with a photograph of a normal 40-year-old eye (Fig. 7.9b). Enhanced fluorescence and/or abnormal fluorescence emission can also occur in patients on PUVA therapy and failure to protect properly such patients from all UV radiation exposure (for at least 24 hrs following ingestion of the drug) can even result in cataract

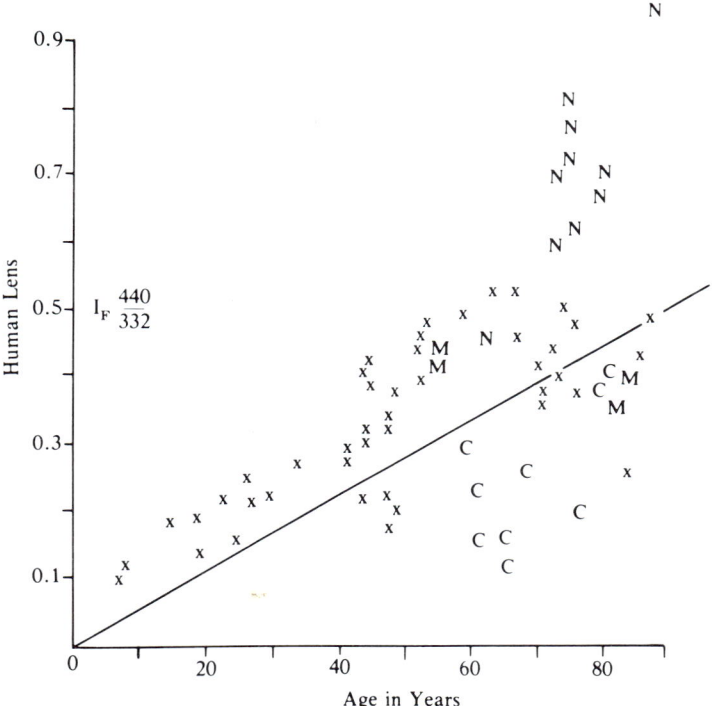

Fig. 7.7 I_F 440 ratios representing whole lens fluorescence intensity at 440 nm (360 nm excitation) divided by tryptophan intensity (in whole lens) at 332 nm (20 nm excitation). The I_F 440 ratio shows age-related increase in the normal lens (X) and solid line, a marked increase in brown nuclear cataracts (N), relatively normal or below normal levels in cortical cataracts (C), and high normal values in mixed cortical and nuclear cataracts (M). Each point represents a single lens.

formation (Fig. 7.10). This 52-year-old patient with Psoriasis was on 4 years of intermittent PUVA treatment (without proper eye protection). Although many dermatology clinics now provide all PUVA patients with proper UV absorbing or reflecting spectacles, data obtained on a series of patients who were treated prior to 1977 (when the potential for photosensitised lens damage from psoralen therapy was first demonstrated [Lerman & Borkman, 1977; Lerman et al, 1977]) show a significant elevation of one of the lens fluorescence peaks (Fig. 7.11). This is in contrast with patients who have been on penicillamine therapy (for a variety of diseases) and tend to have lower lens fluorescence intensities (Fig. 7.11). This is due to the fact that penicillamine (which is an excellent free radical scavenger as well as a chelating agent) is capable of entering the lens, both in vivo as well as in vitro (Lerman, 1976, 1980c; Lerman & Borkman, 1976, 1978; Lerman et al, 1976; Borkman & Lerman, 1977). As a free radical scavenger, penicillamine aborts the UV induced free radical reactions thereby preventing lenticular photodamage.

These studies demonstrate the feasibility of obtaining in vivo lens fluorescence data which are objective, reproducible and can be quantified. Thus, UV slit lamp

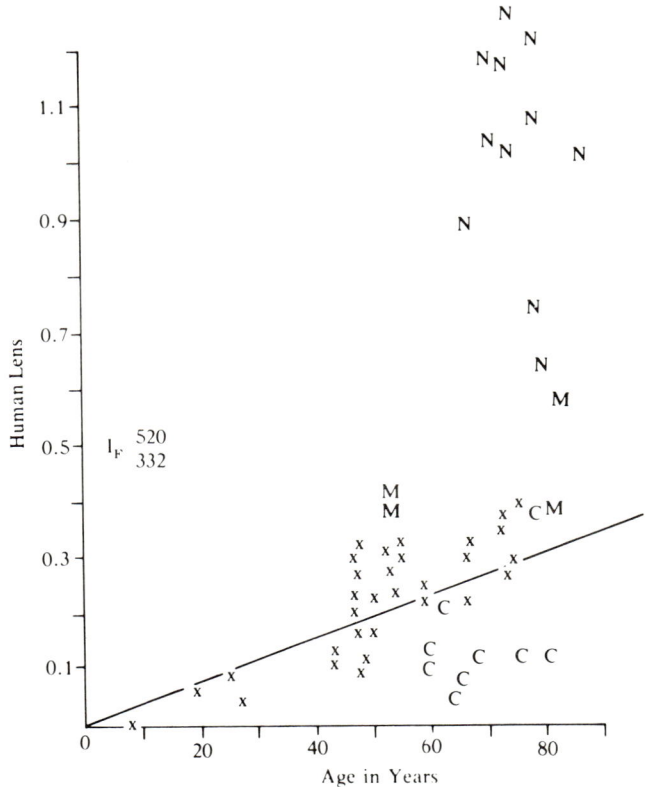

Fig. 7.8 I_F 520 ratios representing fluorescence intensity of second fluorescent region in the lens at 520 nm (420–435 nm excitation) divided by tryptophan fluorescence intensity in the lens at 332 nm (295 nm excitation). Interference filters (295 and 435 nm) were employed in order to decrease the light scattering when cortical and mixed cataracts were examined. Each point represents a single lens.

densitography can be used to monitor objectively one parameter of lens aging (fluorescence), as well as photosensitised lens damage, at a molecular level years before visible opacities become manifest by conventional slit lamp examination and measures can be instituted to at least retard if not prevent such lens opacities.

Aside from detecting abnormal levels (or wavelengths) of lens fluorescence in the living eye, one can now test the hypothesis that the UV filtering capacity of the lens (which can be directly correlated with increasing fluorescence levels) is lower than normal in certain patients with degenerative retinal disease (Lerman, 1980c). That is, the ocular lens in such individuals has not developed sufficient chromophores to enable it to absorb all the UV radiation. In >80% of our population, by the time they

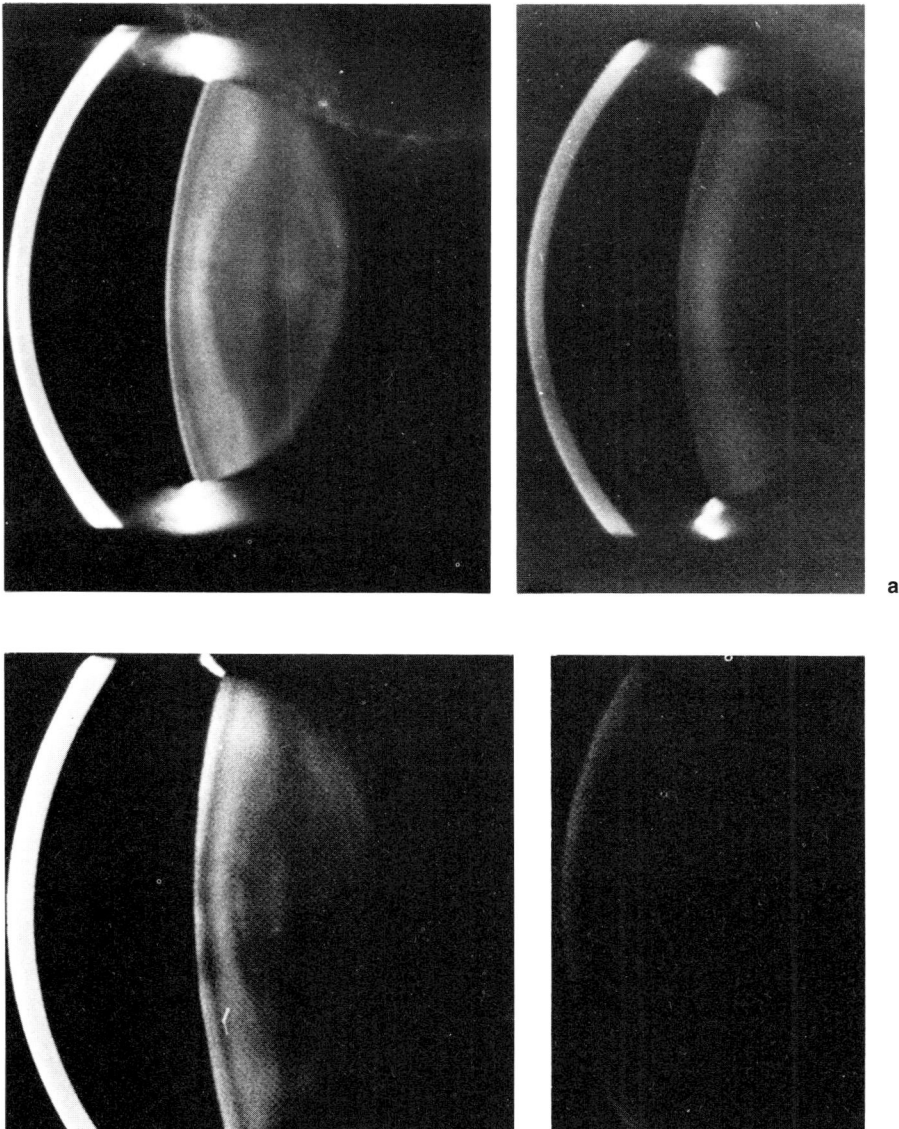

Fig. 7.9   **a** Visible (left) and UV (right) photos of a 40-year-old eye (exposed to excess UV radiation). Note marked enhancement of lens fluorescence compared with a normal 40-year-old eye as shown in **b**. **b** Visible (left) and UV (right) photos of a 40-year-old normal eye.

reach the third to fourth decade, the lens has become a very effective filter of UV and shortwave visible radiation (320–450 nm), thereby protecting the aging (and metabolically less efficient) retina from potential damage (Lerman, 1980c). These wavelengths can cause retinal photodamage as demonstrated by experiments in aphakic primates exposed to 5 mW/cm² UV (325–400 nm) radiation for 1000 sec (which approaches

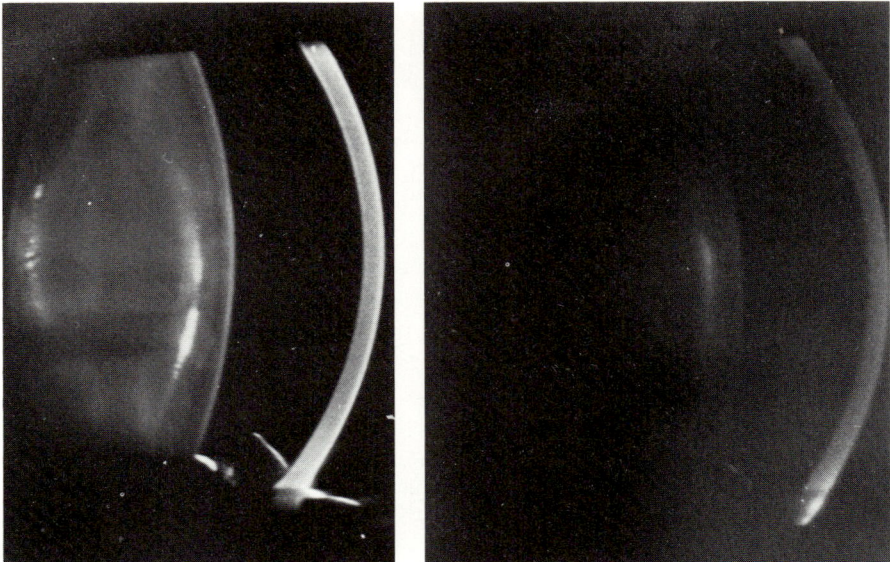

Fig. 7.10 PUVA cataract in a 52-year-old patient on chronic PUVA therapy for 4 years (without adequate eye protection).

ambient solar levels in our area). One can now attempt to determine whether this occurs in the human by measuring lens fluorescence levels. Such studies have demonstrated a significantly lower level (30–50%) of lens fluorescence in patients with retinal degenerative diseases (compared with the usual values for their age groups) indicating that their lenses are less effective filters for the 320–450 nm wavelengths of radiation (Lerman, 1982 & 1983a). These data suggest that photodamage may be a significant factor in the progression (and perhaps pathogenesis) of some retinal

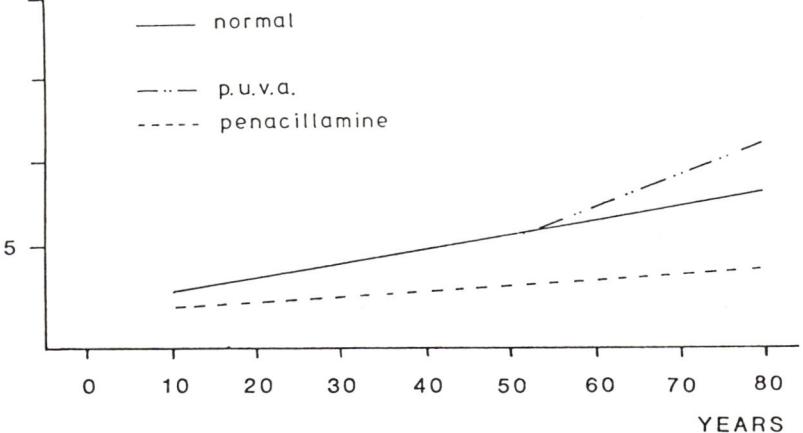

Fig. 7.11 Enhanced fluorescence levels in PUVA patients (treated prior to 1977) compared with normal age-related increase in fluorescence (520 nm region). Note lower lens fluorescence levels in patients on penicillamine therapy.

degenerative diseases and could be particularly relevant for the older pseudophakic patient whose intraocular lens is a very good transmitter of UVB as well as UVA radiation. In view of the increasing use of plastic intraocular lenses, which transmit much more UV radiation than glass (i.e., they even transmit wavelengths shorter than 320 nm), questions have been raised regarding potential UV and shortwave visible (320–450 nm) radiation damage to pseudophakic patients. For example, it has been demonstrated that protecting such patients with UV absorbing glasses significantly reduces the incidence of postoperative cystoid macular oedema.

Because of the confusion and controversial claims regarding the efficacy of commercially available sunglass in protecting the eye from UV photodamage, a large series of such lenses have recently been analysed to determine their transmission characteristics (Lerman et al, 1983b). Their ability to transmit UV and visible radiation (280–750 nm) was measured and these studies are in general agreement with an earlier report (Anderson & Gebel, 1977). There was a wide variation in the UV transmission characteristics of the sunglasses evaluated, ranging from 1.5–40%, with similar transmission values noted when tested for more discrete wavelengths (340–380 nm). Only the NOIR, Spectra-Shield, Silor, Univis, and UV 400 lenses were > 99% effective in filtering all the UV radiation. It should also be noted that visible radiation is significantly decreased in darkly tinted sunglasses, while still permitting some long wavelength UV transmission. In patients with blue, grey and hazel eyes, a 50% or more decrease in visible radiation can result in pupillary enlargement of 0.10–0.25 nm thereby increasing the effective dose of radiation incident on the intraocular tissues.

POTENTIAL HAZARDS FROM OZONE DEPLETION

The foregoing discussion has demonstrated that ambient UV radiation is capable of inducing damage to various ocular tissues, particularly the cornea, lens and retina. The latter two organs are protected from shorter wavelength UV radiation by the cornea which acts as a very effective filter for the 280–300 nm wavelengths. However, longer wavelength UV (above 300 nm) has now been shown to play a significant role in the generation of at least one form of aging cataract, the brown (nuclear) cataract. In the aphakic or pseudophakic individuals (who have lost the filtering protection of their own lenses) the retina might also be susceptible to photochemical damage. The aphakic primate retina can be irreversibly damaged by very low exposure doses (ca. 5 mW/cm²) of UV longer than 325 nm. Furthermore, photochemical damage to ocular tissues is potentiated by certain photosensitising drugs and chemical reagents. Since current levels of solar and man-made UV radiation have already been shown to exert photochemical damage to these ocular tissues, any decrease in the ozone layer could therefore be accompanied by a significant increase in photodamage to the cornea and lens in the phakic individual and retina in the aphake or pseudophake.

VIDEO DISPLAY TERMINALS AND THE EYE

The recent controversy regarding ocular problems which have been reported in workers using video display terminals (VDT) may turn out to be beneficial and opportune. In contrast with the indifference and ignorance with which we embraced the development of the X-ray (in the not too distant past), the community at large, as well as the scientific specialists, are now well aware of the possible dangers in misusing electromagnetic radiation. We now have the ability to monitor radiation emission levels from our technological marvels and obtain reasonably accurate measurements on most wavelength emissions of interest. We also have a considerable body of ever expanding scientific knowledge which enables us to correlate specific radiation emission levels with threshold doses for possible photobiological damage. Such measurements have recently been performed by scientists at the Bureau of Radiological Health, Bell Laboratories and NIOSH (Weiss & Peterson, 1979, An evaluation . . . 1981; NIOSH Research Report 1981). Scientists at the BRH measured ionising radiation (e.g. X-ray) emission levels on 125 VDTs; of these 34 VDTs were also measured for non-ionising radiation emission (UV, visible, infrared (IR), microwave and other radiofrequency (RF) emissions). A smaller number of VDTs were similarly evaluated by the Bell Laboratory scientists. These data indicate that the VDTs 'emit little or no harmful ionising or non-ionising radiation under normal operating conditions' (An evaluation . . . 1981). The specific emissions that were detectable were all well below the current national and international safety standards.

Aside from 'ocular fatigue', questions have been raised regarding a possible relationship between VDT radiation emission and 'organic' ocular photodamage, particularly to the ocular lens. Of the various wavelengths in the electromagnetic spectrum, UV radiation and ocular photodamage have received considerable attention during the last two decades. Although there appears to be a relationship between 'senile' cataracts and total solar (UV) exposure (Lerman, 1980c; Lerman & Borkman, 1976 & 1978; Berler & Peyser, 1983) it should be noted that these types of lens opacity require many years exposure. Furthermore, it has been estimated that sunlight produces between 2 and 5 milliwatts/cm^2 of UV radiation (280–400 nm) depending on geographical location and season (Lerman, 1980c). In the laboratory, the lowest levels of UV radiation (at specific wavelengths) that have been shown to be capable of producing direct UV photodamage to the ocular lens, while considerably lower than ambient (solar) UV radiation, are still significantly larger (at least by a factor of 10) than the UV radiation emission levels emitted by the VDTs. Thus, the best available current experimental and epidemiologic evidence does not indicate that the level of UV radiation emitted by the VDTs is capable of exerting any deleterious effects on the ocular lenses of personnel using these terminals. We should, however, pay more attention to the workplace with respect to the types of lighting (UV emission levels) used in these environments and the reflectance level of work surfaces (including UV reflectance of painted walls, desks, etc.) (Ulrich & Evans, 1976) in order to maintain total ambient UV radiation exposure at minimum levels. Our own ocular lens serves us well as a natural filter for removing the UV radiation that penetrates into the eye, thereby protecting the underlying retina which has been shown to be quite sensitive to rather low levels of UV radiation. Thus particular care must be taken to protect the aphakic and pseudophakic individuals from potential low level UV radiation damage. A similar situation pertains to some patients who are receiving photosensitising drugs. Fortunately the levels of UV radiation emitted by the VDTs are much lower than the amount shown to cause retinal photodamage in experimental primate studies.

In conclusion, measured levels of electromagnetic radiation emitted by VDTs that have been tested are well below the national, international and experimental emission levels compared with the threshold safety levels for each of the specific wavelength regions measured for ionising radiation (e.g. X-rays) and the non-ionising spectrum (UV, visible, IR, microwave and other RF radiation). Further research should be encouraged particularly in the areas relating to non-ionising radiation damage in order to clarify and better define the molecular mechanisms resulting from exposure to UV, IR, microwave (and RF) radiation. It is also important to determine whether damage can result from cumulative low level exposure over a lifetime, and whether a synergistic effect could accrue from low level exposure to broadband radiation (e.g. UV + microwave, ionising + non-ionising).

Finally, it should be noted that we now have the capability of protecting the eye from potential UV photodamage by special eyeglasses and similar UV absorbing materials could be employed at the manufacturing end to prevent UV radiation emission from our ever increasing array of new products.

THERAPY

The best and simplest treatment for direct UV photodamage to ocular tissues is prevention. Lenses which are excellent UV filters have recently been introduced; these include the Spectra-Shield coating for glass lenses and a variety of UV absorbing plastic lenses. Of the latter, the Silor, Univis and UV400 are equally efficient filters and can be ordered with the patient's correction. For those who do not require corrective lenses, plano spectacles made of any of the foregoing materials can be ordered. For patients on phototherapy, goggles (which include sidepieces) are preferred (to prevent reflected radiation). The Blak Ray goggle, and those made from the foregoing materials are recommended. Ordinary commercial sunglasses are not necessarily effective absorbers of UV radiation longer than 320 nm and are not recommended unless their transmission characteristics are such that they remove more than 99% of all UV radiation.

In spite of recent claims by some intraocular lens manufacturers that their lenses absorb UV radiation, there are as yet no proven products available. Since clear glass absorbs UV up to 320 nm, and some intraocular lenses are made of materials which contain some absorbing chromophores, the manufacturers can claim that their lenses are UV filters even though they do not remove the longer wavelengths. In order to be truly effective, the intraocular lens must at least filter all radiation up to 400 nm and preferably a significant percentage of the shorter wavelength visible light (400–450 nm). Such lenses will probably become available in the near future. It is hoped that any lenses claiming to be UV filtering intraocular lenses will have their true absorption and emission characteristics clearly noted as a package insert in order to avoid half truths and questionable claims.

REFERENCES

An evaluation of radiation emission from video display terminals 1981 In: Radiological health, United States Department of Health and Human Services, Food and Drug Administration
Anderson W J, Gebel R K H 1977 Ultraviolet windows in commercial sunglasses. Applied Optics 16: 515–517

Augusteyn R 1975 Distribution of fluorescence in the human cataractous lens. Ophthalmic Research 7: 217–224

Augusteyn R C 1974 Human lens albuminoid. Japanese Journal of Ophthalmology 18: 127–134

Balazs E A, Laurent T C, Howe A F, Varga L 1959 Irradiation of mucopolysaccharides with ultraviolet light and electrons. Radiation Research 11: 149–164

Bando M, Nakajima A, Satoh K 1975 Coloration of human lens protein. Experimental Eye Research 20: 489–492

Berler D, Peyser R 1983 Light intensity and visual acuity following cataract surgery. Ophthalmology 89 (Suppl): 117

Borkman R F, Lerman S 1977 Evidence for a free radical mechanism in aging and UV irradiated ocular lenses. Experimental Eye Research 25: 303–309

Borkman R F, Dalrymple A, Lerman S 1977 Ultraviolet action spectrum for fluorogen production in the ocular lens. Photochemistry and Photobiology 26: 129–132

Brilliant L B 1983 Cataract, altitude and sunlight in the Himalayas. American Journal of Epidemiology (in press)

Castineiras S G, Dillon J, Spector A 1979 Effects of reduction on absorption and fluorescence of human lens proteins. Experimental Eye Research 29: 573–575

Clark B, Johnson M L, Dreher R 1946 The effect of sunlight on dark adaptation. American Journal of Ophthalmology 29: 828–836

Cloud T M, Hakim R, Griffin A C 1960 Photosensitization of the eye with methoxsalen. I. acute effect. Archives of Ophthalmology 64: 346–351

Cloud T M, Hakim R, Griffin A C 1961 Photosensitization of the eye with methoxsalen. II. chronic effects. Archives of Ophthalmology 66: 689–694

Crylin M N, Pedvis-Leftick A, Sugar J 1980 Cataract formation in association with ultraviolet photosensitivity. Annals of Ophthalmology 12: 786–790

Dawson W W, Herron W L 1970 Retinal illumination during indirect ophthalmoscopy: subsequent dark adaptation. Investigative Ophthalmology 9: 89–96

Dilley K J, Pirie A 1974 Changes to the proteins of the human lens nucleus in cataract. Experimental Eye Research 19: 59–72

Dougherty T J, Thoma R E, Boyle D G, Weishaupt K R 1981 Interstitial photoradiation therapy for primary solid tumors in pet cats and dogs. Cancer Research 41: 401–404.

Dowling J E, Sidman R L 1962 Inherited retinal dystrophy in the rat. Journal of Cellular Biology 14: 73–107.

Dragomirescu V, Hockwin O, Koch H R 1978 Development of a new equipment for rotating slit image photography according to Scheimpflug's principle. In: Interdisciplinary topics in gerontology, Karger, Basel, vol 13, p 118–130

Dragomirescu V, Hockwin O, Koch H R 1981 Photo-cell device for slit-beam adjustment to the optical axis of the eye in Scheimpflug photography. Ophthalmic Research 12: 78–86.

Fraunfelder F, Megaw J, Lerman S 1983 Further studies on allopurinol in human cataracts. Investigative Ophthalmology and Visual Science 23: 205–207

Fraunfelder F T, Hanna C, Dreis M W, Cosgrove K W 1982 Possible lens changes associated with allopurinol therapy. American Journal of Ophthalmology 94: 137–140

Freeman R G, Troll D 1969 Photosensitization of the eye by 8-methoxypsoralen. Journal of Investigative Dermatology 53: 449–455

Garner M H, Spector A 1980 Selective oxidation of cysteine and methionine in normal and senile cataractous lenses. Proceedings of National Academy of Science 77: 1274

Ham W T Jr, Muller H A, Williams R C, Geeraets W J 1973 Ocular hazards from viewing the sun unprotected and through various windows and filters. Applied Optics 12: 21–22

Ham W T, Muller H A, Ruffolo J J, Guerry D, Guerry R K 1982 Action spectrum for retinal injury from near ultraviolet radiation in the aphakic monkey. American Journal of Ophthalmology 93: 229–306

Hecht S, Hendley C D, Ross H, Richmond P N 1948 The effect of exposure to sunlight on night vision. American Journal of Ophthalmology 31: 1573–1580

Heller R, Giacometti L, Yuen K 1977 Sunlight and cataract: an epidemiologic investigation. American Journal of Epidemiology 105: 450–459

Henry M M, Henry L M 1977 A possible cause of chronic cystic maculopathy. Annals of Ophthalmology 9: 455–457

Hochheimer B F 1981 A possible cause of chronic cystic maculopathy the operating microscope. Annals of Ophthalmology 13: 153–155

Hockwin O, Lerman S 1982 Clinical evaluation of direct and photosensitized UV radiation damage to the lens. Annals of Ophthalmology 14: 220–223

Hockwin O, Dragomirescu V, Lerman S 1983 In vivo age-related changes in normal and cataractous human lens density. Acta XXIV International Congress of Ophthalmology (in press)

Jose J J, Yielding K L 1978 Photosensitive cataractigens, chlorpromazine and methoxypsoralen cause DNA repair synthesis in lens epithelial cells. Investigative Ophthalmology and Visual Science 17: 687–690

Koch H R, Beitzen R, Kremer F, Chioralia G, Baurmann H, Megaw J, Gardner K, Lerman S 1982 8-Methoxypsoralen and long ultraviolet effects on the rat lens: I. high dosage. Albrect von Graefe's Archives of Clinical and Experimental Ophthalmology 219(4): 193–199

Kuwabara T 1970 Retinal recovery from exposure to light. American Journal of Ophthalmology 70: 187–198

Lanum J 1978 The damaging effects of light on the retina. Empirical findings, theoretical and practical applications. Survey of Ophthalmology 22: 221–249

Lauber J K, Schutze J, McGinnis J 1961 Effects of exposure to continuous light on the eye of the growing chick. Proceedings of Society of Experimental Biology and Medicine 106: 871–872

Lerman S 1972 Lens proteins and fluorescence. Israel Journal Medical Science 8: 1583–1589

Lerman S 1976 Lens fluorescence in aging and cataract formation. Documentia Ophthalmologica Proceedings Series 8: 241–260

Lerman S 1980a Human UV radiation cataracts. Ophthalmic Research 12: 303–314

Lerman S 1980b Lens transparency and aging. In: Regnault F, Hockwin O, Courtour Y (eds) Aging of the lens, Elsevier/North Holland Biomedical Press, New York/London p 263–279

Lerman S 1980c Radiant energy and the eye, MacMillan, New York, ch 2–3

Lerman S 1982a Ocular phototoxicity and PUVA therapy: an experimental and clinical evaluation. FDA photochemical toxicity symposium. Journal of National Cancer Institute 69: 287–302

Lerman S 1982b UV slit lamp densitography of the human lens. An additional tool for prospective studies of changes in lens transparency. In: Ageing of the lens symposium, Strasburg, 1982, Imtegra, Munich, p 139–154

Lerman S 1983a Psoralens and ocular effects in animals and man: in vivo monitoring of human ocular and cutaneous manifestations. Conference on photobiologic, toxicologic and pharmacologic aspects of psoralens. March 1–3, 1982. Journal of National Cancer Institute (in press)

Lerman S 1983b Use of high power lasers in ophthalmology. Journal of Kerato-Refractive Society (in press)

Lerman S, Borkman R 1977 A method for detecting 8-methoxypsoralen in the ocular lens. Science 197: 1287–1288

Lerman S, Borkman R F 1976 Spectroscopic evaluation and classification of the normal aging and cataractous lens. Ophthalmic Research 8: 335–353

Lerman S, Borkman R F 1978 Photochemistry and lens aging. In: von Hahn H P (ed) Interdisciplinary topics in gerontology: gerontological aspects of eye research, S Karger, Basel, vol 13, p 154–183

Lerman S, Hockwin O 1981 UV-visible slit lamp densitography of the human eye. Experimental Eye Research 33: 587–596

Lerman S, Dragomirescu V, Hockwin O 1983a In vivo monitoring of direct and photosensitized UV radiation damage to the lens. Acta XXIV International Congress of Ophthalmology (in press)

Lerman S, Hockwin O, Dragomirescu V 1981a In vivo lens fluorescence photography. Ophthalmic Research 13: 224–228

Lerman S, Jocoy M, Borkman R 1977 Photosensitization of the lens by 8-methoxypsoralen. Investigative Ophthalmology and Visual Science 16: 1065–1068

Lerman S, Megaw J, Gardner K 1982a Allopurinol therapy and human cataractogenesis. American Journal of Ophthalmology 94: 141–146

Lerman S, Megaw J, Gardner K 1982b P-UVA therapy and human cataractogenesis. Investigative Ophthalmology and Visual Science 23: 801–804

Lerman S, Megaw J, Gardner K 1983b Optical spectroscopy as a method to monitor aldose reductase inhibitors in the lens. Investigative Ophthalmology and Visual Science (in press)

Lerman S, Megaw J, Willis I 1980a Potential ocular complications of PUVA therapy and thier prevention. Journal of Investigative Dermatology 74: 197–199

Lerman S, Megaw J, Willis I 1980b The photoreaction of 8-MOP with tryptophan and lens proteins. Photochemistry and Photobiology 31: 235–243

Lerman S, Gardner K, Megaw J, Borkman R 1981b The prevention of direct and photosensitized UV radiation damage to the ocular lens. Ophthalmic Research 13: 284–292

Lerman S, Kuck J F, Borkman R, Saker E 1976 Induction, acceleration and prevention (in vitro) of an aging parameter in the ocular lens. Ophthalmic Research 8: 213–226

Lerman S, Tann T T, Louis D, Hollander M 1970 Anomalous absorption of lens proteins due to a fluorogen. Ophthalmic Research 1: 338–343

Lerman S, Megaw J, Gardner K, Takei Y, Willis I 1981c Localization of 8-methoxypsoralen in ocular tissues. Ophthalmic Research 13: 106–116

Marshall J 1982 Ocular pathology in British VDT studies. Proceedings of IX international ergophthalmological symposium. In: Problems of industrial medicine in ophthalmology, S Karger, Basel (in press)

Megaw J, Lee J, Lerman S 1980 NMR analyses of tryptophan-8-methoxypsoralen photoreaction products. Photochemistry and Photobiology 32: 265–270

Menon I A, Persad S, Haberman H F, Kurian C J, Basu P K 1982 A qualitative study of the melanins from blue and brown human eyes. Experimental Eye Research 34: 531–537

National Institute of Occupational Safety Hazards Research Report 1981 Potential health hazards of video display terminals, DHSS (NIOSH) Publication No 81–129

Noell W K 1965 In: Graymore C N (ed) Aspects of experimental and hereditary retinal degeneration, Biochemistry of the Eye, Academic Press, New York, London p 51–72

Noell W K 1974 Hereditary retinal degeneration and damage by light, Estratto dagli Atti del Simposio di Oftalmologia Pediatrica, Parma, p 322–329

Noell W K, Albrecht R 1971 Irreversible effects of visible light on the retina: role of vitamin A. Science 171: 76–80

Noell W K, Delmelle M C, Albrecht R 1971 Vitamin A deficiency effect on retina: dependence on light. Science 172: 72–76

Noell W K, Walker V S, Kang B S, Berman S 1966 Retinal damage by light in rats. Investigative Ophthalmology 5: 450–473

Organisciak D T, Noell W K 1977 The rod outer segment phospholipid/opsin ratio of rats maintained in darkness or cyclic light. Investigative Ophthalmology and Visual Science 16: 188–190

Parrish J A, Fitzpatrick T B, Shea C, Pathak M A 1976 Photochemotherapy of vitiligo. Use of orally administered psoralens and a high intensity longwave ultraviolet light (UV-A) system. Archives of Dermatology 112: 1531–1534

Parrish J A, Fitzpatrick T B, Tanebaum L, Pathak M A 1974 Photochemotherapy of psoriasis with oral methoxalen and longwave ultraviolet light. New England Journal of Medicine 291: 1207–1211

Penner R, McNair J N 1966 Eclipse blindness. American Journal of Ophthalmology 61: 1452–1457

Persad S, Menon A, Haberman H F 1983 Comparison of the effects of UV visible irradiation of melanins and melanin-hematoporphyrin complexes from human black and red hair. Photochemistry and Photobiology 37: 63–68

Pirie A 1972 Effect of sunlight on proteins of the lens. In: Bellows J (ed) Contemporary Ophthalmology, Williams and Wilkins, Baltimore, p 484–501

Pitts D G, Hacker P D, Parr W H 1977 Ocular ultraviolet effects from 295 nm to 400 nm in the rabbit eye. DHEW (NIOSH) Publication No 77–175

Pomerantzeff P, Govignon J, Schapens C L 1961 Indirect ophthalmoscopy: is the illumination level dangerous. Transactions of the American Academy of Ophthalmology and Otolaryngology 73: 246–251

Satoh K, Bando M, Najajima A 1973 Fluorescence in human lens. Experimental Eye Research 16: 167–172

Sliney D H 1976 In: Landers M B (ed) Retinitis pigmentosa, Plenum Press, New York, p 211–220

Spector A, Roy O, Stauffer J 1975 Isolation and characterization of an age-dependent polypeptide from human lens with non-tryptophan fluorescence. Experimental Eye Research 21: 9–24

Takei Y, Franks Y, Megaw J, Gardner K, Gammon A, Lerman S 1984 Photobinding of labeled 8-methoxypsoralen to monkey intraocular tissues. Investigative Ophthalmology and Visual Science 25, in press

Thomas D M, Schepler K L 1980 Raman spectra of normal and ultraviolet-induced cataractous rabbit lens. Investigative Ophthalmology and Visual Science 19: 904–912

Tso M O M 1973 Photic maculopathy in rhesus monkey: a light and electron microscopic study. Investigative Ophthalmology and Visual Science 12: 17–34

Tso M O M 1982 The effects of light of the retina in health and disease. Ophthalmology 89 (Suppl): 117

Tso M O M, Fine B S, Zimmerman L E 1972 Photic maculopathy produced by the indirect ophthalmoscope. I. Clinical and histopathic study. American Journal of Ophthalmology 3: 686–699

Ulrich O A, Evans R M 1976 Ultraviolet reflectance of paint. American Welding Society Report, August 6

Weiss M M, Petersen R C 1979 Electromagnetic radiation emitted from video computer terminals. Bell Telephone Laboratories Incorporated. American Industrial Hygiene Association Journal 40: 300–309

Wulf H C, Andreasen M P 1981 Distribution of ^{3}H-8-MOP and its metabolites in rat organs after a single oral administration. Journal of Investigative Dermatology 76: 252–257

Wulf H C Andreasen M P 1982 Concentration of ^{3}H-8-methoxypsoralen and its metabolites in the rat lens and eye after a single oral administration. Investigative Ophthalmology and Visual Science 22: 32–36

Yu N-T, Kuck J F R, Askren C C 1979 Red fluorescence in older and brunescent human lenses. Investigative Ophthalmology and Visual Science 18: 1278–1280

Zigman S 1971 Eye lens color formation and function. Science 171: 807–809

Zigman S, Vaughn T 1974 Near UV light effects on the lenses and retinas of mice. Investigative Ophthalmology 13: 462–465

Zigman S, Datiler M, Torozynshi E 1979 Sunlight and human cataract. Investigative Ophthalmology and Visual Science 18: 462–467

8. Vitreous surgery

R. J. Cooling

INTRODUCTION

There have been many important developments and changes of emphasis in the field of pars plana vitreous surgery since its introduction into clinical practice in 1970 by Robert Machemer. Remarkable technical improvements have rapidly extended the capabilities of vitreous surgery which have become increasingly exploited in the treatment of a wide range of ocular disorders. A considerable body of surgical experience has now accumulated clarifying the major benefits and limitations of vitreous surgery and literally shedding new light upon the patho-physiology of vitreo-retinal disease.

It is the intention of this brief review to focus upon those aspects of vitreous surgery which have been the subject of recent development and to consider the major posterior segment applications of closed vitrectomy in current practice.

INSTRUMENTATION AND TECHNIQUES

Common gauge microsurgery

One of the most influential developments in modern vitreous surgery was the advent of common gauge instrumentation. This system, devised by Connor O'Malley (1975) and popularised by Charles, embodied a number of ingenious concepts which have since become incorporated into most commercially produced vitrectomy instruments. The method represented a significant departure from the original concept of a single intraocular instrument subserving all basic functions of suction-cutting, infusion and illumination (full-function probes). These various functions are divided between instruments of uniform shaft diameter introduced through three self-sealing, custom-made sclerotomies of less than 1 mm in diameter. The method provides an infusion facility independent of the suction cutter using an indwelling 20-gauge cannula (Fig. 8.1). This enables maintenance of the intraocular pressure irrespective of the rate of fluid outflow and following the withdrawal of all other intraocular instruments. Location of infusion remote from the aspiration system reduces turbulence and dispersion of debris, diminishes the total volume of fluid replaced and facilitates a wide range of manoeuvres, in particular exchange techniques.

With common gauge systems, two instrument techniques of vitreous surgery have become standard practice employing separate fibreoptic endoillumination to provide focal or diffuse illumination. The disturbing reflexes accompanying extraocular illumination are avoided and the variable positioning of illumination with respect to other instruments offers superlative visualisation. With the adoption of a standard gauge, a variety of instruments including scissors, microforceps and dissectors may be

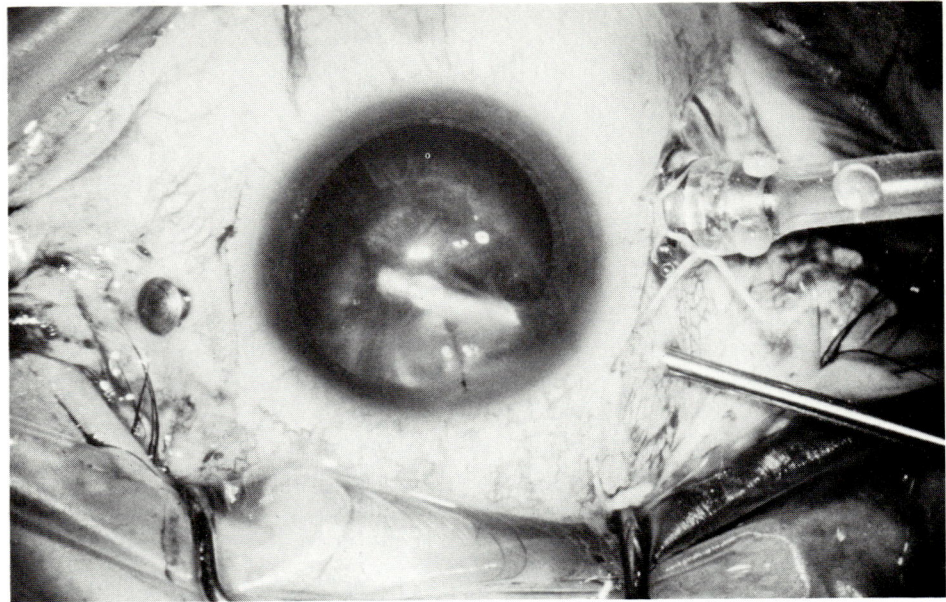

Fig. 8.1   Pars plana lensectomy using 20 gauge suction-cutter and independent infusion.

interchanged in rapid fashion and transposed with the endoilluminator such that intraocular manipulations can be performed with greater precision. It was this inherent versatility of the common gauge system that prompted the development of an ever-expanding range of accessory instrumentation that has come to play such an important part in modern vitreous surgery. Fears expressed that multiple pars plana incisions would significantly increase the risk of entry site complications have not been substantiated.

Recent developments in the designs of fundus contact lenses and endoilluminators have substantially improved visualisation (Fig. 8.2). A number of lightweight plano-concave lenses constructed of scratch-resistant quartz have recently been introduced. Handheld designs afford excellent central and peripheral observation, in part related to the experience and endurance of the surgical assistant (Ho et al, 1983). Constant fluid infusion beneath the lens eliminates air bubbles and the accumulation of blood. High output continuous fibre endoilluminators are now routinely used providing an intensity of illumination far in excess of previous designs. With the increased risk of cumulative light toxicity to the retina and the likelihood of damage by light below 500 nm, the use of a 505-nm wavelength pass filter during periods of highest risk has been suggested (Meyers & Bonner, 1982).

Recent interest has focused upon methods of generating and controlling suction force, obligatory for any mechanical method of vitreous removal. Besides the obvious requirements of simplicity and reliability, the aspiration system must offer a wide range of suction force and be capable of constant variation. It is desirable that the application and termination of suction force be instantaneous with no residual vacuum or regurgitation, although facilities for reflux are necessary. In addition, it is preferable that suction be under the direct control of the surgeon.

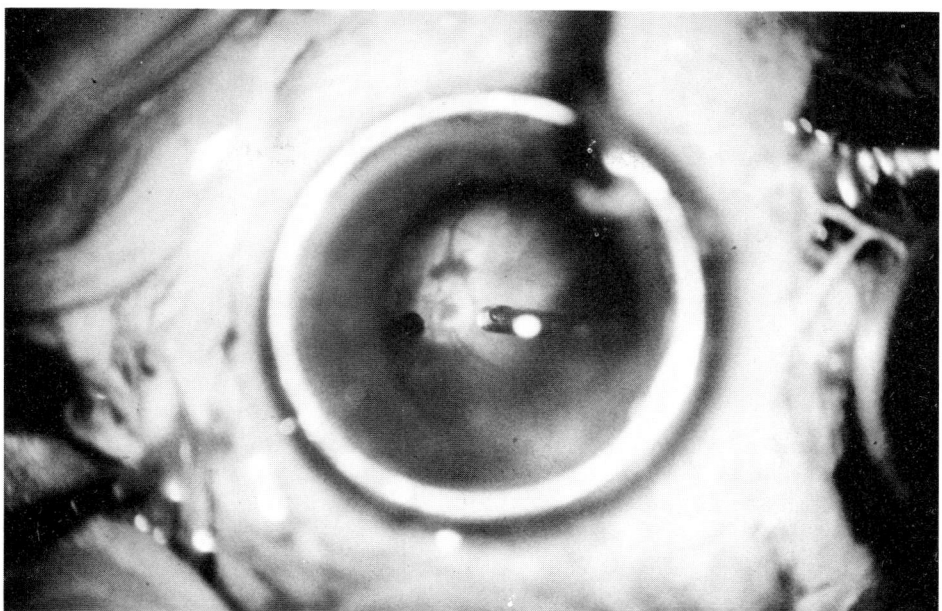

Fig. 8.2   Bi-manual vitrectomy with common gauge instrumentation visualised through irrigating fundus contact lens.

In the early days, the use of manual syringe suction controlled by the assistant was common to most vitrectomy systems. This method has persisted in certain disposable vitrectors capable of generating considerable force in a relatively uncontrolled manner. Increasingly, automated suction units have been adopted, offering a number of important advantages. The requisite level of suction force can be reduced by the use of an automated system with decreased fluctuation of intraocular pressure and an overall reduction in the total volume of fluid exchanged. Some of the earlier systems provided activation of the suction system by a venting port located on the hand piece but, as in most vitreous instrumentation, control has now been delegated to single or multi-stage foot-switches. With the need for constant variation in the level of suction, linear suction control has been developed and incorporated into most commercial systems (Fig. 8.3). Linear suction offers a far more controlled and safer method of aspiration by the use of a stepless foot pedal control in which suction can be varied from zero to a pre-selected maximum. Interestingly, such a system was first developed many years ago by workers at the Jules Stein using simple vacuum and a regulated manifold but the system did not reach commercial production. Linear suction allows the level of suction force to be tailored to the consistency of tissues being excised. Suction force is minimised and sudden vacuum avoided to reduce the risk of creating retinal tears within the region of the vitreous base. It should not be forgotten that the design of the suction cutter also has an influence upon the level of suction, experience showing that a rapid guillotine action requires a reduced level of suction (Charles, 1981a).

Epiretinal membrane dissection
The development of surgical techniques whereby fibrocellular membranes can be

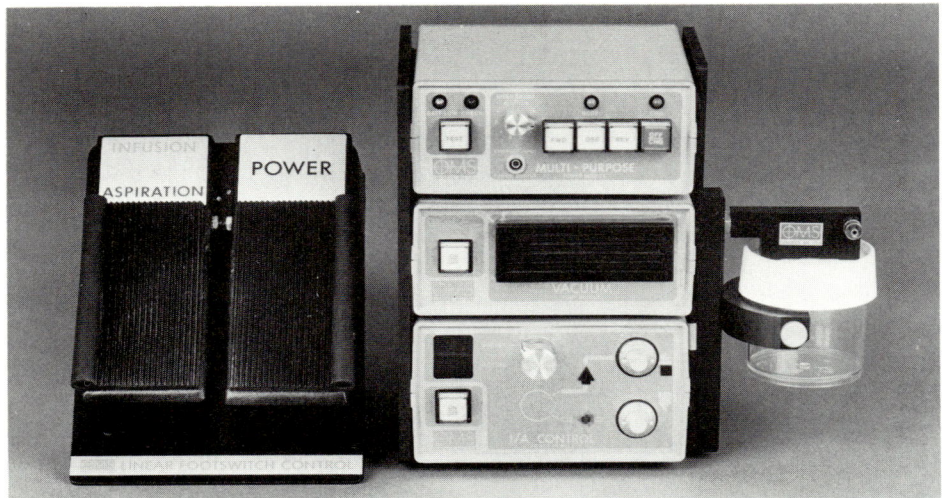

Fig. 8.3 Modular console design with linear suction facility (OMS).

dissected from the retinal surface represents a major advance in vitreous surgery. In general, these technically demanding procedures carry significant risk of iatrogenic retinal damage and the possibility of recurrent membrane formation. Nevertheless, epiretinal dissection is frequently an essential surgical objective in terms of visual restoration and stabilisation of the underlying condition.

Epiretinal membranes develop as a consequence of cellular migration and proliferation on the surface of the retina. Cell-mediated contraction causes tangential traction on the underlying retina to produce distortion, detachment or extracellular fluid accumulation. As an index of maturity, in situ collagen synthesis occurs, stabilising the effects of cellular contraction. Despite their extraretinal location, epiretinal membranes have variable attachments to the retina chiefly at sites of glial outgrowth through dehiscences in the internal limiting lamina. Epiretinal membranes may arise as an idiopathic phenomenon or in association with a wide range of ocular conditions including vasoproliferative retinopathies, rhegmatogenous retinal detachment, posterior segment inflammatory disorders and intraocular trauma.

Non-vascularised epiretinal membranes, which do not depend upon the presence of cortical gel for their development, can readily be separated from the retinal surface by membrane peeling. The tip of a bent hypodermic needle engages the edge of the membrane and traction is applied parallel with the retinal surface. On occasions, minor capillary bleeding occurs and resistance may be encountered at sites of glial outgrowth. In the absence of a discrete edge, central incision of the membrane is required before peeling can be accomplished. Concomitant removal of the internal limiting lamina is a frequent finding on histopathological study of excised epimacular membranes which in some way may account for the very low incidence of membrane recurrence in this situation.

In massive periretinal proliferation (MPP), extensive non-vascularised cellular proliferation and subsequent contraction leads to progressive immobilisation of the detached retina. The extent and distribution of surface proliferation shows considerable variation with a gradation of clinical appearances ranging from posterior eversion of retinal tears or isolated, full-thickness star folding, to a rigid funnel-shaped detachment obscuring the optic disc. Attempts to excise broad areas of epiretinal membrane are thought to be counterproductive by inducing further damage to the internal limiting lamina with increased risk of glial reproliferation. Relief of tangential traction to mobilise the retina (particularly in the region of retinal breaks) is accomplished by the division of bridging membranes and segmentation of star folds employing right angled intraocular scissors.

In long-standing retinal detachments, accessory retinal glia or pigment epithelial cells may proliferate in the subretinal space to produce retroretinal star folding or fibrocellular bands in various configurations. Techniques to divide subretinal strands have been described by Machemer (1980) including the introduction of intraocular scissors into the subretinal space through a convenient retinal break. It is, however, unusual for such subretinal bands to prevent retinal reattachment.

Vascularised epiretinal proliferation, as seen in the vasoproliferative retinopathies, depends upon gel-retina contact (McLeod & Restori, 1981). Multiple fibrovascular outgrowths pervade the cortical gel and the resulting intimate adhesion between the vitreous and retina precludes gel separation at this site. This forms the locus of subsequent traction forces with variable effects upon the underlying neuroretina. In this situation, membrane peeling is inappropriate in view of the intimate connection with the retina and the risk of creating breaks in adjacent atrophic retina. Consequently, intraocular scissors with a right-angled configuration are used to dissect a cleavage plane between the membrane and retina with meticulous segmentation to isolate individual epicentres (Fig. 8.4). All potential bleeding sites are coagulated prior to sectioning since fresh haemorrhage produces an adherent fibrin clot obscuring further dissection. The alternative technique of delamination, favoured by Charles, aims to completely resect the epiretinal plaque. Sites of fibrovascular attachment are divided by Sutherland scissors in which the cutting blades are orientated parallel with the surface of the retina. It is possible that delamination may reduce the risks of retinal damage during extensive epiretinal dissection and lower the risk of non-vascularised reparative gliosis. Whichever method is employed, it may be difficult on occasions to determine the end-point of epiretinal dissection and adequate release of tangential traction. Complete dissection in areas of grossly adherent and heavily vascularised membrane may be impossible to accomplish although the facility with which dissection can be achieved is often difficult to predict prior to surgery.

Intraocular coagulation
Methods of intraocular delivery of various forms of destructive energy for tissue coagulation have been in use over many years. Certain techniques have been refined and used in conjunction with vitreous surgery whilst others have largely fallen into disuse.

Originally employed in the treatment of posterior retinal breaks, endodiatherapy is mainly used to prevent or arrest haemorrhage from vascularised epiretinal tissues. Bimanual bipolar endodiathermy is the safest and most convenient method. A low frequency bipolar unit is connected to two separate conductive intraocular instruments and current flow between the instrument tips coagulates intervening tissues.

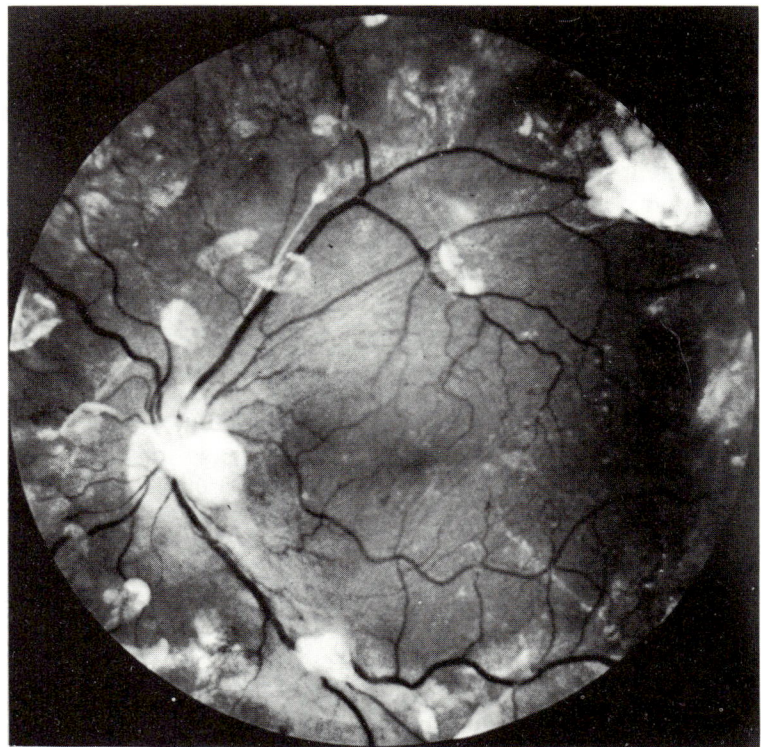

Fig. 8.4   Multiple segmented fibrovascular complexes following surgery for proliferative diabetic retinopathy.

As a method of sealing posterior retinal breaks, transvitreal cryotherapy is a difficult technique with considerable risks of choroidal haemorrhage and tear enlargement and is no longer used by most vitreous surgeons.

Intraocular techniques of photocoagulation have recently been introduced, representing an important advance in the capabilities of vitreous surgery. This facility has a number of important applications but currently its principal use is in the treatment of patients with active proliferative retinopathy. The presence of hazy media either before or after surgery and especially in phakic eyes often precludes conventional methods of photocoagulation. Pan-retinal endophotocoagulation is undertaken with the aim of reducing the level of vasoproliferative activity to cause regression or prevent the development of rubeosis iridis in the postoperative period.

A method of endophotocoagulation has been developed by Charles using a short multifilament fibreoptic probe attached to a portable xenon-arc light coagulator (1981b). Unlike transvitreal cryotherapy or carbon dioxide endolaser photocoagulation, direct retinal contact is not required to achieve coagulation. However, the exit beam is widely divergent and the tip of the probe must be positioned within 1 mm of the attached retina to achieve burns of 800–1000 nm diameter. Lesions of uniform size and intensity are difficult to achieve especially in more peripheral areas. Unfortunately, the fibreoptic probe is easily damaged by a build-up of heat and can therefore only be fired in a fluid medium. Despite these inherent drawbacks, the system has proved effective in practice being used principally for pan-retinal ablation and the treatment of flat posterior breaks or peripheral tears elevated on a scleral buckle. Perhaps the most important disadvantage is the production of full-thickness burns by absorption of longwave infra-red energy by fluid in the inner retinal layers with an increased risk of reparative gliosis.

Facilities for laser endophotocoagulation have recently been described (Landers et al, 1982; Fleischman et al, 1981). These systems offer a number of important advantages over current methods of xenon endophotocoagulation and are likely to become more widely available in the near future. A single low-loss fibre is used and coupled to a standby or remotely located laser providing either argon or krypton energy. Minimal beam divergence enables 600 micron burns to be achieved at a distance of 3 mm from the surface of the retina. Burns of more even size and intensity over a wider area of the fundus can be applied in rapid succession, providing a more efficient method of operative pan-retinal ablation. Possibly the most important advantage is the ability to undertake treatment in the presence of air, gas or liquid silicone so enabling treatment of reattached retina following simultaneous exchange.

Intraocular tamponade

Following vitreous removal, internal tamponade of retinal breaks is achieved by exchanging the fluid content of the vitreous cavity for air, other inert gases or liquid silicone. Due to the high surface tension of these materials, recruitment of subretinal fluid by passage of fluid through the retinal break is prevented. Despite complete exchange of the preretinal space, the duration of temporary tamponade with the use of air is rather short lived. As an alternative, sulphur hexafluoride gas with low aqueous solubility provides twice the duration of gas tamponade. However, with complete exchange, a 20% SF_6/air mixture should not be exceeded to avoid uncontrolled elevation of intraocular pressure from postoperative expansion of the bubble. It is advisable to discontinue nitrous oxide anaesthesia 10 minutes prior to gas exchange and throughout the remainder of surgery to prevent marked postoperative reduction in the size of the gas bubble. Alternatively, an entirely intravenous technique of general anaesthesia may be used.

Prior to gas exchange, subretinal fluid is evacuated by internal drainage through an accessible retinal break. A flute needle or linear suction device is positioned over the tear and viscous subretinal fluid readily flows through the retinal break. Employing the same instrument, vitreous replacement fluid is exchanged for a gas mixture insufflated through the indwelling infusion terminal. In the aphakic eye, this procedure can be visualised using the operating microscope whilst in phakic eyes indirect ophthalmoscopy is necessary, or alternatively, a high powered bi-concave contact lens can be used. A single intraocular gas bubble filling the pre-retinal space allows excellent visualisation of the entire fundus. Gas exchange may displace residual subretinal fluid posteriorly which can in turn be drained trans-vitreal or externally to achieve a complete fill. Recently, several mechanical devices have been introduced to provide constant intraocular pressure during gas infusion so allowing various complex manoeuvres to be undertaken through the gas-filled cavity (Hueneke & Aaberg, 1983).

Trans-scleral cryotherapy is carried out subsequent to fluid/gas exchange. This may prevent dissemination of viable pigment epithelial cells and so reduce the risks of epiretinal membrane formation. In addition, retinal freezing is more rapid in onset and slower to dissipate with the thermal insulation of a gas bubble. Appropriate postoperative posturing is of crucial importance in the immediate and early postoperative period. Immediate prone-positioning allows reformation of the anterior chamber angle and prevents prolonged gas contact with the lens or corneal endothelium. The development of posterior subcapsular vacuolation of the lens may result from prolonged contact with any inert gas but fortunately is almost always reversible.

Because of the limited duration of gas tamponade and the early reopening of retinal breaks from ongoing traction, wider interest has been shown in the use of liquid silicone to provide prolonged intraocular tamponade. Silicone oil of 1000 centistokes viscosity can be injected via a standard infusion line using a compressed/air powered syringe operated by a foot switch (Leaver et al, 1984). Fluid/silicone exchange is slow and readily controlled and the high refractive index of silicone oil enables continued visualisation using the operating microscope, even in the phakic eye. Because of the low density of silicone oil, the need for operative and postoperative posturing is reduced and there is little tendency for oil to enter the subretinal space unless the tear is rigidly held open by surface traction. Since intraocular silicone appears relatively inert in the short term, it is possible that the delayed effects upon the lens and outflow pathways may be avoided by removal of silicone oil with cessation of epiretinal membrane proliferation and contraction.

PROLIFERATIVE DIABETIC RETINOPATHY

The complications of proliferative diabetic retinopathy in the form of vitreous haemorrhage and retinal detachment remain the leading posterior segment indications for vitreous surgery.

Bleeding into the vitreous gel or more commonly the retrohyaloid space originates from fenestrated capillaries within epiretinal membranes or from related trunk vessels. Whilst this may be a consequence of hypoxic damage to the vascular endothelium, it has been postulated that mechanical forces may be responsible due to contraction of fibrocellular epiretinal membranes (Machemer, 1978). Contraction leads to compression and reduced blood flow as shown by fluorescein angiography with resultant hypoxia and further stimulus to fibrovascular proliferation. By implication, isolation of all posterior vascular proliferations reduces the propensity for haemorrhage and the stimulus for vascular proliferation. The long term results of surgery appear to support this hypothesis. Whilst there is no evidence that vitreous haemorrhage directly influences surface fibrosis, it seems likely that intragel haemorrhage potentiates the development of incomplete posterior vitreous detachment, precluding further epiretinal vascular proliferation. However, new vessels may subsequently extend forwards along the surface of the detached posterior hyaloid boundary.

The presence of tangential traction brought about by the contraction of epiretinal membranes is largely responsible for the development of traction retinal detachment. The distribution of retinal detachment therefore reflects the characteristic development of multifocal epiretinal membranes along the temporal vascular arcades and nasal to the optic disc. Additional traction forces may develop between the vitreous base and posterior epiretinal membranes along the separated posterior hyaloid face and between individual fibrovascular complexes (bridging traction). In the presence of extensive areas of confluent epiretinal membranes with gross contraction, a plateau configuration or 'table-top' detachment will be seen. However, in a significant proportion of cases, traction detachment remains localised or undergoes slow progression and on occasions may spontaneously reattach with avulsion of fibro-vascular membranes from the retinal surface.

In the presence of extensive surface traction or the development of a full-thickness retinal break, retinal detachment may progress to involve the macula. With the development of a posterior retinal break, the detachment often becomes more extensive and assumes a bullous configuration. Although rhegmatogenous detachment is more likely to extend to the ora serrata, the area of detachment may be confined posteriorly by the scars of previous photocoagulation. A familiar clinical sequence is the development of a fresh vitreous haemorrhage which within a short period undergoes rapid clearance only to reveal a rhegmatogenous retinal detachment. Typically, there is a single retinal break which is often small and extremely elusive. Retinal breaks are usually located in atrophic retina immediately adjacent to areas of posterior fibrovascular proliferation. Less commonly breaks may arise at the posterior vitreous base border or rarely at the macula. It is now thought that retinal detachment gives rise to an increased production of vasoproliferative factor(s) from reduced choroidal oxygenation of the retina.

In the light of these considerations, there are certain surgical objectives that should be achieved at the time of vitreous surgery.

1. Excision of blood-stained vitreous gel and retrohyaloid haemorrhage; simultaneous lens removal for pre-existent or intraoperative opacity precluding adequate visualisation or to facilitate peripheral epiretinal dissection.
2. Removal of the entire posterior vitreous cortex with relief of antero-posterior and bridging traction.
3. Dissection of selected epiretinal membranes by segmentation or delamination and relief of tangential traction.
4. Identification and closure of all retinal breaks (pre-existent or iatrogenic); creation of a chorio-retinal adhesion by trans-scleral cryotherapy, temporary gas tamponade and possibly scleral buckling.
5. Prevention and control of intraocular haemorrhage.

In former years, it was common practice to remove even clear lenses during vitrectomy in diabetic eyes. Lensectomy was largely undertaken to improve visualisation of membrane dissection, to facilitate fluid/gas exchange or to promote postoperative clearance of residual opacity in the vitreous cavity. Lens removal often proved necessary with the development of intra-operative cataract particularly during lengthy procedures. However, this problem appears to have been significantly reduced by improved infusion fluids providing supplemental glucose. Clinical impressions of an increased incidence of rubeosis iridis in eyes that were rendered aphakic were first mooted in the late 1970s. Studies undertaken by Blankenship (1980) and Rice (1983) have now demonstrated a significant increase in the postoperative incidence of both iris neovascularisation and neovascular glaucoma in those eyes in which the lens was removed during vitrectomy compared to those in which the lens was retained. These findings endorse current practice of avoiding lensectomy wherever possible. However, this carries an increased risk of persistent post-operative haemorrhage at a time when scatter photocoagulation may be required for the treatment of rubeosis iridis, thereby placing greater importance on the use of operative photocoagulation.

The decision to undertake vitreous surgery in any patient with proliferative diabetic retinopathy depends upon a wide variety of factors. In broad terms, the potential for useful visual recovery must be balanced against the risks of irreversible visual loss from surgery in the light of the complexity of the surgical pathology.

Although a prescribed minimum period of 6 months for spontaneous resolution of vitreous haemorrhage has been advocated, the need for surgical intervention is often determined by other factors including the possibility of coexistent progressive retinal detachment or potentially treatable maculopathy.

Macular detachment identified by ophthalmoscopy or diagnostic ultrasound, necessitates immediate surgical intervention depending on the duration of detachment. Although the potential for visual recovery may be greater with shallow traction detachment of the macula, the likelihood of visual recovery after a period of 6 months does not usually justify surgical intervention. However, in many patients it is often difficult to be certain of the precise onset of macular detachment in the presence of concomitant vitreous haemorrhage. As might be expected, the extent of pre-operative fibrovascular epiretinal proliferation is an important factor governing surgical prognosis, largely reflecting complications associated with complex epiretinal dissection. Surgery should not be undertaken for extramacular detachment since the risks of visual loss following surgery exceed the likelihood of macular involvement (Charles & Flinn, 1981).

Whilst rubeosis with secondary glaucoma contraindicates surgery, the presence of early rubeosis does not preclude intervention provided intra-operative photocoagulation can be undertaken.

The question of surgery must also take into account the life-expectancy and psychological status of the patient and the natural history or response to surgery of the fellow eye.

Considerable experience has now been reported in the treatment of severe diabetic eye disease indicating significant visual improvement in a high percentage of cases of persistent vitreous haemorrhage or traction macular detachment (Aaberg, 1981; Barrie et al, 1982; Blankenship & Machemer, 1978; McLeod et al, 1980). Extended observations have also revealed that in those cases successful at 6 months following surgery, visual improvement appears to be maintained over a prolonged period in the majority of patients (Blankenship, 1978; Rice & Michels, 1980).

SELECTED RETINAL DETACHMENTS

Vitrectomy techniques have come to play an important role in the management of certain types of complex retinal detachment known to respond unfavourably to conventional scleral buckling techniques. Vitrectomy techniques may be used to achieve the following objectives:

1. Clearance of intraocular opacities e.g. opaque lens, dense vitreous haemorrhage, asteroid hyalosis, pupillary membranes.

2. Relief of vitreo-retinal or surface traction to mobilise the retina and allow closure of retinal breaks.
3. Creation of a large fluid space to provide more efficient gas tamponade of retinal breaks.
4. Various manoeuveres including internal drainage of subretinal fluid, internal methods of chorio-retinal adhesion or direct manipulation of the retina.

Macular breaks

Of the various methods used in the treatment of retinal detachment associated with a macular break, those employing an internal approach have obvious appeal. Macular buckling is often technically demanding with risks of choroidal haemorrhage and optic nerve compression. To avoid these complications and the need for macular coagulation, liquid silicone injection has been used to provide prolonged internal tamponade (Scott, 1974). However, there is a significant risk of long term complications which do not appear to justify the use of this procedure.

Gonvers & Machemer (1982) have recently described the use of vitrectomy and fluid/gas exchange to provide temporary internal tamponade with prone positioning for 12–18 hours postoperatively. This method is based upon the concept that retinal detachment results from residual vitreo-retinal adhesion in the perimacular region following posterior gel detachment. Temporary closure of the macular break is accompanied by rapid absorption of subretinal fluid and no direct macular coagulation is applied to preserve visual function. Although the reported results of this technique are encouraging, redetachment has occurred in eyes with a posterior staphyloma and in these circumstances it may be preferable to apply discrete laser endophotocoagulation to the perifoveal area with no detrimental effect upon the functional outcome.

Giant retinal tears

Giant retinal tears are difficult to treat because of the circumferential extent of the tear, the independent mobility of the posterior flap with folding and inversion and their propensity to develop ultimately massive periretinal proliferation.

The development of closed vitrectomy techniques has provided a solution to some of the problems associated with closure of the retinal tear. Vitrectomy enables gel to be removed from behind the posterior flap which is a frequent cause of failure to unroll the flap by preoperative positioning. With direct access to the retinal surface, the retina may be simply unfolded or in the presence of epiretinal membrane contraction require mobilisation. Circumferential traction at the posterior edge of the tear may require multiple radial incisions to facilitate reapposition. Complete vitrectomy enables the entire preretinal space to be exchanged for a non-expanding gas bubble or liquid silicone. Following repositioning of the retina, posterior slippage of the flap may occur, particularly following incomplete exchange, during subsequent manipulation of the globe or from the effects of residual traction on the posterior flap. To overcome this problem, various methods of fixation of the flap have been described including interrupted trans-scleral retinal suturing with monofilament nylon (Federman et al, 1982) or the intraocular insertion of a retinal tack composed of polyacetal (Ando & Kondo, 1983). Since posterior slippage commonly arises during trans-scleral cryotherapy with the patient supine, McCuen employs postoperative photocoagulation to create a chorio-retinal adhesion in conjunction with complete intraocular gas tamponade.

Various authors (Machemer & Allen, 1976; Freeman & Castillejos, 1981) have reported improved anatomical results in the short term with the use of vitreolensectomy and temporary gas tamponade with operative prone-positioning. Unfortunately, the long term anatomical and functional results are less encouraging with the frequent development of macular pucker or massive periretinal proliferation. Indeed, there is no firm evidence to indicate that the prognosis for useful vision has been significantly improved by these methods in comparison with previous treatments.

Recently, there has been mounting interest in the use of liquid silicone in conjunction with vitrectomy in the hope of improving long term results by the prevention of massive periretinal proliferation. The efficacy of this method has been shown in a recently reported consecutive series of 73 eyes with giant retinal tears (Leaver et al, 1984). An initial anatomical success rate of 97% was achieved with the retina remaining attached 6 months following surgery in 86% of cases. The visual acuity at 6 months was 6/60 or better in 70% of eyes, the causes of reduced vision appearing to be intrinsically related to the features of the detachment rather than as a direct consequence of silicone oil tamponade.

Massive periretinal proliferation
Massive periretinal proliferation complicating rhegmatogenous retinal detachment is seen as occupying one end of a spectrum of conditions termed nonvascular proliferative extraretinal retinopathies by Foos (1978). This condition remains the greatest challenge in vitreo-retinal surgery and is the principal reason for ultimate failure in retinal detachment surgery. Once considered attributable to changes in the vitreous gel (massive vitreous retraction), it is now known that this condition in all its various manifestations is the product of cellular proliferation, fundamentally affecting the retinal surfaces. This is reflected in the new terminology of proliferative vitreoretinopathy, a classification which seeks to facilitate direct comparison of various treatment methods and yet largely ignores the key element of the rhegmatogenous component.

In the early stages of the condition with localised star folds confined to a single quadrant, conventional scleral buckling procedures may achieve permanent reattachment of the retina. With progression, the use of vitrectomy, membrane peeling techniques and gas tamponade as proposed by Machemer appeared to be a logical solution to the problem. Although the results were encouraging in the short term, approximately two thirds of these cases ultimately failed from recurrent epiretinal membrane formation with reopening of retinal breaks.

An alternative approach to this problem in the form of silicone oil tamponade was introduced by Cibis in 1962 and advocated by Scott over many years. Recently, methods have been described combining vitrectomy techniques with silicone oil exchange in an attempt to prevent or limit the effects of recurrent membrane formation (Lean et al, 1982) Microsurgical epiretinal dissection is necessary to mobilise retinal breaks to prevent passage of silicone oil into the subretinal space and following partial exchange, further dissection can be readily accomplished under biomicroscopic control. Liquid silicone may continue to tamponade the retinal break and reduce the extent of reproliferation or limit the extent of recurrent detachment by restricting fluid space in the preretinal compartment. Although the use of liquid silicone as a temporary intraocular tamponade is attractive, in cases of MPP removal of the silicone oil at variable intervals following retinal reattachment is often accompanied by rapid redetachment of the retina with reopening of the retinal break(s).

To date, there is no firm evidence that any of these described methods has any direct inhibitory effect upon epiretinal cellular proliferation. Considerable interest has therefore centred upon the use of pharmacological methods to suppress cellular proliferation, in particular the use of triamcinolone acetonide (Tano et al, 1980) and most recently fluorouracil, a synthetic pyrimidine analogue (Blumenkranz et al, 1982). In experimental models of massive periretinal proliferation, a single intravitreal injection of fluorouracil has been shown to produce a prolonged inhibitory effect upon intraocular fibrocellular proliferation. Although pharmacological therapy as an adjunct to vitreous surgery appears a promising approach, the question of potential toxicity and appropriate treatment regimes remain to be established before its value in the clinical situation can be determined. It is possible that more specific agents aimed at inhibiting cellular contraction may ultimately provide a more rational approach.

Retrolental fibroplasia
Encouraging results have recently been reported with the use of vitreo-lensectomy in advanced cicatricial retrolental fibroplasia during the first 2 years of life (Machemer, 1983). Treatment was confined to those eyes with total retinal detachment which does not undergo spontaneous reattachment. Extremely anterior sclerotomies are necessary and protracted anterior dissection required to mobilise the retina. The risks of reproliferation giving rise to recurrent detachment appear high but the initial anatomical results are encouraging and some patients appear to have achieved navigating vision.

POSTERIOR PENETRATING TRAUMA

There can be little doubt that modern vitreous surgery has transformed our approach to the management of posterior penetrating trauma. However, a number of outstanding issues have yet to be resolved including the precise indications, timing and extent of surgery. Because of the wide variation in the nature and degree of ocular damage and the individual response to injury, reliable statistical evidence to support the various approaches has been difficult to obtain. Nevertheless, it has long been recognised that responsibility for the development of complications and ultimate visual loss following penetrating trauma often rests with the reparative response to intraocular damage rather than the initial structural damage per se. The policy of early intraocular reconstruction to reduce the inflammatory response and forestall complications was introduced many years ago. With the development of modern vitreo-retinal surgery, it has become possible to implement this policy in a more controlled and definitive manner.

A number of factors have been identified which appear to enhance the level of inflammation following injury and whose effects may be minimised by surgical management. Clinically, circumstantial evidence has indicated the importance of vitreous haemorrhage acting in concert with vitreous incarceration within the wound or disruption of the lens. Experimental models of posterior penetrating trauma in the primate eye (Cleary & Ryan, 1979) have also shown that intravitreal haemorrhage is a potent stimulus to fibrocellular proliferation and the development of traction retinal detachment. Cellular proliferation may be derived from several sources depending upon the tissues involved and the location of the wound. A variety of traction forces may develop, the prevailing elements being largely determined by the characteristics of the individual injury. Transvitreal traction may occur along the tract of a penetrating missile with the development of a localised posterior traction detachment. Diffuse vitreous haemorrhage commonly leads to complete vitreous detachment in the absence of direct posterior retinal damage and thereby gives rise to dynamic vitreous traction. However, circumferential or radial traction in the vitreous base is the most common type of vitreo-retinal traction likely to be encountered following posterior segment trauma.

That diffuse fibrocellular proliferation may rapidly involve the retinal surface within a short period of injury has been identified in the primate model and in histopathological studies of severely injured eyes. However, our knowledge of the acute surgical pathology in severely injured eyes with visual potential is somewhat limited. It is significant that early clinical vitrectomy has not revealed widespread surface proliferation in the absence of extensive retinal detachment or major retinal incarceration within the wound. Furthermore, although pure traction retinal detachment from transgel or vitreous base traction may be seen, the vast majority of retinal detachments occurring in eyes with dense vitreous haemorrhage are found to be rhegmatogenous in nature.

The responsible retinal break is rarely located at the site of primary retinal damage due to the development of spontaneous chorio-retinal adhesion. However, an exception to this rule is the development of a retinal break at sites of foreign body ricochet involving the posterior retina. In most instances, retinal breaks occur in the region of the vitreous base as described by Cox (1978). Breaks most commonly arise in immediate relationship to sites of basal gel incarceration in the form of a traction tear or disinsertion. On occasions, breaks may occur within the opposing vitreous base following massive vitreous loss and gross incarceration. Oral tears may also develop in relation to areas of localised traction retinal detachment giving rise to progressive detachment with a typical convex configuration. Tears may also occur at the time of posterior vitreous detachment including giant tear formation which is usually related to the site of gel incarceration.

The principal aims of vitrectomy in the treatment of posterior penetrating trauma can therefore be stated as follows:

1. Clearance of intraocular opacity to restore form vision.
2. Reduction of the inflammatory response by the removal of vitreous haemorrhage or a disrupted lens.
3. Complete removal of the vitreous gel to prevent or relieve certain types of vitreo-retinal traction, e.g. trans-gel traction; to influence indirectly vitreous base traction.
4. Identify and control associated retinal detachment or prevent the development of retinal breaks.
5. The removal of retained foreign material.
6. Restore normal aqueous dynamics.

Vitrectomy techniques have also provided unique opportunities in the management of posterior segment intraocular foreign bodies. The long term results of traditional methods of treatment are disappointing even with small ferro-magnetic fragments with an initially favourable prognosis. Despite successful removal of the foreign body by pars plana or direct trans-scleral routes, a significant incidence of retinal detachment is likely to be encountered especially in those eyes with vitreous haemorrhage.

Vitrectomy techniques are principally used to facilitate the removal of non-magnetic foreign bodies or ferrous fragments impacted in the post-equatorial retina. Opaque media precluding direct visualisation of the foreign body requires the removal of associated cataract or diffuse vitreous haemorrhage to allow controlled extraction of the foreign body. Impacted foreign bodies are mobilised from the retina and subsequently removed by intraocular microforceps through an enlarged pars plana sclerotomy.

With regard to the timing of vitreous surgery, there is general agreement that intervention is often required within the first few weeks of injury to prevent the development of irreversible complications. However, it must be emphasised that no blanket policy can be adopted and that each case must be judged on its individual merits.

Some authorities continue to advocate posterior vitrectomy within the first 24–48 hours and have presented results which claim to support this policy (Coleman, 1982). It is possible that intraocular microsurgery at the time of primary repair may be necessary with lens disruption, gel incarceration within anterior wounds or with primary displacement of the retina. However, the surgical risks are considerable at this stage although certain recent technical developments including intracameral Healon are extending the possibilities of primary posterior vitrectomy. However, it is considered that in the majority of injuries the stated objectives of vitreous surgery are more readily accomplished by early secondary intervention. This interval may, however, be extremely short in eyes with extensive intraocular disruption or retinal incarceration with the rapid development of surgically irreversible sequelae.

Certain factors influencing the timing of vitreous surgery are listed in Table 8.1 with an indication of the priority which may be accorded each of these factors in any individual injury. Factors may be identified requiring immediate or early intervention that clearly take precedence over those criteria arguing for delay. Establishment of retinal detachment by clinical or ultrasonic means usually necessitates prompt intervention with the likelihood of widespread epiretinal membrane formation of

Table 8.1 Timing of vitreous surgery in posterior penetrating trauma (Factors listed according to priority)

Criteria for intervention	Criteria for delay
Infectious Endophthalmitis	Ocular Hyperaemia
Established Retinal Detachment	Impaired Corneal Clarity
Toxic IOFB	Choroidal Haematoma
Secondary Glaucoma	Vitreous Attachment
Suspected Oral Break	Uncomplicated Vitreous Opacity
Ciliary Body Traction	
? Wound Integrity	
Age	

rapid onset. Similarly, certain toxic intraocular foreign bodies inducing an acute inflammatory response, e.g. copper containing foreign bodies, should be considered for immediate surgery. In the presence of dense vitreous haemorrhage and evidence of basal gel incarceration within the wound and attached retina on ultrasound (Fig. 8.5a,b), the principal risk appears to be that of oral break formation and the development of retinal detachment of unpredictable latency.

The major factors that argue for a period of delay concern impaired visualisation due to accompanying anterior segment wounds or corneal decompensation and the occurrence of intraoperative haemorrhage from extensive scleral wounds or the effects of severe contusion. In addition, haemorrhage into the suprachoroidal space can only be evacuated with spontaneous haemolysis after seven to ten days so allowing controlled access to the vitreous cavity. Complete vitrectomy is facilitated by the development of posterior vitreous detachment which may occur pre-operatively or during the course of delayed vitrectomy. Finally, in eyes with vitreous opacity uncomplicated by significant incarceration or other factors, vitreous surgery may be postponed perhaps indefinitely and alternative measures including anterior encirclement and cryotherapy alone employed to prevent future retinal detachment.

COMPLICATIONS

Corneal damage

The incidence and severity of corneal changes following closed vitrectomy have been significantly reduced. Various factors appear responsible including reduced fluid exchange and the use of more physiological replacement fluids, improved techniques of lensectomy and shorter duration of surgery. Corneal problems are now largely confined to diabetic eyes in the form of delayed resurfacing following spontaneous or intentional epithelial debridement. Diabetic corneal epithelium readily becomes oedematous during surgery necessitating removal and this may be related to the osmotic effects of accumulated sugar alcohols as identified in the diabetic lens. Impaired reepithelialisation is caused by defective adhesion of regenerated epithelium to the underlying stroma. That the basement membrane may be defective is suggested by recent ultrastructural studies of excised diabetic corneal epithelium in which concomitant removal of the basement membrane has been identified (Kenyon et al, 1978). Should removal of the epithelium prove necessary, post-operative topical therapy is limited to once daily cycloplegics and antibiotics with avoidance of phenylephrine. Recourse to a bandage contact lens rarely proves necessary.

With improved surgical techniques, the occurrence of permanent corneal oedema from endothelial decompensation is a rare event. Damage to the endothelium is most likely to occur during pars plana ultrasonic phaco-emulsification. There is now experimental (Talbot et al, 1981) and clinical evidence from prospective specular microscopic studies (Diddie & Schanzlin, 1983) to show that preservation of the anterior lens capsule during phaco-emulsification appears to exert a protective effect upon the corneal endothelium presumably as a mechanical barrier.

Lens damage

Lens touch is most likely to occur at the time of instrument insertion particularly into a soft eye, during excision of retro-lental gel or when removing peripheral vitreous

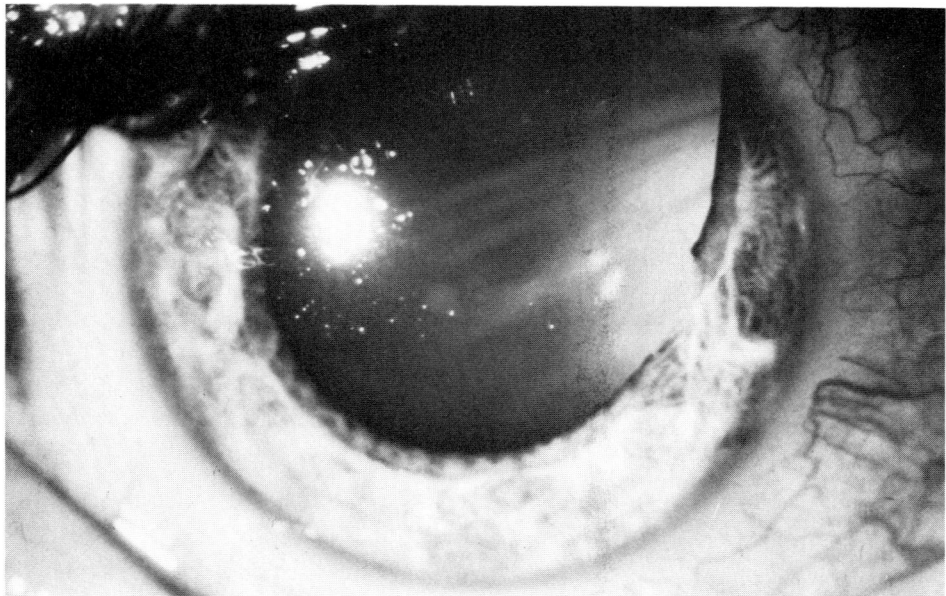

a

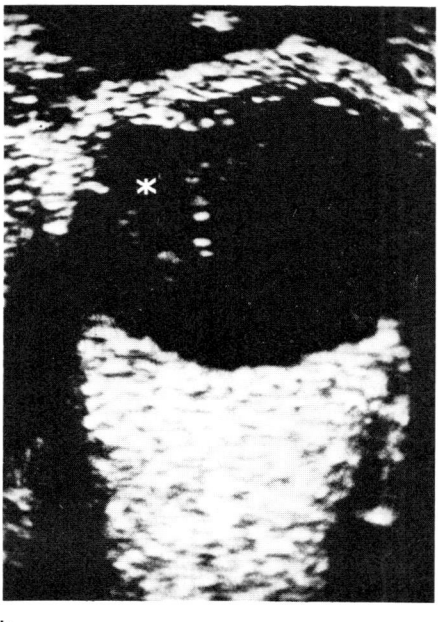

b

Fig. 8.5   **a** Vitreous gel incarceration into anterior scleral perforating wound (not shown) with orientation of blood-stained retrolental gel towards the wound. **b** Horizontal B-scan ultrasound showing major anterior gel incarceration (asterisk).

from the opposite side of the vitreous base. Defects in the posterior capsule may also arise in young patients with strong vitreo-lenticular adhesions during attempted removal of retro-lental gel with high suction. In most instances of inadvertent lens damage and especially if changes are observed in the underlying cortex, removal of the lens at the time of vitrectomy is undertaken with the likelihood of progressive cataract formation postoperatively.

The development of fine posterior subcapsular opacification during lengthy procedures and usually in diabetic eyes was a significant complication in early series. Experimental studies have shown that the addition of carbohydrate and bicarbonate buffer to irrigating solutions helps preserve lens clarity (Christiansen et al, 1976). With the use of improved formulations of replacement fluid (Graham & Hodson, 1980), this problem appears to have been significantly reduced.

The effects of vitrectomy in the phakic eye upon the long term risk of cataract formation has not yet been determined. However, Michels (1981) has described an increased incidence of nuclear sclerosis and cataract in eyes undergoing epimacular membrane peeling for idiopathic pucker.

Ocular hypertension

Transiently raised intraocular pressure following vitrectomy is a relatively common problem caused by a variety of mechanisms.

Elevated intraocular pressure within the first 24 hours may result from the use of expansile concentrations of intraocular gas or be due to the development of angle closure with inappropriate posturing.

In the first few days, elevation is most commonly related to obstruction of the aqueous outflow pathways by erythrocytes, ghost cells or inflammatory cells particularly in the aphakic eye. Medical management usually suffices but, if intractable, washout of the vitreous cavity may prove necessary. This problem is best avoided by thorough clearance of blood products and the removal of as much peripheral opaque gel as possible. The development of persistent glaucoma often occurs upon a background of decreased outflow facility directly related to the underlying condition.

The development of neovascular glaucoma, virtually restricted to eyes with vasoproliferative retinopathy, continues to be one of the principal causes of visual failure following vitreous surgery. The incidence has been shown to be reduced by preservation of the lens (Blankenship, 1980) and in those eyes that have undergone pan-retinal photocoagulation. In addition, iris neovascularisation is an almost invariable consequence in eyes with extensive retinal detachment arising or persisting postoperatively. Early rubeosis may be arrested by retinal photocoagulation or reattachment of the retina. The established condition rarely responds to medical treatment and surgical measures rarely prevent progression to phthisis bulbi.

Pars plana entry sites

The creation of entry site tears of the oral retina during instrument insertion is now much less of a problem with smaller gauge instrumentation, improved tip designs and location of the sclerotomies through the anterior pars plana. Entry sites are routinely prepared using a sharp instrument such as the disposable microvitreoretinal blade to avoid detachment of the ciliary epithelim and to ensure penetration of the vitreous base. Instruments should be slowly advanced into the vitreous cavity and the tip of the instrument observed through the microscope to confirm unimpeded passage through the vitreous base. Should a tear be created, considerable care must be exercised with reintroduction of instruments and during vitrectomy to avoid enlargement of the tear. Of instruments in current use, right-angled vitreous scissors are particularly prone to induce entry site tears by the engagement of basal vitreous and should be introduced in a closed position through an enlarged sclerotomy. However, all entry sites should be examined by indirect ophthalmoscopy at the completion of vitrectomy to exclude a possible tear which should be treated by trans-scleral cryotherapy and supported on a circumferential scleral explant.

Withdrawal of vitrectomy instruments in the presence of retinal detachment carries the risk of retinal incarceration or prolapse through the entry site. Raised intraocular pressure causes expulsion of basal gel and forward tenting of the peripheral retina towards the entry site. The development of retinal incarceration and impending prolapse is often indicated by the appearance of radial folding of the retina towards the sclerotomy. This problem, which is far more common than is appreciated, can be avoided by discontinuing infusion and lowering intraocular pressure below normal prior to instrument withdrawal. In the event of retinal prolapse, the retina may be reposited and fluid/gas exchange performed to relieve the incarceration.

Delayed complications involving pars plana entry sites may occur as a consequence of the inevitable incarceration of basal gel within the sclerotomies. This potential source of static traction may be exacerbated by subsequent fibrocellular proliferation giving rise to localised traction retinal detachment or rhegmatogenous detachment from a tear at the posterior border of the vitreous base. Fibrovascular proliferation may also occur and be responsible for recurrent postoperative vitreous haemorrhage (Kreiger et al, 1977). Various factors appear to increase the local inflammatory response and the potential for fibrocellular proliferation. Experimentally, incomplete vitrectomy has been shown to potentiate this proliferative process (Gregor & Ryan, 1982) and it would therefore seem rational to achieve as complete a vitrectomy as possible. Further measures include avoidance of diathermy or cryotherapy to the entry sites and secure wound closure with non-absorbable materials. Since this problem cannot be entirely eliminated, routine cryotherapy to the post-oral retina in the vicinity of all entry sites is undertaken and on occasions supplemented by prophylactic anterior encirclement.

Retinal detachment

The majority of retinal detachments occurring after vitreous surgery are rhegmatogenous in nature. In addition to entry site tears, breaks may develop at the posterior border of the vitreous base during vitreous removal, or as a complication of epiretinal dissection. On occasion, previously treated posterior breaks may reopen as a consequence of reparative gliosis. Posterior tears arising in atrophic and ischaemic retina or at photocoagulation scars may be extremely difficult to identify and may only be discovered by an intraocular search with an extrusion device. Fortunately, the majority of detachments will respond favourably to scleral buckling, cryotherapy and internal gas tamponade.

Endophthalmitis

Bacterial endophthalmitis is a fortunately rare but devastating complication of vitreous surgery with a reported incidence of 0.2% (Blankenship, 1977). The early features include severe orbital pain, decreased vision and hypopyon. Upon suspicion of bacterial endophthalmitis, immediate samples of intraocular fluid are aspirated for microbiological studies. Systemic and intraocular broad-spectrum antibiotics are administered together with topical and systemic corticosteroids. Despite these measures, visual function is rarely salvaged.

Sympathetic ophthalmitis

The possibility of sympathetic ophthalmitis following vitreous surgery has occupied the attention of vitreous surgeons for many years. Of the various reported cases, vitreous surgery has generally followed previous surgery or penetrating trauma (Lewis et al, 1978). In a recent survey undertaken by Gass (1982), an incidence of sympathetic ophthalmitis of 0.06% was reported in a total of approximately 15 000 vitrectomies. By excluding those cases in which vitrectomy was preceded by other surgical procedures or penetrating wounds, the incidence of sympathetic ophthalmitis was reduced to 0.01%, approximating figures previously reported for sympathetic ophthalmitis induced by surgery. The findings suggest that the risk of sympathetic ophthalmitis following vitrectomy alone does not exceed that of other surgical procedures involving the anterior uveal tract. However, the risk of sympathetic ophthalmitis is undoubtedly increased when vitrectomy is undertaken following previous accidental or surgical penetration of the globe.

The author has encountered three cases of sympathetic ophthalmitis following vitrectomy and in all cases changes predominantly affected the posterior segment. This posterior form of sympathetic ophthalmitis is said to occur in less than 5% of all cases and, as suggested by Gass, it is possible that vitreous surgery may have a particular role in the causation of this pattern of disease.

REFERENCES

Aaberg T M 1981 Pars plana vitrectomy for diabetic traction retinal detachment. Ophthalmology 88: 639–642

Ando F, Kondo J 1983 A plastic tack for the treatment of retinal detachment with giant tear. American Journal of Ophthalmology 95: 260–261

Barrie T, Feretis E, Leaver P K, McLeod D 1982 Closed microsurgery for diabetic traction retinal detachment. British Journal of Ophthalmology 66: 754–758

Blankenship G W 1977 Endophthalmitis after pars plana vitrectomy. American Journal of Ophthalmology 84: 815–817

Blankenship G W 1980 The lens influence on diabetic vitrectomy results: a report of a prospective randomized study. Archives of Ophthalmology 98: 2196–2198

Blankenship G W, Machemer R 1978 Pars plana vitrectomy for the management of severe diabetic retinopathy. An analysis of results five years following surgery. Ophthalmology 85: 553–559

Blumenkranz M S, Ophir A, Claflin A J, Hajek A 1982 Fluorouracil for the treatment of massive periretinal proliferation. American Journal of Ophthalmology 94: 458–467

Charles S 1981a Vitreous microsurgery. Williams and Wilkins, Baltimore, p 26–28

Charles S 1981b Endophotocoagulation. Retina 1: 117–120

Charles S, Flinn C E 1981 The natural history of diabetic extramacular traction retinal detachment. Archives of Ophthalmology 99: 66–68

Charles S, Wang C 1981 A linear suction control for the vitreous cutter (Ocutome). Archives of Ophthalmology 99: 1613

Christiansen J M, Kollarits C R, Fukui H, Fishman M L, Michels R G, Mikuni I 1976 Intraocular irrigating solutions and lens clarity. American Journal of Ophthalmology 82: 594–597

Cleary P E, Ryan S J 1979 Method of production and natural history of experimental posterior penetrating injury in the rhesus monkey. American Journal of Ophthalmology 88: 212–220

Coleman D J 1982 Early vitrectomy in the management of the severely traumatised eye. American Journal of Ophthalmology 93: 543–551

Cox M S, Freeman H M 1978 Retinal detachment due to ocular penetration: 1. Clinical characteristics and surgical results. Archives of Ophthalmology 96: 1354–1361

Diddie K R, Schanzlin D J 1983 Specular microscopy in pars plana vitrectomy. Archives of Ophthalmology 101: 408–409

Federman J L, Shakin J L, Lanning R C 1982 The microsurgical management of giant retinal tears with trans-scleral retinal sutures. Ophthalmology 89: 832–838

Fleischman J A, Swartz M, Dixon J A 1981 Argon laser endophotocoagulation — an intraoperative trans-pars plana technique. Archives of Ophthalmology 99: 1610–1612

Foos R 1978 Nonvascular proliferative extraretinal retinopathies. American Journal of Ophthalmology 86: 723–725

Foulks G N, Thoft R A, Perry H D, Tolentino F I 1979 Factors related to corneal epithelial complications after closed vitrectomy in diabetics. Archives of Ophthalmology 97: 1076–1078

Freeman H M, Castillejos M E 1981 Current management of giant retinal breaks: results with vitrectomy and total air fluid exchange in ninety-five cases. Transactions American Ophthalmological Society 79: 89–102

Gass J D M 1982 Sympathetic ophthalmia following vitrectomy. American Journal of Ophthalmology 93: 552–558

Gonvers M, Machemer R 1982 A new approach to treating retinal detachment with macular hole. American Journal of Ophthalmology 94: 468–472

Graham M V, Hodson S 1980 Intraocular irrigating and replacement fluid. Transactions of the Ophthalmological Societies of the United Kingdom 100: 282–285

Gregor Z, Ryan S J 1982 Pars plana vitrectomy entry sites. Transactions of the Ophthalmological Societies of the United Kingdom 102: 461–467

Ho P C, Mainster M A, Dieckert J P, Tolentino F I 1983 Fundus contact lenses for closed pars plana vitrectomy. Ophthalmology, Instrument and Book Supplement 106–114

Hueneke R L, Aaberg T M 1983 Instrumentation for continuous fluid/air exchange during vitreous surgery. American Journal of Ophthalmology 96: 547–548

Kenyon K R, Wafai Z, Michels R G et al 1978 Corneal basement membrane abnormality in diabetes mellitus. Investigative Ophthalmology 17a (supplement): 245

Kreiger A E, Straatsma B R, Foos R Y 1977 Incisional complications in pars plana vitrectomy. Modern Problems in Ophthalmology 18: 210–223

Landers M B, Trese M T, Stefansson E, Bessler M 1982 Argon laser intraocular photocoagulation. Ophthalmology 89: 785–788

Lean J S, Leaver P K, Cooling R J, McLeod D 1982 Management of complex retinal detachment by vitrectomy and fluid/silicone exchange. Transactions of the Ophthalmological Societies of the United Kingdom 102: 203–205

Leaver P K, Cooling R J, Feretis E B, Lean J S, McLeod D 1984 Vitrectomy and fluid/silicone–oil exchange for giant retinal tears: results at six months. British Journal of Ophthalmology (in press)

Lewis M L, Gass J D M, Spencer W M 1978 Sympathetic uveitis after trauma and vitrectomy. Archives of Ophthalmology 96: 263–267

Machemer R 1978 Pathogenesis of proliferative neovascular retinopathies and the role of vitrectomy: a hypothesis. International Ophthalmology 1: 1–3

Machemer R 1980 Surgical approaches to subretinal strands. American Journal of Ophthalmology 90: 81–85

Machemer R 1983 Closed vitrectomy for severe retrolental fibroplasia in the infant. Ophthalmology 90: 436–441

Machemer R, Blankenship G 1981 Vitrectomy for proliferative diabetic retinopathy associated with vitreous haemorrhage. Ophthalmology 88: 643–646

Machemer R, Laua H 1978 A logical approach to the treatment of massive periretinal proliferation. Ophthalmology 85: 84–93

Machemer R, Allen A W 1976 Retinal tears 180° and greater. Archives of Opthalmology 94: 1340–1346

McLeod D, Restori M 1981 Rapid B-scanning in diabetic eye disease. Ultrasonography in Ophthalmology. Documenta Ophthalmologica Proceedings Series, The Hague, Dr W Junk Publishers 19: 21–31

McLeod D, Leaver P K, Feretis E 1980 Vitrectomy for severe diabetic eye disease. Transactions of the Ophthalmological Societies of the United Kingdom 100: 291–298

Meyers S M, Bonner R F 1982 Yellow filter to decrease the risk of light damage to the retina during vitrectomy. American Journal of Ophthalmology 94: 677

Michels R G 1981 Vitreous surgery for macular pucker. American Journal of Ophthalmology 92: 628–639

O'Malley C, Heintz R M 1975 Vitrectomy with an alternative instrument system. Annals of Ophthalmology 7: 585–594

Rice T A, Michels R G, Maguire M G, Rice E F 1983 The effect of lensectomy on the incidence of iris neovascularisation and neovascular glaucoma after vitrectomy for diabetic retinopathy. American Journal of Ophthalmology 95: 1–11

Rice T A, Michels R G 1980 Long-term anatomic and functional results of vitrectomy for diabetic retinopathy. American Journal of Ophthalmology 90: 297–303

Scott J D 1974 Macular holes and retinal detachment. Transactions of the Ophthalmological Societies of the United Kingdom 94: 319–324

Talbot J F, Marshall J, Sherrard E, Kohner E M, McLeod D 1981 Experimental phaco-emulsification: effects on the corneal endothelium. The Cornea in Health and Disease (6th Congress of the European Society of Ophthalmology), Academic Press Inc. London. 805–810

Tano Y, Chandler D, Machemer R 1980 Treatment of intraocular proliferation with intravitreal injection of Triamcinolone Acetonide. American Journal of Ophthalmology 90: 810–816

9. The management of diabetic retinopathy

R. K. Blach

INTRODUCTION

The challenge of diabetic retinopathy remains a formidable one to the ophthalmologist for the following reasons:

1. Up to 5% of the general population may be diabetic (National Commission on Diabetes, 1973).

2. The incidence of retinopathy among diabetics is about 50% (Cullen, 1972).

3. It has been estimated that 5% of people with retinopathy are blind and about 10% of the blind population in the United Kingdom and in the United States of America is diabetic (Caird et al, 1968).

4. Diabetes is the commonest cause of newly registered blindness under the age of 65. In the United Kingdom, according to the latest figures, it accounts for about a quarter of new registrations in this age group (DHSS, 1979).

5. Diabetic retinopathy is, by and large, a treatable condition so that blindness can be prevented by treatment. Indeed, of all the major complications of diabetes, diabetic retinopathy is the most amenable to therapy.

6. The sheer additional workload to the ophthalmologist, representing a profession which is small in size and modest in prestige and yet one which already has a huge commitment in trying to keep an ageing population functional, is creating major problems in the organisation of ophthalmic care in the community and in the selection of priorities for medicine generally (Blach & Bloom, 1978).

DIABETIC RETINOPATHY

In order to apportion medical care most effectively, it is desirable to identify both those groups of patients most likely to be at risk of blindness and those cases suffering from the type of retinopathy which is the most effective to treat in terms of preventing visual deterioration. It is, therefore, necessary (1) to identify risk factors and (2) to classify diabetic retinopathy.

Risk factors

Non-ocular factors in the development of diabetic retinopathy include diabetic control, hypertension, pregnancy, renal disease, age and sex.

Diabetic control

The arguments for and against the maintenance of good diabetic control in the prevention of diabetic complications have been well summarised by Tchobroutsky (1978). However, the recent advances in the quality of diabetic control have as their rationale the concept that good control must be beneficial, and powerful backing for this concept is obtained from the work of Pirart (1977).

Hypertension
There is evidence but no proof that co-existing hypertension worsens the prognosis for diabetic retinopathy (Harrold, 1971).

Pregnancy
There has been no controlled study of the effects of pregnancy on diabetic retinopathy although there is a clinical impression that pregnancy and the oestrogen pill have a deleterious effect especially on proliferative diabetic retinopathy. This group of patients has to be especially carefully watched (Casser et al, 1978).

Age and sex
Although no type of diabetic retinopathy is confined to one age group or sex nevertheless proliferative diabetic retinopathy tends to occur in the younger age group and has an equal sex incidence, whereas background diabetic retinopathy is commonest in the elderly and commoner in females than in males (Little & Jack, 1983).

A therapeutic classification of diabetic retinopathy
From the practical point of view it is most convenient to classify diabetic eye disease into early, established and advanced.

Early diabetic retinopathy
Early retinopathy exists in diabetics with either no visible retinopathy or minor changes consisting of haemorrhages, micro-aneurysms and exudates, but with normal vision. Changes in retinal structure and function which are not readily visible have been detected by a number of investigative techniques such as electrodiagnostic tests, colour vision, vitreous fluorometry and, most important, fluorescein angiography, although the value of these investigations is greater for the research worker than to the clinician. Many of these tests are of speculative value in trying to determine the pathogenesis of diabetic retinopathy—whether it is basically a vascular, neurocellular, or pigment epithelial condition. Fluorescein angiography can, however, be of practical use to the ophthalmologist in that it can define the type of maculopathy which is present and can often resolve the question of the possible presence of new vessels suspected ophthalmoscopically.

Established diabetic retinopathy
Features of established diabetic retinopathy have been described repeatedly and enthusiastically since the 1850s (Desmarres, 1858). These features are common to all other retino-vascular diseases but their spatial and temporal distribution is unique to diabetes. On the one hand, there are the consequences of abnormal vascular permeability with the development of haemorrhages, fatty hard exudates and retinal oedema which are the features of background diabetic retinopathy and, where the macula is involved, diabetic maculopathy. On the other hand, there are the consequences of retinal capillary non-perfusion giving rise to ischaemia which, in

turn, is the basic stimulus to neovascularisation. These two responses are not mutually exclusive in the same eye.

BACKGROUND DIABETIC RETINOPATHY

Background diabetic retinopathy or maculopathy may cause blindness as a result of a variety of features each of which may be dominant in particular cases. Thus focal or exudative diabetic maculopathy is chiefly associated with the development of hard exudates or haemorrhage in the foveal region. Exudates usually form a ring or part of a ring which, itself, is centred on a vascular malformation. Where oedema is the dominant feature cystic or oedematous diabetic maculopathy is the cause of visual loss. Where ischaemic changes occur the condition may eventually lead to ischaemic or proliferative diabetic retinopathy.

PROLIFERATIVE DIABETIC RETINOPATHY

Pre-proliferative retinopathy. In pre-proliferative diabetic retinopathy intra-retinal micro-vascular abnormalities (IRMA) lead to reduced perfusion of the retina. Abnormally enlarged capillary loops, arteriovenous shunts and venous loops, blot haemorrhages and the development of cotton wool spots are common features of this stage of diabetic retinopathy (Fig. 9.1).

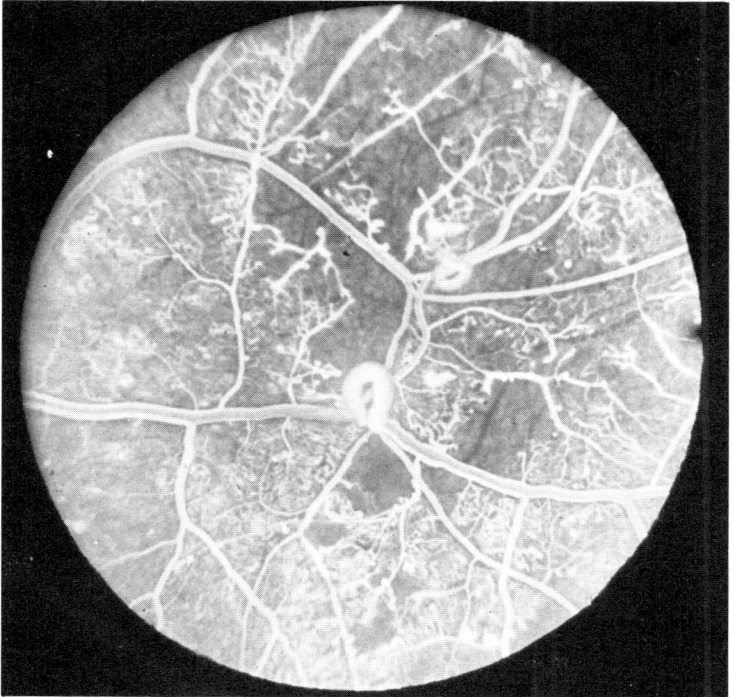

Fig. 9.1   A fluorescein angiogram showing features of pre-proliferative diabetic retinopathy with prominent venous loops.

Proliferative diabetic retinopathy. Proliferative diabetic retinopathy is the result of retinal capillary non-perfusion. The subsequent neovascularisation gives rise to vitreous detachment, haemorrhage, fibrosis, retinal traction and traction retinal detachment. When neovascularisation occurs in the anterior segment neovascular glaucoma may eventually ensue. Some recent fluorescein angiographic studies by Shimizu & Kobayaashiy (1981) have related the degree of capillary non-profusion in the entire fundus to peripheral retinal new vessels, disc new vessels and anterior segment neovascularisation. They found that capillary occlusion was modest where there were only peripheral retinal vessels, increased with disc new vessels and massive where there was anterior segment neovascularisation.

Advanced diabetic eye disease
Advanced diabetic eye disease consists of intra-ocular haemorrhage, pre-retinal traction, retinal detachment and neovascular glaucoma, all the result of ischaemic or proliferative diabetic retinopathy.

THE MANAGEMENT OF DIABETIC RETINOPATHY

Different treatment options dominate at various stages of the disease. In early diabetic retinopathy medical therapy, especially diabetic control and possibly photocoagulation, need to be considered. In established diabetic retinopathy photocoagulation, with the appropriate techniques for the individual conditions, and possibly vitrectomy, are the most important. In advanced diabetic eye disease surgery, photocoagulation and sociological management are important.

Early diabetic eye disease

Good diabetic control
Evidence has accumulated over the years that good diabetic control, certainly in the early stages of diabetes, tends to delay and reduce the severity of diabetic retinopathy. Whatever the associations of diabetes, hyperglycaemia must be the dominant element and normo-glycaemia under physiological circumstances must have a beneficial effect on secondary metabolic abnormalities. However, once irreversible features have developed as a result of diabetes, normalisation may not have beneficial results, and indeed, under certain circumstances, may have adverse effects. The more recently introduced aids towards normalisation include the assessment of control by HBA 1c, more sophisticated self-monitoring instruments, and the introduction of insulin pumps. While all these might be expected to have a good effect in early diabetes, they have led to occasional surprising results in the established disease. Thus a few patients on the insulin pump with existing diabetic retinopathy have been found to develop a mass of cotton wool spots on starting the pump (Krock Multicentre Study, 1984).

Drugs
Whether the huge amount of research on blood constituents and blood vessel abnormalities in diabetes can be related to diabetic retinopathy in terms of cause or

effect is an open question. It has failed to clear the shadow of doubt over the many forms of medical treatment that have been advocated for early diabetic eye disease. Certainly such drugs as Lipotriad and Doxium are much too expensive to be used as mere placebos. The role of aspirin, however, by virtue of its effects on prostaglandin synthesis and, therefore, platelet aggregation, is the subject of a number of studies including the Early Treatment Diabetic Retinopathy Study at present being undertaken under the aegis of the National Eye Institute in Washington. Clofibrate, although it has been shown by clinical trials to reduce hard exudates in diabetic retinopathy, is not so free from side effects as photocoagulation, which is more effective.

Photocoagulation
The role of photocoagulation in early diabetic eye disease was first advocated by Meyer-Schwickerath himself who suggested that all visible lesions should be treated. There is certainly evidence, for example in Coats' disease, that abnormal haemodynamics within the retina can have a deleterious effect on the mechanisms of retinal blood flow in adjacent areas of retina and to this degree destruction of retino-vascular abnormalities in the early stages of diabetic retinopathy might be a logical procedure. However, the visual prognosis for very early diabetic retinopathy untreated is, in fact, very good and it is entirely correct that a major but complicated clinical trial on early treatment of diabetic retinopathy is being undertaken in America. However, this trial is very complicated, the protocol alone weighing 10 pounds, and whether it will resolve our problems or confirm our doubts on the value of early treatment is as yet unknown.

Established diabetic retinopathy
The treatment of established diabetic retinopathy was the subject of intensive study during the 1970s. The corner stone of treatment is undoubtedly photocoagulation and its place in the treatment of proliferative diabetic retinopathy is now fully established both as a result of clinical trials and clinical conviction. The treatment of background retinopathy and pre-proliferative retinopathy remain less certain.

Background diabetic retinopathy
The best treatment for background diabetic retinopathy or maculopathy is still not fully established. A number of studies in the early 1970s especially those of Patz (1973) and Spalter (1977) suggested that photocoagulation for diabetic maculopathy is effective although the presence of some features of this condition such as macular ischaemia have a bad prognostic significance. The randomised controlled clinical trial using Xenon Arc photocoagulation for diabetic maculopathy by the British Multicentre Study Group has recently published its final report (1983). This showed too that treatment was more effective than no treatment, but the effect was greatest in those whose initial vision was good and was not significant in those with a vision of 6/36 or worse. On these grounds it can be argued that, unless there is a danger of developing proliferative changes, treating those cases with diabetic maculopathy with a vision of 6/36 or worse is not justified. However, the different types of maculopathy were not considered in this trial and the study of Whitelock et al (1979) attempted to

differentiate the various types of maculopathy so as to bring some order into this confused picture. They divided maculopathy into three groups:

(a) focal or exudative diabetic maculopathy;
(b) cystic or oedematous diabetic maculopathy;
(c) ischaemic diabetic maculopathy.

The suggested treatment for these three types of maculopathy was described. For exudative diabetic retinopathy, focal photocoagulation to the centre of the circinate excudates was advocated. Although initially it was thought that the treatment here should be rather intense to destroy the vascular malformation, recent studies by Glover (1983) have suggested that gentle treatment of the pigment epithelium in the same region may have the same effect. The results of treatment for this group in Whitelocke's study were particularly good. This group indeed responds so readily to treatment that it may well be that the good results here carried the rather poor response for the oedematous and ischaemic groups. Attempts to reduce macular oedema by photocoagulation have led to the trial of various techniques such as grid photocoagulation whereby a very gentle photocoagulation is carried out as a grid over the oedematous area. In the case of ischaemic maculopathy both focal and panphoto-coagulation have been considered.

The treatment of macular oedema in diabetes remains the single most important problem in the management of diabetic retinopathy. Apart from the various techniques of photocoagulation, antiprostaglandin drugs such as Indomethacin (Miyake et al, 1983) have been advocated. None of the results of present studies, including grid photocoagulation, has been shown to give rise to any improvement in vision although sometimes improvement of diabetic control, control of hypertension and grid photocoagulation will reduce the amount of macular oedema (Bresnick, 1983). This, however, also occurs spontaneously. Macular oedema remains the most serious cause of visual loss in the elderly diabetic with background retinopathy but is also found in ischaemic diabetic eye disease.

Proliferative diabetic retinopathy
PRE-PROLIFERATIVE DIABETIC RETINOPATHY
The management of the pre-proliferative phase of diabetic retinopathy is similar to that of ischaemic or proliferative eye disease, that is to say good diabetic control, control of hypertension and the management of associated risk factors. Photocoagulation, as gentle pan-photocoagulation, can be applied, or, if it is felt that this is not justified in the absence of frank new vessels, careful and repeated observation is required so that photocoagulation can be given as soon as true pre-retinal neovascularisation occurs.

PROLIFERATIVE RETINOPATHY
Early treatment of proliferative diabetic retinopathy is one of the most important sight-saving procedures that is open to the ophthalmologist. The results of treatment are now so good, as has been proved in both the British and American controlled clinical trials (Hercules et al, 1977; Asher et al, 1981; Diabetic Retinopathy Study Research Group, 1981; British Multicentre Study Group, 1984), and the results of no treatment are so disastrous in terms of complete visual loss, that the failure of supervision of diabetics from the ocular point of view and failure to treat cases of pro-

liferative retinopathy are being regarded as negligence. The treatment of this group of patients is far more urgent than those with cataract and open-angle glaucoma and is equivalent in urgency to the treatment of rhegmatogenous retinal detachment.

The techniques of photocoagulation for proliferative diabetic retinopathy have been described in many accounts elsewhere (Blach, 1977; Blach & Hamilton, 1978). It will be remembered that although it is not known how photocoagulation works, the general aim of treatment is not to destroy vessels directly but to reduce the metabolic needs of the retina so that the vessels will disappear within 2 or 3 weeks. This applies both to retinal new vessels, where so-called localised pan-photocoagulation is applied around the area of the new vessels without any attempt being made to close them, and to disc neovascularisation. A gadget to hasten the application of pan-photocoagulation has been described for the Lasertek laser (Hamilton & Dolan, 1981), (Fig. 9.2). The scheme of treatment at Moorfields Eye Hospital is given in

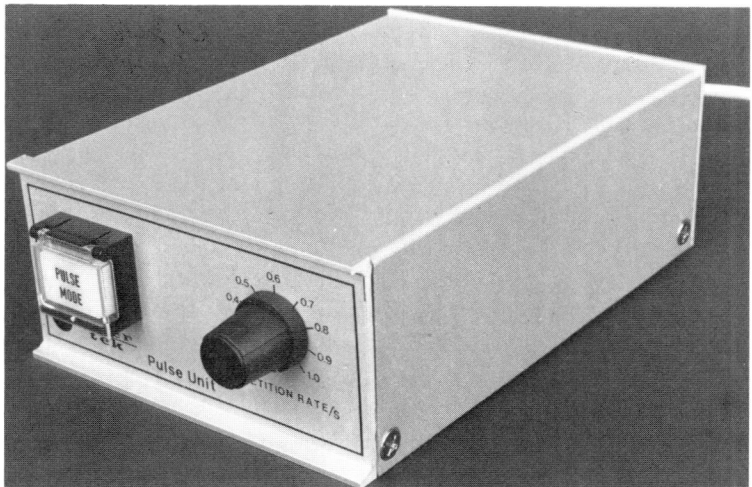

Fig. 9.2   A gadget that can be used with the Lasertek machine for semi-automatic pan-photocoagulation.

Table 9.1. The evidence for the beneficial effects of photocoagulation especially pan-photocoagulation is overwhelming. Asher (1981), in reviewing the Moorfields treated cases, found that the regression rate of disc neovascularisation following photocoagulation was 79% compared with the published reports of the risks of blindness from untreated disc new vessels of 70% within 5 years. The treatment of

Table 9.1

Panphotocoagulation of disc new vessels (NV)
1/12 after completion of 2000 burns:
(a) No NV — Check 6/12
(b) Attenuated NV — Check 3/12
(c) NV present — Repeat R_λ
(d) NV present — Repeat R_λ (? + Xenon)
(e) NV present — Direct R_λ

If repeated laser pan-photocoagulation is not effective, Xenon photocoagulation may be tried and the difficult technique of direct occlusion of disc new vessels can be used.

proliferative diabetic retinopathy, therefore, is much more clear-cut and effective than of background diabetic retinopathy, and this, of course, is especially important since the complications of proliferative retinopathy are so much more devastating than those of background retinopathy. Indeed, advanced diabetic eye disease is entirely the result of proliferative diabetic retinopathy.

When fibrosis associated with neovascularisation develops, traction of the retina becomes a threat. Certainly photocoagulation, while dangerous, will still deal with the neovascular element of the condition but direct traction of the retina can only be prevented by means of vitrectomy and membranectomy operations. At what stage such major procedures should be undertaken remains an open question, although the results of the Early Vitrectomy Trial, which is at present being undertaken in America, with all the difficulties involved, are awaited with interest. In advanced diabetic eye disease, however, there are specific indications and contra-indications for vitrectomy which will be considered.

Advanced diabetic eye disease
Advanced diabetic eye disease consists of intraocular haemorrhage, retinal traction phenomena and neovascular glaucoma.

Intraocular haemorrhage
The occurrence of vitreous or sub-hyaloid haemorrhages is a most frightening event for the patient and it is correct that his doctor should have both a humane and logical approach. The patient should rest with his head up in the sitting position for a period of 24 hours and this will often allow the blood to settle at the bottom of the eye. If he lies flat in bed it will simply rest over the macula. It may be correct to admit him to hospital provided the facilities for stopping such a haemorrhage, i.e., photocoagulation, are available since the journey itself will often shake up the blood within the eye, rather like snow in a paper weight. If the blood clears sufficiently, treatment may be given. If there is no change the patient may be discharged and a B-scan ultrasonogram subsequently undertaken. If some clearance occurs, then resting may be prolonged.

Retinal traction
Retinal traction is important (a) if there are associated retinal holes and (b) if the macula itself is threatened or affected.

(a) If retinal holes exist the threat of further retinal detachment is great and vitrectomy, membranectomy and retinal detachment surgery should be undertaken.

(b) Where the macula is not threatened, localised traction retinal detachment may be left untreated as it can remain localised for very long periods of time. However, if the macula is threatened or the macula has been off for only a short period of time then urgent vitrectomy and membranectomy should be undertaken (Fig. 9.3a,b).

The various techniques involved in this fascinating branch of ophthalmic surgery are described elsewhere in this book. It should, however, be remembered: (1) that the very fact that these cases come to this advanced stage of the disease is a criticism of our medical community, since, by and large, advanced diabetic eye disease is preventable; (2) this type of surgery is dramatic and expensive with poor results in functional terms, perhaps the ophthalmological equivalent of cardiac transplantation. It should, therefore, only be undertaken in centres which are likely to benefit from their

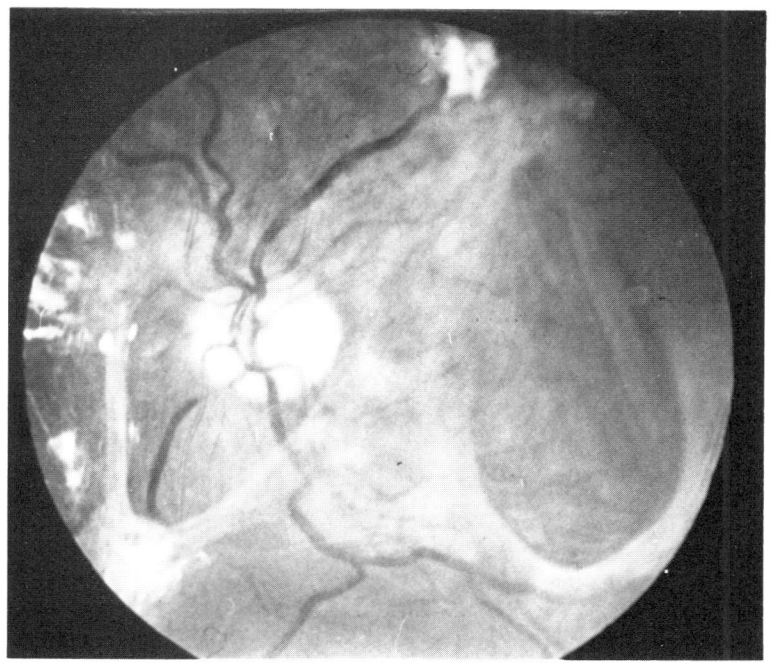

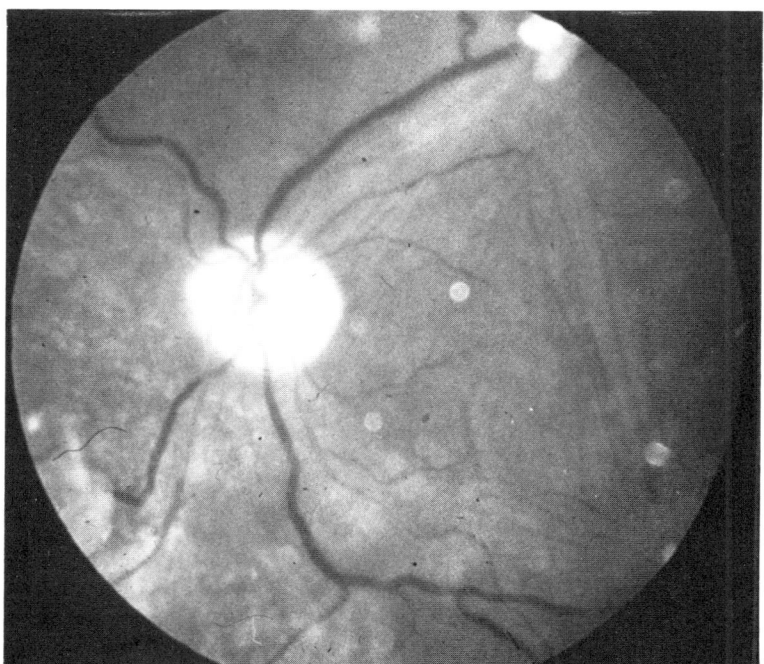

Fig. 9.3   **a** Retinal traction before vitrectomy and membranectomy.
b The same case postoperatively.

experience. Such centres will not only have the surgical expertise but the required infra-structure that has such an important influence on ultimate success.

Neovascular glaucoma

The most horrifying complication of diabetic eye disease is neovascular glaucoma. This condition, however, is now during its various stages amenable to therapy. A logical approach to the management of all stages of this condition is indicated in Figure 9.4 but, in order to understand the logic of this sequence, an understanding of the development of neovascular glaucoma is essential (Blach et al, 1977).

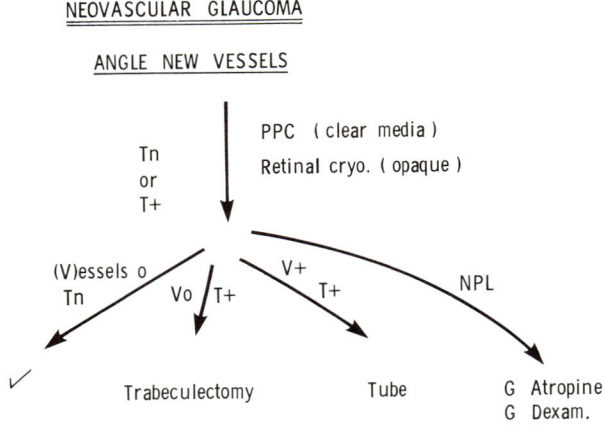

Fig. 9.4   Treatment options for neovascularisation for the anterior chamber angle. The options are described in the text.

Neovascular glaucoma occurs as a result of neovascularisation of the anterior chamber angle as a response to retinal ischaemia. Pan-photocoagulation of the retina causes regression of the vessels in the angle with a restoration to normality. However, the real cause of the rise in intraocular pressure is not the new vessels themselves, but the associated fibrosis which causes the iris to contract on the cornea, thus blocking the trabecular meshwork and creating a false angle (Fig. 9.5a,b). Unfortunately, if traditional glaucoma surgery is undertaken in this sort of case the new vessels will simply grow into the filtering bleb. However, photocoagulation at this stage, while not affecting the fibrous tissue or the synechiae, will still affect the neovascular element and, if this has been obliterated, then traditional glaucoma surgery is effective (Flanagan & Blach, 1983). If, due to opaque media, photocoagulation cannot be undertaken, then retinal cryotherapy may be considered. This can be conveniently undertaken using an amoylette cryotherapy machine through two stab incisions in the conjunctiva, one in each upper quadrant with three or four radial applications of cryotherapy under direct vision of the indirect ophthalmoscope. Cyclo-cryotherapy according to the technique illustrated, will reduce aqueous production (Fig. 9.6).

If treatment is still not successful and neovascularisation persists, then the insertion of a Molteno tube (Molteno et al, 1977) may be considered. Some feel that this should be associated with lensectomy and vitrectomy in order to reduce the chances of the tube blocking and facilitating treatment of the retina.

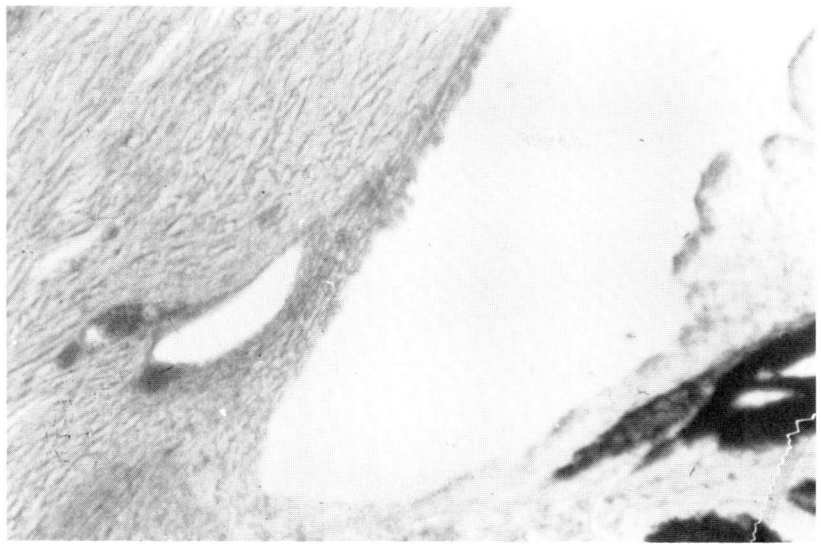

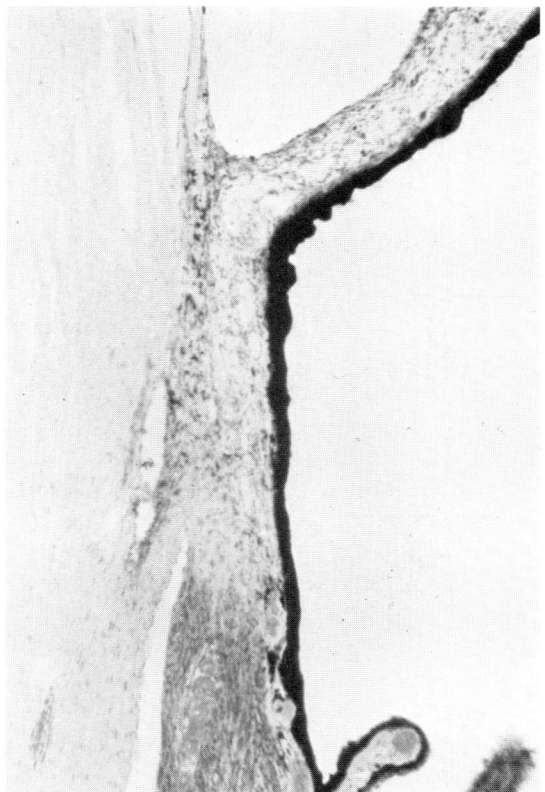

Fig. 9.5   **a** A normal angle. **b** Peripheral anterior synechiae showing a false angle.

CYCLOCRYOTHERAPY

1) 2.5mm FROM LIMBUS
2) 1st ℞ =   2 QUADRANTS
                4 APPLICATIONS/QUADRANT
               60 SECONDS/APPLICATION
3) 2nd ℞ SOS = 1 QUADRANT
4) LOCAL ANAESTHESIA

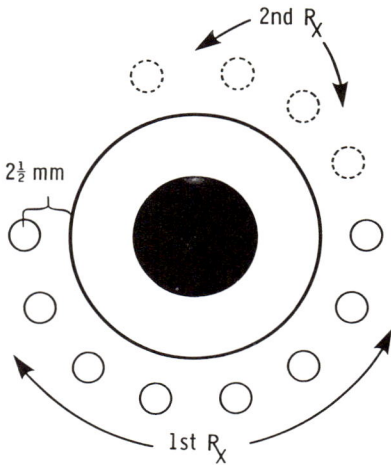

Fig. 9.6   The technique of cyclocryotherapy.

If all else fails and the eye is both blind and painful then, rather than enucleation or the retro-bulbar injection of alcohol, it is more considerate to give the patient atropine and steroid drops for a period of 2 or 3 months so as to make the eye comfortable and white.

SOCIOLOGICAL ASPECTS

The management of a visually handicapped diabetic in the community depends on the degree of his visual loss, his associated problems and his age. Those who have lost detailed vision as a result of background diabetic retinopathy tend to maintain their visual field, their navigational vision and, therefore, their social independence. The younger members of this group can often be greatly helped professionally by means of the skilled use of low vision aids. The more elderly seldom have the motivation to persist in their use.

Those who have lost their vision as a result of ischaemic or proliferative diabetic retinopathy go blind as a result of advanced diabetic eye disease. These people not only lose their detailed vision but also their field of vision — in other words they lose their navigational vision and become dependent on other people. Even this group, with the help of an active spouse and an intelligent memory, can sometimes maintain their professional lives. This, however, is the exception rather than the rule and much commoner is the onset of depression and fear.

Much can be done to alleviate the lot of the blind and practical help, for example click or pre-set syringes for the diabetic, can be obtained both from local blind associations and the British Diabetic Association. It is, however, not possible to adapt to blindness so that practical help and understanding will always be a primary function of society.

CONCLUSION

In conclusion, therefore, effective management of diabetic eye disease is available at most of its stages. The application of available knowledge, however, is not always forthcoming, although with enthusiasm and sensible organisation this can be achieved. The fact that excellent services are available in certain countries and in certain parts of our own country suggests that this is not a problem for which bureaucrats and Government can be blamed but is a problem where the solution is in our own hands. Some serious gaps in our knowledge in the management of diabetic eye disease remain. Specifically these include the underlying cause of diabetes, the management of macular oedema, the application of photocoagulation in the early stages of the disease, and the place of vitrectomy in the earlier stages of diabetic retinopathy. Nevertheless, with sufficient energy, enthusiasm and skill it has been repeatedly shown that both the knowledge and the facilities exist to treat our large population with diabetic eye disease.

REFERENCES

Asher R, Hunt S et al 1981 International Ophthalmology 3: 79
Blach R K 1977 Scientific Foundations of Ophthalmology, Perkins and Hill, ch 40, Heinemann, London
Blach R K, Bloom A 1978 Health Trends 10: 88
Blach R K, Hamilton A M 1978 International Ophthalmology 1: 119
Blach R K, Hitchings R A, Laatikainen L 1977 Transactions of the Ophthalmological Societies of the UK
    97: 275
Bresnick G U 1983 Ophthalmology 90: 1301
British Multicentre Study Group 1983 Diabetes 32: 1010
British Multicentre Study Group 1984 Diabetologica (in press)
Caird F I, Burdett A F, Draper J 1968 Diabetes 17: 121
Casser J, Kohner E M et al 1978 Diabetologica 15: 105
Cullen J F 1972 Transactions of the Ophthalmological Societies of the UK 92: 59
Cullen J F, Town S M, Campbell C J 1974 Transactions of the Ophthalmological Societies of the UK
    94: 544
Desmarres L A 1858 Maladies des yeux, 2nd edn, Gernier, Paris p 523
DHSS 1979 A report of public health medical subject No. 129 London, HMSO
Diabetic Retinopathy Study Research Group 1981 Ophthalmology 88: 583
Flanagan DW, Blach R K 1983 British Journal of Ophthalmology 67: 526
Glover R G 1983 Transactions of the Ophthalmological Societies of the UK (in press)
Hamilton A M, Dolan R 1981 British Journal of Ophthalmology 65: 718
Harrold E P P 1971 British Journal of Ophthalmology 55: 225
Hercules B L, Gayed IR et al 1977 British Journal of Ophthalmology 61: 555
Krock Multicentre Study 1984 New England Journal of Medicine (in press)
Little H, Jack R L et al 1983 Diabetic retinopathy, Thieme Stratton, New York, p 14
Miyake K, Miyake Y et al 1983 American Journal of Ophthalmology 95: 415
Molteno A C B, von Rooyem N B, Bartholomew R S 1977 British Journal of Ophthalmology 61: 120
National Commission on Diabetes to the Congress of the United States 1973
Patz A, Schatz H et al 1973 Transactions of the American Academy of Ophthalmology and Otolaryngology
    77: 34
Pirart J 1977 Diabete et Metabolisme 3: 97, 173, 245

Schott K 1965 Ber Deutsch Ophthal Ges 66: 349
Shimizu K, Kobayaashiy et al 1981 Ophthalmology 88: 601
Spalter H F 1977 American Journal of Ophthalmology 71: 242
Tshobroutsky G B 1978 Diabetologica 15: 143
Whitelocke R A F, Kaerns M, Blach R K et al 1979 Transactions of the Ophthalmological Societies of the
    UK 99: 314

10. Current treatment of malignant melanomas of the posterior uvea *

J. A. Shields

DEFINITION

Malignant melanoma of the uvea is the most common primary intraocular malignancy. This tumour arises from the uveal melanocytes, which are derived embryologically from the neural crest. Melanomas which occur in the ciliary body and peripheral choroid frequently attain a large size before they are diagnosed clinically. Tumours arising in the macular region are usually smaller at the time of diagnosis because they produce visual symptoms earlier. The clinical features, differential diagnosis, and diagnostic approaches to posterior uveal melanomas are discussed in the literature (Shields, 1983). This section reviews the controversy regarding treatment and discusses the current available alternatives in the management of malignant melanomas of the ciliary body and choroid.

CURRENT CONTROVERSY REGARDING TREATMENT

The traditional treatment for malignant melanoma of the posterior uvea was enucleation of the involved eye as soon as the diagnosis was believed to be certain. Some investigators have pointed out that patients with small melanomas have a very good prognosis following enucleation (Flocks et al, 1955; Shammas & Blodi, 1977). More recently, other authorities have questioned the value of enucleation, and have even speculated that this procedure may worsen the patient's prognosis (Zimmerman et al, 1978). As a result, a rather heated controversy has erupted among clinicians who manage patients with intraocular melanomas (Shields & Augsburger, 1980).

Although this controversy is not resolved, I believe that the goal of the ophthalmic clinician in the management of a patient with a posterior uveal melanoma is to control the tumour and to salvage the patient's vision when this can be achieved without endangering the patient's systemic health. The method of treatment should be carefully selected so as to meet these goals.

Alternatives in management

Important considerations which the author and his colleagues take into account in recommending specific management of a patient with a malignant melanoma of the posterior uvea include: (1) the size of the tumour; (2) the location of the tumour; (3) the activity of the tumour; (4) the condition of the opposite eye; (5) the age of the patient; (6) the general health of the patient; and (7) the psychological status of the patient (Shields, 1983).

*Modified with kind permission of the publisher from Shields J A 1983 Diagnosis and management of intraocular tumors. The C V Mosby Co, St Louis, ch 10, p 210–254.

Once all of the factors which influence the therapeutic choice have been thoroughly assessed, the patient with a posterior uveal melanoma can be managed by any of several methods, depending upon the overall clinical situation (Shields, 1983).

PERIODIC OBSERVATION

In recent years, many authorities have begun to recommend only periodic observation to manage initially selected melanomas of the posterior uvea. This approach seems to be particularly justifiable in the case of many small or medium-sized melanocytic tumours which are presumably malignant melanomas, but which have the dormant characteristics on ophthalmoscopic examination (Shields, 1983).

Indications
The author believes the relative indications for managing a posterior uveal melanoma by periodic observation are as follows:

1. Any small melanoma which appears dormant on the initial examination and which has not been documented with fundus photography or ultrasonography to have grown.

2. Most medium-sized melanomas which appear dormant on the initial examination.

3. Most small or medium-sized melanomas in elderly or seriously ill patients, even though the tumour shows signs of slow growth.

4. Most small- or medium-sized melanomas if the tumour is located in the patient's only useful eye, even though the tumour shows signs of slow growth.

Technique
The diagnostic tests used and the frequency of follow-up examinations depend upon the size category and the apparent activity of the tumour (Shields, 1983). If a patient has a tumour which is classified as a suspicious naevus, he should have fundus photographs and be re-examined in 3 months. If no growth is detected, he should be examined every 6 months thereafter. If a lesion is classified as a small melanoma which has dormant characteristics, the patient should have baseline 45-degree fundus photographs, fluorescein angiography, and A-scan and B-scan ultrasonography. The photographs should be repeated in 3–4 months. If the lesion shows no apparent change at that time, fundus photography should then be repeated every 6 months. If growth is suspected on the basis of clinical examination and fundus photography, then fluorescein angiography and ultrasonography can be repeated to confirm any change, and the patient should be considered for one of the therapeutic methods to be described.

Medium-sized melanomas which have dormant characteristics, especially if they are found in elderly patients, can usually be safely managed by periodic observation. Because of the greater tendency to show subsequent growth, they should have initial 45 degree and equator-plus photographs, fluorescein angiography and ultrasonography. The photographs and ultrasonography should be repeated every 3–6 months, and therapy considered if the growth is documented.

Complications

There appears to be little or no danger in simply observing periodically small- to medium-sized melanomas which show dormant features. Most of these tumours have little, if any, tendency to grow, and a low potential to metastasize. Lesions located within 2 mm of the optic disc or foveola should be followed more frequently. If growth toward either of these structures is documented, then photocoagulation or other applicable treatment should be considered.

Results

No long term data are yet available concerning periodic observation of choroidal melanomas. It does appear to be quite safe simply to observe most small- to medium-sized melanomas which have dormant features. Between 1974 and 1978, about 150 patients with small melanomas who were evaluated on the Oncology Service at Wills Eye Hospital were managed initially by periodic observation. Most of these lesions remained dormant as documented by fundus photography. Only 10–15% of such lesions were documented to grow during a 2–5 year follow-up. Of medium-sized melanomas which are initially managed by observation, only about 25–30% can be documented to grow. Although these figures may change as further cases are collected, our preliminary observations on most small- and many medium-sized melanomas have led us to agree with other authors that the prognosis for life is not worsened by periodic observation of such lesions until growth is documented before initiating treatment.

PHOTOCOAGULATION

Photocoagulation, using the Xenon arc or the Argon laser, is a useful method of treating selected small choroidal melanomas. It cannot be used in the treatment of ciliary body melanomas.

Indications

The relative indications for treatment of a choroidal melanoma by photocoagulation are as follows:

1. A small melanoma which shows unequivocal evidence of growth by both serial photography or ultrasonography.

2. Some small melanomas which have not necessarily been documented to grow but which show features of progressive growth on the initial examination, particularly if the tumour margin is located within 2 mm of the foveola or optic disc margin. If a course of continued observation is pursued in such cases, the tumour can eventually extend to the disc margin or to the foveola, thus decreasing the chance of a good visual result following photocoagulation.

3. Selected medium-sized melanomas which are within 3 mm of the optic disc or fovea. In such cases, radiotherapy may result in visual loss due to radiation vasculopathy and an attempt at photocoagulation seems justified.

To utilise photocoagulation, the ocular media should be clear. In most cases, I do not utilise photocoagulation to treat a growing pigmented tumour unless fluorescein angiography and ultrasonography show features of a melanoma and unless the P-32 test is positive.

Photocoagulation is difficult to impossible when the growing tumour has a peripapillary or subfoveal location. In these instances, enucleation is sometimes the only acceptable therapeutic option. If it is obvious that such a tumour will eventually necessitate enucleation, the eye should be removed while the tumour is still small. If the tumour grows to a large size prior to enucleation, the prognosis is worse.

Technique

Most melanomas are treated with either Argon laser or Xenon photocoagulation. If the Xenon arc is used, retrobulbar anaestheia is preferable. When one uses the Argon laser, topical anaesthesia will usually suffice.

The Rodenstock panfunduscope contact lens facilitates photocoagulation of a choroidal melanoma because the wide-angle view enables the physician to visualise the entire lesion in one field. During the first treatment session, burns are applied in two confluent rows around the margins of the tumour. The settings necessary to obtain adequate burns aound the tumour vary with the degree of fundus pigmentation. Using the Argon laser, however, a spot size of 200–500 microns, an intensity of 500–1000 milliwatts, and duration of 0.5 second, will usually suffice.

About 3 weeks later, the tumour is surrounded again using similar settings. After 2–3 surrounding treatments, most of the choroidal vessels around the tumour become obliterated or incorporated into scar tissue. In subsequent sessions about 3–5 weeks apart, the surrounding area is retreated and the surface of the tumour is treated heavily. It may require up to 1500 milliwatts with a duration of 1.0–1.5 seconds to obtain sufficient destruction of the tumour. After 4–10 treatments, the area of the tumour is usually replaced by a depressed scar consisting of a thin layer of fibroglial tissue overlying the bare sclera. In many cases treated by this method, a central area of flat pigmentation is often left in the centre of the scar. It is not necessary to continue treatment once the central pigment is flat, less than 1.5 mm in diameter, and hypofluorescent with fluorescein angiography.

Complications

The complications of photocoagulation for choroidal melanomas include branch retinal vascular obstruction, cystoid macular oedema, pre-retinal membrane formation, choroidovitreal neovascularisation, vitreous haemorrhage, and retinal detachment. In the author's experience, all of these complications are more frequent following Xenon arc photocoagulation and are relatively uncommon or less severe when Argon laser is used.

Results

Photocoagulation of a choroidal melanoma can be successful when the indications previously outlined are followed. We have follow-up data on 35 patients treated between 1974 and 1979. The first 18 were treated with Xenon arc and the latter 17 with Argon laser. Twenty-five of the patients have useful vision in the involved eye, five have poor vision (less than 6/60) and five eyes in the earlier group were enucleated, usually because of persistent growth of the melanoma. During that follow-up period, there were no tumour-related deaths in the overall group of 35 patients with choroidal melanomas who were treated with photocoagulation. We have seen two metastatic deaths, however, in subsequent patients treated by this technique. Treatment of choroidal melanomas by photocoagulation is most often successful if the tumour is in the small size category, being less than 3 mm in thickness as measured by A-scan ultrasonography.

DIATHERMY

Diathermy has been occasionally used to treat selected choroidal melanomas. Unfortunately, this method of treatment weakens the sclera over the tumour and theoretically creates a route for extrascleral extension of tumour cells. Because of this complication, diathermy has been largely abandoned in the treatment of uveal melanomas.

CRYOTHERAPY

Although cryotherapy can be effective, in the treatment of retinoblastomas and retinal capillary hemangioma, it has not been used extensively for the management of uveal melanomas. The author has treated one peripheral choroidal melanoma by the triple freeze–thaw technique and achieved a favourable result, although it required eight treatments to control the tumour clinically.

RADIOTHERAPY

Although once believed to be ineffective in the treatment of uveal melanomas, radiotherapy has recently become more widely accepted in the management of melanomas of the choroid and ciliary body (Brady et al, 1982; Shields et al, 1982).

Indications
In view of the recent controversy regarding enucleation for posterior uveal melanomas, the indications for radiotherapy are increasing. The relative indications will probably continue to change as more follow-up data on treated patients becomes available. Since the most widely employed method of radiotherapy has been the application of a radioactive episcleral plaque, only the indications for that technique will be presented. Other techniques of radiotherapy, which are still undergoing clinical trials, will most likely prove to have similar indications (Char et al, 1980; Gragoudas et al, 1980; Packer et al, 1980).

Between April 1976 and December 1983, we treated more than 450 patients with episcleral plaque radiotherapy on the Oncology Service at Wills Eye Hospital. The particular type of radioactive plaque which we employ depends upon several factors, but mostly upon the thickness of the tumour as measured with A-scan ultrasonography. At present, we generally use cobalt-60 plaques for melanomas greater than 5 mm in thickness, iridium-192 plaques for melanomas 3–5 mm in thickness and iodine-125 plaques for growing melanomas 2–3 mm in thickness. We rarely use radiotherapy for growing tumours less than 2 mm in thickness, because photocoagulation is often quite successful in such instances. We currently employ cobalt plaque therapy rather than enucleation as the initial therapeutic modality for most large choroidal and ciliary body melanomas in which the patient still has useful vision in the involved eye. When the tumour is greater than 15 mm in basal diameter and/or 10 mm in thickness, however, we are more inclined toward enucleation.

Technique
The technique for application of a radioactive plaque to treat an intraocular tumour is discussed in the literature (Shields, 1983). Particularly in the case of uveal melanomas, the procedure should be performed as gently as possible to minimise the theoretical possibility of systemic dissemination of tumour cells during the surgical manipulations. The procedure is generally done under retrobulbar anaesthesia. A conjunctival peritomy is performed and the rectus muscles are isolated with silk traction sutures. The sclera in the quadrant of the tumour is inspected to detect any extrascleral extension of the tumour and then to localise the lesion with transcleral transillumination. The sclera is marked with several light diathermy applications around the shadow of the tumour 1 mm from its margin. A radioactive phosphorus uptake (P-32) test can then be performed if desired and, if positive, the plaque is sutured to the sclera.

Complications
There are very few early complications of episcleral plaque radiotherapy. Transient diplopia can occur, particularly if a rectus muscle is disinserted to properly position the plaque. It is rarely necessary, however, to disinsert a rectus muscle to do this. Later complications of plaque radiotherapy include radiation retinopathy, radiation papillopathy, vitreous haemorrhage, radiation cataract, punctal occlusion with epiphora, keratoconjunctivitis sicca, radiation anterior uveitus, scleral necrosis and persistent diplopia.

Between April 1976 and December 1983, about 450 patients with a posterior uveal melanoma were treated with episcleral plaque radiotherapy on the Oncology Service at Wills Eye Hospital. Tumours treated by plaque radiotherapy can sometimes show a rather dramatic response to treatment. Although treatment of tumours located in the macular area can eventually lead to visual loss due to radiation retinopathy, many cases show a favourable regression of the tumour with minimal radiation damage. Treatment of tumours located near the optic disc frequently result in radiation papillopathy. However, we have occasionally treated lesions immediately adjacent to the optic disc with minimal radiation damage to the retina adjacent to the tumour.

Patients treated with plaque radiotherapy are followed with serial 45 degree and wide-angle fundus photography and ultrasonography to document tumour regression. Rather typical regression patterns can be noted following radiotherapy of a posterior uveal melanoma. Ophthalmoscopically, shrinkage of the tumour results in conversion of the lesion from a smooth, dome-shaped configuration to a shrunken mass with an irregular surface. The change in shape can be best documented with B-scan ultrasonography and the change in thickness can be best confirmed with A-scan ultrasonography.

Most patients with posterior uveal melanoma treated by episcleral plaque radiotherapy show a decrease in size of their tumour during the first year. In general, the visual results have been satisfactory although complications do occur. The preliminary data suggest that the mortality rate may be as low as or lower for patients treated with cobalt plaques than for patients with comparable-sized tumours treated with enucleation (Shields, 1983; Shields et al, 1982).

LOCAL RESECTION

Theoretically, an ideal approach to the management of a melanoma of the ciliary body or choroid is to remove surgically the tumour and salvage the eye, particularly if this can be achieved without worsening the patient's prognosis for life.

Indications
The relative indications for local resection of a posterior uveal melanoma are as follows:
1. A growing ciliary body melanoma or a ciliochoroidal melanoma which does not cover more than 4 clock hours of the pars plicata;
2. A choroidal melanoma which is not greater than 8 mm in diameter which is centred near the equator and is documented to be growing.

It should be stressed that melanomas which meet these criteria can also be managed by episcleral plaque radiotherapy in most instances. The preferred method of therapy in these instances is unresolved, and each case must be evaluated individually.

Techniques
The techniques for local excision of the posterior uveal melanomas are described in the literature (Shields, 1983). These techniques include iridocyclectomy and sclero-chorioretinal resection and the various modifications of these procedures.

Complications
There are a number of early complications which can occur from local resection for posterior uveal melanomas. Complications of iridocyclectomy or iridocyclochorio-retinectomy include subluxated lens, cataract, vitreous bleeding and retinal detachment. In many cases, removal of the tumour necessitates removal of a large portion of the zonular support to the lens. This can lead to postoperative shifting of the lens, with inflammation, corneal oedema, or glaucoma. To avoid this complication, the lens should generally be removed at the time of surgery when the tumour covers more than three clock hours of the pars plicata.

The most important surgical complications of sclerochorioretinal resection are vitreous bleeding and retinal detachment. Postoperative or late complications of local resections include vitreous fibrosis, cataract, and ischaemic inflammation in the anterior segment. The vitreous fibrosis can lead to chronic traction on the retina and a delayed retinal detachment.

Results
Very few surgeons have had extensive experience with local resection of posterior uveal melanomas. About 25 patients had iridocyclectomy or iridotrabeculectomy on the Oncology Service between 1974 and 1982. The initial results appear favourable.

Sclerochorioretinal resection for purely choroidal melanomas also provided fairly good visual results and rare fatalities (Peyman & Raichand, 1978). There were about 10 cases of eye wall resections for choroidal melanomas performed on the Oncology

Service between 1974 and 1979. One patient developed clinically apparent metastasis about 2 years after surgery and the other patients are alive and well, in spite of the fact that epithelioid cells were present in a number of the tumours. The early complications of sclerochorioretinal resection, however, are greater than those following episcleral plaque therapy, which usually is not associated with immediate visual morbidity. As a result, we have more recently advocated episcleral plaque radiotherapy for a number of patients who would have been treated by sclerochorioretinal resection in the past. If long term follow-up of patients treated by episcleral plaque radiotherapy should prove to be discouraging, then we may treat more patients with local resection of the melanoma.

ENUCLEATION

As mentioned earlier, the role of enucleation in the management of patients with posterior uveal melanomas remains controversial. The author currently believes that there are definite indications for enucleation, although the indications for this procedure are fewer than they were in the past.

Indications
Our current indications for enucleation to treat a posterior uveal melanoma are as follows:
1. Any ciliary body or choroidal melanoma which has produced visual loss but is too large to manage with either radiotherapy or local resection.
2. Any posterior uveal melanoma which has produced total retinal detachment or severe secondary glaucoma. In most instances, such tumours cannot be reasonably managed with any method other than enucleation.
3. Small and medium-sized choroidal melanomas which are documented to be growing and involve the optic nerve head.

Techniques
The technique of enucleation in the treatment of intraocular tumours is described in the literature (Shields, 1983). In the case of uveal melanomas, the author currently employs the so-called 'no-touch' technique for most cases (Fraunfelder et al, 1977). The value of this technique in reducing the mortality rate from uveal melanomas remains unproven, although some workers believe that adherence to this technique does reduce the mortality rate.

C•nplications
When enucleation is performed carefully, major surgical complications are rare. Bleeding at the time of surgery can be controlled by pressure in the socket. Late extrusion of the ball implant has not yet occurred in the series of more than 400 enucleations performed by the author and his colleagues. We believe that careful closure of Tenon's capsule is responsible for preventing this complication.

Results
Unfortunately, the mortality rate for patients with posterior uveal melanomas remains

rather high following enucleation. It is well-known that 30–45% of patients who undergo enucleation for choroidal melanoma will die of metastasis within 5 years, in spite of the fact that no evidence of metastasis is detected on the systemic evaluation prior to enucleation. The mortality rate for patients treated with the so-called 'no-touch' technique are still not available, but we have had a number of patients who developed metastases in spite of careful utilisation of this technique.

EXENTERATION

Exenteration of the orbital contents is considered by most authorities to be an acceptable method of treating uveal melanomas with extraocular extension into the orbit. Other physicians believe that exenteration does not improve the patient's prognosis for life in such cases (Shields, 1983).

Indications

The author's current indications for orbital exenteration for a uveal melamoma are as follows:

1. *Extensive* extraocular involvement by the melanoma at the time of initial presentation, provided there is no evidence of systemic metastasis.
2. *Extensive* orbital recurrence of a uveal melanoma sometime after enucleation, provided there is no evidence of systemic metastasis.

With improved diagnostic techniques and earlier recognition of uveal melanomas, it is now less common for patients to present initially with extensive extraocular involvement.

Techniques

The technique of exenteration is described and illustrated in the literature (Shields, 1983). Some surgeons prefer to use a skin graft to cover the exposed orbital bones, but most allow the socket to undergo healing by granulation. Eventually, any of several available prostheses may be employed to minimise the cosmetic deformity.

Complications

There are few major complications of orbital exenteration. Potential surgical complications include extensive bleeding which may rarely necessitate a blood transfusion. The thin ethmoid bones can be fractured during the procedure, leaving an opening between the orbit and nasal cavity. Postoperative infection can be controlled with appropriate antibiotics. Sloughing of the skin graft, if one is used, is of little consequence because the socket can be allowed to undergo granulation.

Results

The value of orbital exenteration in preventing local recurrence and distant metastases is unknown at this time. Some clinicians believe that it should be done on almost all cases with extrascleral extension, while others believe it should rarely, if ever, be performed (Shields, 1983). No reported series is large enough to draw meaningful conclusions.

MANAGEMENT OF SYSTEMIC METASTASES FROM UVEAL MELANOMAS

Once metastases to liver, lung, and other organs have occurred, the patient's prognosis is poor. Treatment of such patients is limited to palliative radiotherapy, chemotherapy, and perhaps immunotherapy. Such treatment should be administered by the appropriate specialists.

Radiation therapy has its greatest value in relieving pain from osseous metastases and in relieving the neurological symptoms from brain metastases, although bone and brain metastases are uncommon except in terminally ill patients. There is little information available on the effectiveness of chemotherapy.

Immunotherapy has had no clinical trial in the *primary* management of uveal melanomas. *Postoperative* immunotherapy following enucleation, however, theoretically seems to be a rational approach. A recent collaborative study has been undertaken to determine the role of intradermal injections of MER (methanol extracted residue of BCG) in patients who are considered at a high risk to develop metastases following enucleation. This study has been in progress for several years, but long term results are pending a review of the cases.

SUMMARY

The management of malignant melanoma of the posterior uvea has recently become a topic of great controversy. The traditional treatment of enucleation of the tumour-containing eye has recently been challenged by a number of authorities, and clinicians are more frequently using alternative methods of management when possible. Current management can range from periodic observation and fundus photography of selected small lesions which appear dormant, to photocoagulation, radiotherapy, or local resection in the case of growing tumours in eyes with useful or salvageable vision. In cases where the tumour is far advanced and there is no hope of useful vision, enucleation is often inevitable.

The choice of therapy is a complex issue and each case must be individualised. In selecting a therapeutic approach, certain factors must be carefully weighed. These include the size of the melanoma, its extent and location, its apparent activity, the status of the opposite eye and the age, general health and psychological status of the patient.

Periodic observation is believed by the author to be the treatment of choice for most small and many medium-sized melanomas of the posterior uvea which have not been documented to grow. If such lesions are documented to grow or if they show ophthalmoscopic evidence of progressive growth on the initial examination, then photocoagulation may be employed, provided the tumour is not greater than 10 mm in diameter or 3 mm in thickness. In the case of medium-sized or large tumours which are growing, the patient can be managed with either episcleral plaque radiotherapy or local resection of the tumour. Because it has less immediate visual morbidity than local resection, more patients are being managed today by radiotherapy, most commonly in the form of cobalt-60 plaque.

Patients with large tumours which have produced severe visual loss are currently managed by enucleation. Recently, authorities have advocated the so-called 'no-touch' technique of enucleation, although its true value remains undetermined. If there is extrascleral extension on initial examination, or if there is orbital recurrence following enucleation, then exenteration of the orbit or one of its modifications seems advisable.

Patients who have known systemic metastases, either before or after enucleation or other treatment, have a poor prognosis. In such cases, palliative irradiation, chemotherapy or immunotherapy may be employed.

It is expected that the management of posterior uveal melanomas will remain controversial for several years. It is hoped that with the accumulation of further knowledge of the various therapeutic alternatives, the physician will be able to recommend, with more certainty and confidence, a specific form of therapy in an individual case. Randomised clinical trials will be helpful in achieving this goal. Until such studies are done and the data tabulated, each case should be evaluated independently and the physician should choose the form of therapy which seems most appropriate in view of the overall clinical situation.

REFERENCES

Brady L W, Shields J A, Augsberger J J, Day J L 1982 Malignant intraocular tumors. The Janeway Lecture, American Radium Society. Cancer 49: 578–585

Char D, Castro J R, Quivey J M et al 1980 Helium ion charged particle therapy for choroidal melanoma. Ophthalmology 87: 565–570

Flocks M, Gerende J H, Zimmerman L E 1955 The size and shape of malignant melanomas of the choroid and ciliary body in relation to the prognosis and histological characteristics: A statistical study of 210 tumours. Transactions of the American Academy of Ophthalmology and Otolaryngology 59: 740–758

Fraunfelder F T, Boozman F W, Wilson R S, Thomas A H 1977 No-touch technique for intraocular malignant tumors. Archives of Ophthalmology 95: 1616–1620

Gragoudas E S, Goitein M, Verhey L et al 1980 Proton beam irradiation. An alternative to enucleation for intraocular melanomas. Ophthalmology 87: 571–581

Packer S, Rotman M, Fairchild R, Albert D M, Atkins H L, Chan B 1980 Irradiation of choroidal melanoma with iodine-125 ophthalmic plaque. Archives of Ophthalmology 98: 1453–1457

Peyman G A, Raichand M 1978 Resection of choroidal melanomas. In: Jakobiec F A (ed) Ocular and adnexal tumors. Aesculapius, Birmingham, p 61

Shammas H F, Blodi F C 1977 Prognostic factors in choroidal and ciliary body melanomas. Archives of Ophthalmology 95: 63–69

Shields J A 1977 Current approaches to the diagnosis and management of choroidal melanomas. Survey of Ophthalmology 21: 443–463

Shields J A 1978 Accuracy and limitation of the P-32 test in the diagnosis of ocular tumors. An analysis of 500 cases. Ophthalmology 85: 950–966

Shields J A 1983 Diagnosis and management of intraocular tumors. Mosby, St Louis

Shields J A, Augsburger J J 1980 The management of choroidal melanomas. American Journal of Ophthalmology 90: 266–268

Shields J A, Augsburger J J, Brady L W, Day J L 1982 Cobalt plaque therapy for posterior uveal melanomas. Ophthalmology 89: 1201–1207

Zimmerman L E, McLean I W, Foster W P 1978 Does enucleation of an eye containing a malignant melanoma prevent or accelerate the dissemination of tumor cells? British Journal of Ophthalmology 62: 420–425

11. Macular disease with serious retinal detachment

A. C. Bird

Retinal detachment due to functional changes in the subretinal structures has been recorded for many years but it was not until the advent of fluorescein angiography with stereoscopic imaging and the more widespread use of stereo-biomicroscopy that some understanding was brought to the nature of these disorders. In 1967, Gass produced his monograph which is a landmark since for the first time disease entities became well defined and the distinction was made between lesions with and without subretinal neovascularisation. The crucial role of proliferation of vessels derived from the choroid in the subretinal space in the pathogenesis of disciform macular disease was emphasised in subsequent publications (Teeters & Bird, 1973a,b). The importance of disciform degeneration in ophthalmology has been underlined by appreciation that this disorder is now the commonest cause of registered blindness in England (Sorsby, 1966) and by the recent publication of controlled clinical trials showing undoubted benefit to the patient with laser photocoagulation.

During the last few years major efforts have been made in research to gain a better understanding of the pathogenesis of disciform macular disease to determine the best treatment techniques.

RESEARCH

It is acknowledged that the behaviour of subretinal blood vessels determines the outcome of a disciform lesion. Evidence from histopathological studies suggests that subretinal neovascularisation is multifocal and may occur at any retinal location. By contrast clinically evident disciform lesions are confined very largely to the macular area. To resolve this apparent dilemma it is important to understand the behaviour of subretinal new vessels. Histopathological studies have shown that perforation of Bruch's membrane occurs throughout the fundus (Brown, 1940) and is a constant finding in the pre-equatorial region (Friedmann et al, 1963; Riechling & Klemens, 1940). Perforation of Bruch's membrane is also commonly seen histopathologically in the posterior fundus in patients in whom it had not been recognised clinically (Green & Key, 1977). These studies indicate that perforation of Bruch's membrane alone does not give rise to a clinically recognisable lesion and may not result in visual disability. It is evident that such neovascular complexes must undergo rapid proliferation before they can become evident during life and that such rapid proliferation occurs in only a very small percentage of subretinal new vessel complexes.

It has become evident recently that blood vessel behaviour is determined very largely by its environment. The fact that choroidal blood vessels are fenestrated allowing free passage of small molecules from the lumen to the extracellular space, and that retinal blood vessels have tight intercellular junctions and endothelial cells which modify metabolically the passage of molecules across the lumen is determined by the environment within the choroid and retina. The separation of these two circulations by Bruch's membrane and the retinal pigment epithelium must somehow be a reflection of metabolic influences preventing proliferation of blood vessels in these regions. The responsiveness of vascular systems to changes of environment have been well illustrated (Folkman et al, 1971; Folkman, 1974; Silver, 1980). It has been shown that diffusible agents derived from tumour cells and activated macrophages implanted into the cornea will stimulate invasion of the cornea by new blood vessels and that cartilage blocks this response. These experiments illustrate that blood vessel behaviour is determined by the balance of environmental influences: growth occurring when there is an excess of stimulatory over inhibitory stimuli and closure when the balance is reversed.

In order to identify the possible changes in tissue environment occurring with age which may be responsible for inducing new vessel proliferation from the choroid several studies are available. These have concentrated on changes in Bruch's membrane which occur with age.

For many years it was thought that a fracture in Bruch's membrane was essential for blood vessels to grow into the subretinal space and that calcification of Bruch's membrane may render it brittle allowing fractures to occur (Hogan, 1967). However, it has yet to be shown that fractures in Bruch's membrane are an essential prerequisite for perforation of this membrane by choroidal blood vessels. Furthermore, as was argued by Hagerdoorn (1939) and by Ashton & Sorsby (1951), ruptures of Bruch's membrane are alone insufficient to cause subretinal neovascularisation, since angioid streaks and traumatic ruptures are not inevitably followed by disciform degeneration. It has also been suggested that closure of choroidal capillaries may play a role in the stimulus to new vessel growth because of the consequent ischaemia (Klein, 1951). Recent histopathological studies have shown a relatively intact choriocapillaris beneath some disciform lesions (Kornsweig et al, 1966) and Sarks (1973) showed that subretinal new vessels did not occur at sites of choroidal ischaemia. It appears now that gradual age changes at the level of Bruch's membrane which are accompanied by formation of drusen are crucial to the pathogenesis of subretinal neovascularisation.

PATHOGENESIS OF DRUSEN

Progressive thickening of Bruch's membrane has been recorded with age (Hogan, 1967; Hogan et al, 1971). Changes have been noted in the collagen and elastic fibres and there is progressive deposition of abnormal material in the inner part of Bruch's membrane. All the evidence now indicates that the material is derived from the pigment epithelium and is related to disordered photoreceptor outer segment handling by the pigment epithelium. During life there appears to be progressive disorder of this system. After the age of 30 years accumulation of long term phagosomes has been seen in the retinal pigment epithelial cells as lipid deposits (liposomes) (Feeney, 1978; Feeney-Burns, 1980) suggesting decreasing ability of the lysosomal enzymes to degrade phagosomal material. By the age of 50 years deposits of amorphous material appear between Bruch's membrane and the basement membrane of the retinal pigment epithelium. Sarks (1976) and Hogan suggested this to be accumulation of debris voided by the pigment epithelial cell which was then being incompletely cleared via the choriocapillaris. Hogan also inferred that progression of this progress leads to the formation of dense deposit which displaced the pigment epithelium from the inner surface of Bruch's membrane thus forming drusen. Sarks (1976) documented this as a progressive phenomenon histologically and has recently described the evolution of drusen with age (1980). The drusen initially are small (50 μm), dense in consistency and basophilic. With time they become less dense, larger and acidophilic, and finally they become confluent. During the development of drusen a second layer of abnormal material accumulates which Sarks termed the basal linear deposit. It is fibrillary in nature (Hogan et al, 1971) and appears to consist of basement membrane material. Within the abnormal material there is an ingress of macrophages (Sarks, 1980) and the fibrous layers of Bruch's membrane become thinned, particularly at the sites of macrophage accumulation.

It is likely that the combined effect of deposition of abnormal material derived from the pigment epithelial cells due to disturbance of outer segment handling, and abnormal basement membrane production, cause disruption of the structure of Bruch's membrane which may in turn allow choroidal blood vessels to grow towards the retina. The presence of activated macrophages may cause thinning of the fibrous layers and their presence stimulate blood vessel growth.

The second dilemma apparent when comparing histopathological findings and clinical findings in disciform macular degeneration relate to the site of new vessel proliferation. Why is it that perforation of Bruch's membrane by choroidal blood vessels occurs throughout the fundus and yet rapid proliferation of such new vessel complex is only rarely seen outside the macular region (Silva & Brockhurst, 1976; Mazow & Ruiz, 1973)? No striking qualitative difference can be identified histopathologically between the peripheral fundus and the central fundus concerning the deposition of phakosomal material and basement membrane change, although clinical evidence suggests that drusen are much more common in the posterior pole than in the periphery. Further studies may imply that there are fundamental differences between age change in different parts of the fundus. An alternative explanation may be a difference in tissue reactivity in different parts of the eye. It is possible that the response to age change at Bruch's membrane differs between the macula and the peripheral retina. Research into putative differences in responsiveness might be important in giving further understanding of the disciform process. Such research may also give some clue as to the cause of racial differences of disciform macular disease, since it has been clearly demonstrated that disciform degeneration is common in Caucasian societies but is rare amongst Negroes and Mongoloid races (Gregor & Joffe, 1978). Negroes do have age-related changes at the level of Bruch's membrane but the neovascular response causing visual loss only rarely takes place. This may be comparable with low incidence of disciform lesions in blacks with the presumed ocular histoplasma syndrome (Baskin et al, 1980).

Ryan (1982) has been very successful in developing an animal homologue of disciform macular disease. High intensity laser lesions have been placed at various sites in the fundus of rhesus monkeys. In about one-third of lesions near the foveola there has been subsequent proliferation of blood vessels derived from the choroid in the subretinal space. These neovascular complexes show rapid proliferation during the early period following photocoagulation and during this early period the blood vessels leaked fluorescein during angiography and were shown on histopathological examination to have fenestrated endothelial cells. During the subsequent weeks the proliferation became progressively slower and the leakage less evident. Finally there was some reduction in the capillary content of the new vessel complexes and the blood vessels lost their fenestrations. Thus in the old lesion the blood vessels had characteristics more similar to retinal vessels than choroidal vessels. The response to peripheral lesions was in marked contrast to central lesions. In only 1 out of 290 non-macular laser burns did proliferation of blood vessels occur.

This animal model of disciform macular disease is extremely valuable since the behaviour of the neovascular complex is very similar to that observed in man. The time course of the lesion is somewhat shorter than seen in senile disciform macular disease in that the sequence of growth stability and resolution of the neovascular process occurred wihin 8–12 weeks whereas in senile macular degeneration it may be 3 years before the vascular complex becomes stable. On the other hand the intervals do not differ markedly from that seen in myopia or presumed ocular histoplasma syndrome in man. This model provides a good substrate to investigate the differential behaviour of lesions in the central fundus and peripheral fundus. It is conceivable that the initial lesion is different in that defocusing of the laser beam will reduce the energy density of light incident at Bruch's membrane and therefore change the pattern of damage. However, the difference in reactivity is so marked that it is unlikely that variations of the laser lesions alone would explain the difference in behaviour characteristics.

TREATMENT

In 1982 three randomised control trials were published in which it as shown that laser photocoagulation confers significant benefit to visual prognosis in the treatment of senile disciform macular disease (Moorfields Macular Study Group, 1982; Coscas & Soubrane, 1982; Macular Photocoagulation Study Group, 1982). All three studies used very similar protocols, the patients being limited to those over 50 years who had clinical evidence of age-related change in the ocular fundus recognisable as drusen and who had subretinal neovascular complexes which were well defined and which approached within 200 μm of the foveola in the American study and 100 μm of the foveola in the two European studies. All three tested the potential benefit of Argon blue/green energy. Benefits of treatment appeared to be somewhat greater in the American study than the British study. This difference might be due to the slight differences in protocol between the two studies. In the American study all patients treated were given retrobulbar anaesthesia and the levels of energy used were somewhat greater than the British study. Differences may also be accounted for by the differences in patients admitted to the two trials; there were more patients with neovascular tissue distant from the fovea and more older patients in the American than the British study and in the American study it was shown that it was precisely in these patients that the therapy conferred most benefit.

Ophthalmologists and their patients will be heartened by the positive results of these prospective randomised clinical trials. However, this form of treatment will not be of great benefit to the patient community without some modification of clinical practice. It is a universal experience amongst ophthalmologists that only a minority of patients with senile disciform macular disease are suitable for treatment when first seen. No more than 5–10% of patients presenting with senile disciform macular degeneration to the ophthalmologists have lesions in which the neovascular complex does not underlie the fovea. In the remainder laser destruction of the neovascular tissue would also destroy the foveola and defeat the object of therapy. There is little doubt that the low percentage of patients with treatable lesions is due to the length of time between the presenting symptom and the first visit to an ophthalmologist. It is during this critical period that there is rapid growth of the subretinal new vessels towards the foveola. On one study 80% of patients who presented to an ophthalmologist within 2 weeks of their initial symptom were treatable but the percentage fell to 40% when the interval was 1 month and was less than 10% when the interval was 4 months (Grey et al, 1979). Another useful attribute of treatable lesions was identified. It was shown that patients with a visual acuity of 6/18 of better had a good chance of having a treatable lesion whereas those with 6/36 or worse had a very small chance of being suitable for photocoagulation. This study is encouraging in that it implies that if patients were seen early in the course of their disorder, most could be treated but clearly demonstrates that a change in clinical practice is needed if the full potential benefit of this treatment is to be realised. The onus will fall upon those in primary care to initiate rapid referral but there are important implications in respect of working habits and work load of ophthalmologists.

The information derived from behavioural studies suggests that certain guidelines can be laid down concerning the management of senile disciform macular degeneration in the community. The presenting symptoms are distortion and blurring of central vision. If a patient is recognised in practice with a short history of progressive visual blurring, distortion and good visual acuity, the likelihood of the causative lesion being treatable is high. Recognition of such patients should be followed by urgent assessment by fluorescein angiography. This condition should be managed with the same degree of urgency as a potential retinal detachment.

Within the last few months two further controlled studies have been published demonstrating that argon laser photocoagulation for disciform macular lesions as part of presumed ocular histoplasmosis and in patients with no other ocular disease, so-called idiopathic neovascularisation, also confers benefit on the visual prognosis (Macular Photocoagulation Study Group, 1983a, b). The constraints on treatment are very similar to those in senile macular disease. It is unlikely that controlled trials will be undertaken on uncommon disorders since it would be impossible to achieve large enough numbers for such trials to be helpful. It is interesting that treatment has been helpful in conditions causing disciform degeneration which are quite different from one another. In senile macular disease the changes at the level of Bruch's membrane are diffuse, whereas in ocular histoplasmosis it may be assumed that the disease is multifocal. The difference in the basic disorders almost certainly explains the different untreated visual prognosis and the different patterns of growth of neovascular tissue. Whilst proof does not exist the combined studies imply that most if not all conditions with subretinal neovascularisation threatening central vision should be treated if the description of the new vessel complex conforms to the criteria laid down within the controlled trials.

It is quite clear that while this form of treatment is better than no treatment, it is not ideal. Argon laser photocoagulation, as it has been assessed in clinical trials, is relatively ineffective when the neovascular complex is nearer than 200 μm from the foveola. It has been demonstrated that a very large proportion of the shorter wavelength blue line energy from the argon laser is absorbed within the luteal pigment such that most of the laser energy will be absorbed in the neuroretina rather than at the level of the pigment epithelium (Marshall & Bird, 1979). This would prevent adequate exposure of the subretinal neovascular tissue near the foveola and also cause damage to centrifugal neurons such that the foveola may be denervated by parafoveolar lesions. This disadvantage may be avoided by using the green line only of the argon laser since only 10% of this wavelength is absorbed in the luteal pigment. Longer wavelength such as the yellow line or the red line of krypton may prove even more helpful although the greater absorption of the longer wavelengths within the choroid rather than the pigment epithelium may prove to be a disadvantage. These potential advantages and disadvantages can be identified theoretically but can only be tested by further controlled trials. Several controlled trials are already underway comparing different wavelengths of laser energy and hopefully within the next 2–3 years further results will give us additional guidance as to the ideal wavelength for laser photocoagulation of disciform macular disease; it is to be hoped that the longer wavelengths will increase the number of patients suitable for treatment as well as the visual results of treatment.

It is clear that the basic disorder, namely the deposition of abnormal material beneath the retina, has not been modified and a risk of recurrent growth of new vessels exists. It has also been shown that elderly patients with detachment of the pigment epithelium but without subretinal new vessel formation do not benefit significantly from photocoagulation as used by the Moorfields Macular Study Group (1979). In this trial argon blue/green energy was used and the lesions were coagulated more than once if persistent detachment was identified on the first post-treatment visit. This study demonstrated that the visual prognosis for those patients treated was worse for those patients left untreated during the early part of the study. The differential behaviour between the two groups can be accounted for by a combination of three factors. Although tearing of the pigment epithelium was no more common in one group than the other, it occurred immediately after photocoagulation in the treated group whereas it occurred some time after photocoagulation in the untreated group. It was also identified that in untreated patients the presence of subretinal new vessels did not necessarily prejudice visual acuity for several months. In such patients the neovascular tissue was identified to be growing on the outer surface of the pigment epithelium such that the metabolic relationship between the pigment epithelium and the receptors was not altered. This was in marked contrast to treated patients who all lost vision if subretinal neovascularisation occurred. Finally it was recorded that many patients who were successfully treated from the morphological standpoint lost vision. It is conceivable that flattening of the pigment epithelium itself may induce visual loss but it was thought much more likely that absorption by blue/green energy in the neuroretina around the foveola caused denervation of the foveola and consequent loss of visual acuity.

If a further controlled trial is to be undertaken these factors should be borne in mind in the designed trial. Patients likely to suffer a tear of the pigment epithelium could be excluded since this complication is limited largely to patients with big pigment epithelial detachments which have a homogenous appearance and in which fluorescein appears to accumulate slowly. Choice of a wavelength other than blue/green may also avoid visual loss occurring following apparently successful treatment.

REFERENCES

Ashton N, Sorsby 1951 A fundus dystrophy with unusual features, a histological study. British Journal of Ophthalmology 35: 751
Baskin M A, Jampol L M, Huamonte F U, Rabb M F, Vygantas C M, Wyhinny G 1980 Macular lesions in blacks with the presumed ocular histoplasmosis syndrome. American Journal of Ophthalmology 89: 77–83
Brown E V L 1940 Retroretinal tissue from the choroid in Kuhnt-Junius degeneration of the macula. Archives of Ophthalmology 23: 1157
Coscas G, Soubrane G 1982 Photocoagulation de neovaisseaux sous-retiniens par le laser a argon dans la degenerescence maculaire senile: resultats de l'etude randomisee de 60 cas. Bulletins et Memoires de la Société Francaise d'Ophtalmologie 83: 102–105
Feeney L 1978 Lipofuscin and melanin of human retinal pigment epithelium. Investigative Ophthalmology and Visual Science 17: 583–607
Feeney-Burns L 1980 Lipofuscin of pigment retinal human epithelium. American Journal of Ophthalmology 90: 783–791
Folkman J, Merler E, Abernathy C 1971 Isolation of a tumour factor responsible for angiogenesis. Journal of Experimental Medicine 133: 275–288
Friedmann E, Smith T R, Kuwabara T 1963 Senile choroidal vascular patterns and drusen. Archives of Ophthalmology 69: 220
Gass J D M 1967 The pathogenesis of disciform detachment of the neuroepithelium. American Journal of Ophthalmology 63: 575
Green W R, Key S N 1977 Senile macular degeneration; a histopathological study. Transactions of the American Ophthalmological Society 75: 180
Gregor Z, Joffe L 1978 Senile macular degeneration in Black African. British Journal of Ophthalmology 62: 8, 547–550
Grey R H B, Bird A C, Chisholm L H 1979 Senile disciform macular degeneration; features indicating suitability for photocoagulation. British Journal of Ophthalmology 63: 85–89
Hagerdoorn A 1939 Angioid streaks. Archives of Ophthalmology 21: 746
Hogan M J 1967 Bruch's membrane and disease of the macula; the role of elastic tissue and collagen. Transactions of the Ophthalmological Societies of the United Kingdom 87: 113
Hogan M J, Alverado J, Weddell J E 1971 Histology of the human eye: an atlas and textbook. Saunders, Philadelphia, p 334
Klein B 1951 Macular lesions of vascular origin. American Journal of Ophthalmology 34: 1279
Kornsweig A L, Eliasoph I, Feldstein M 1966 Retinal vasculature in macular degeneration. Archives of Ophthalmology 75: 224
Macular Photocoagulation Study Group 1982 Argon laser photocoagulation for senile macular degeneration; results of a randomised clinical trial. Archives of Ophthalmology 100: 912
Macular Photocoagulation Study Group 1983a Argon laser photocoagulation for ocular histoplasmosis. Archives of Ophthalmology 101: 1347–1357
Macular Photocoagulation Study Group 1983b Argon laser photocoagulation for idiopathic neovascularization. Archives of Ophthalmology 101: 9, 1358–1361
Marshall J, Bird A C 1979 A comparative histopathological study of argon and krypton laser irradiations of the human retina. British Journal of Ophthalmology 63: 657–668
Mazow M L, Ruiz R S 1973 Eccentric disciform degeneration. Transactions in American Ophthalmology and Otolaryngology 77: 68
Moorfields Macular Study Group 1979 Retinal pigment epithelial detachments in the elderly: a controlled trial of laser photocoagulation. British Journal of Ophthalmology 63: 669
Moorfields Macular Study Group 1982 Treatment of senile disciform macular degeneration: a single-blind randomised trial by argon laser photocoagulation. British Journal of Ophthalmology 66: 745–753
Riechling W, Klemens F 1940 Uber eine gefabfduhrende bindegewebsschicht zeischen dem pigment epithel der retina und der lamina vitrea. Albrecht von Grafes Archiv für Klinische und Experimentelle Ophthalmologie 141: 500
Ryan S J 1982 Subretinal neovascularization: natural history of an experimental model. Archives of Ophthalmology 100: 1804–1809

Sarks S H 1973 New vessel formation beneath the retinal pigment epithelium in senile eyes. British Journal of Ophthalmology 57: 951

Sarks S H 1976 Ageing and degeneration in the macular region: a clinico-pathological study. British Journal of Ophthalmology 60: 324

Sarks S H 1980 Drusen and their relationship to senile macular degeneration. Australian Journal of Ophthalmology 8: 117–130

Silva V B, Brockhurst R J 1976 Hemorhagic detachment of the peripheral retinal pigment epithelium. Archives of Ophthalmology 94: 1295–1299

Silver I A 1980 Physiology of wound healing. In: Hunt T K (ed) Wound healing and wound infection: theory and surgical practice. Appleton-Century-Crofts, p 11

Sorsby A 1966 The incidence and causes of blindness in England and Wales 1948–1962. Reports on public health and medical subjects, No 144. Her Majesty's Stationery Office, London, p 14

Teeters V W, Bird A C 1973a A clinical study of vascularity of senile disciform degeneration. American Journal of Ophthalmology 75: 53

Teeters V W, Bird A C 1973b The development of neovascularization of senile disciform degeneration. American Journal of Ophthalmology 76: 1

12. Glaucoma

R. Mapstone

An association between diabetes and primary open angle glaucoma is generally accepted together with the notion that, the co-existence of diabetes and ocular hypertension delineates an individual at particular risk of developing field loss. This section begins by looking at the evidence for the putative association between glaucoma and diabetes.

DIABETES AND RAISED PRESSURE

Diabetes and primary open angle glaucoma

Published data refer to the prevalance of open angle glaucoma in patients with diabetes and, to the prevalence of diabetes in patients with open angle glaucoma. For the former Armstrong et al (1960) reported that, in a group of unselected diabetics, the prevalence of open angle glaucoma was 40/1000 compared with a rate of 13/1000 in a control group. The other side of the coin — the prevalence of diabetes in patients with open angle glaucoma — is around 80/1000 (Lieb et al, 1967; Davies, 1980). It is difficult to determine the significance, and the relevance, of these findings and for the following reasons. In affluent societies published prevalence rates for diabetes are numerous, but few allow age specific and sex comparisons to be made. Hamman (1983) has taken this into account and constructed a table of age adjusted prevalence rates from various sources.

This reveals wide variations — from 8.4/1000 to 78/1000 in females and, from 11.8/1000 to 113.4/1000 in males. In developing countries the rates are even more variable, from 3/1000 in a township in Zimbabwe to 344/1000 in a Micronesian population in the South Pacific (Zimmet et al, 1978). So, while there may be an increased prevalence of open angle glaucoma in diabetes there is no compelling reason for asserting that there is an increased prevalence of diabetes in open angle glaucoma. Any relationship that exists between diabetes and open angle glaucoma is not therefore as clear-cut as has been claimed (Becker, 1971).

Diabetes and primary closed angle glaucoma

Becker (1968) wrote that there "appeared" to be no association between diabetes and closed angle glaucoma prevalence. An observation that seems to be confirmed by a population study (Nielsen, 1983) which found one patient with closed angle glaucoma in a diabetic population. However, because there is a low prevalence of closed angle glaucoma in diabetes, it is not a necessary consequence that there is a low prevalence of diabetes in closed angle glaucoma, neither is there any published evidence to show that the question has been investigated.

Diabetes and ocular hypertension

Armaly (1969), during the follow-up of a group of patients with ocular hypertension, discovered four who had developed field loss, and all four demonstrated abnormal glucose tolerance test results. Wilensky et al (1974) reported a similar experience. Consequently it became accepted that a combination of diabetes and ocular hypertension represented an individual at particular risk.

Bankes (1967), using data obtained from the Bedford glaucoma survey, found that the intra-ocular pressure in diabetics and "pre-diabetics" was no different from that in the general population. Becker (1971) however recorded an increased mean intra-ocular pressure in diabetics with no retinopathy. More recently Klein & Klein (1984) investigated a population of 2103 diabetics in Wisconsin and, below age 30, the prevalence of ocular hypertension was 68/1000 in females and 59/1000 in males. Above age 30 the rates were 96/1000 and 73/1000 respectively — little different from the prevalence rates in the population at large (Hollows & Graham, 1966).

Bankes (1967) also looked at the rate of diabetes in ocular hypertension and recorded a figure of 16.6/1000. So, again, any relationship that may exist between ocular hypertension and diabetes is unremarkable. This does not imply that a relationship is absent. There may exist within a glaucomatous population subgroups in which there is a relationship but, because of the way in which the glaucomas are classified, the relationship is obscured.

The diagnostic difficulty

One of the major problems involved in evaluating the prevalence of diabetes in glaucoma samples concerns the question of diabetes diagnosis. In North America the usual oral glucose load is 100 g whereas, in Europe, a 50 g load is preferred. Again, the National Diabetes Data Group (1979) placed emphasis upon a raised plasma fasting glucose concentration, the European Association for the Study of Diabetes however, based diagnosis upon blood glucose concentrations after an oral glucose load. In 1980 the WHO Expert Committee on Diabetes Mellitus made recommendations for diagnosis which were similar to those proposed by both European and North American study groups. It proposed a standard glucose load of 75 g for adults with fasting and 2-hour post-ingestion glucose values being of major diagnostic value. They also recognised two abnormal states, diabetes and impaired glucose tolerance, the latter state removing the dubious terms latent, chemical, suspect, borderline and sub-clinical diabetes. If a fasting venous plasma value ≥ 8 mmol/l was found, that was classed as diabetic. If the 2-hour venous plasma sample was ≥ 11 mmol/l that too was classed as diabetic. If the fasting level was < 8 mmol/l, but the 2-hour sample ≥ 8 mmol/l but, < 11 mmol/l, then that response was classed as impaired glucose tolerance.

The relationship between diabetics/impaired glucose tolerance and the primary glaucomas/ocular hypertension.

Mapstone & Clark (1984) following the criteria suggested by the WHO (see above), looked at the prevalence of diabetes/impaired glucose tolerance in 316 patients with open angle glaucoma, closed angle glaucoma or ocular hypertension. The patients were divided into three groups, those with open angle glaucoma or ocular hypertension and wide angles; those with open angle glaucoma or ocular hypertension and narrow angles and, those with closed angle glaucoma. Their table records the results and shows that there was a preponderance of diabetes/impaired glucose tolerance in patients with narrow angles — no matter whether the clinical diagnosis was open angle glaucoma, closed angle glaucoma or ocular hypertension. If the proportion of patients with *narrow* angle eyes, who developed an abnormal response to an oral glucose load, was compared with the proportion in patients with *wide* angle eyes, then there was a highly significant difference between the two ($\chi^2 = 12.12$, p = 0.0005). The anterior chamber depth of each patient was also known and, if the clinical diagnosis was ignored and, the probability of demonstrating an abnormal glucose tolerance test response plotted against anterior chamber depth, then the result was as shown in Figure 12.1. There was a highly significant negative linear correlation between the

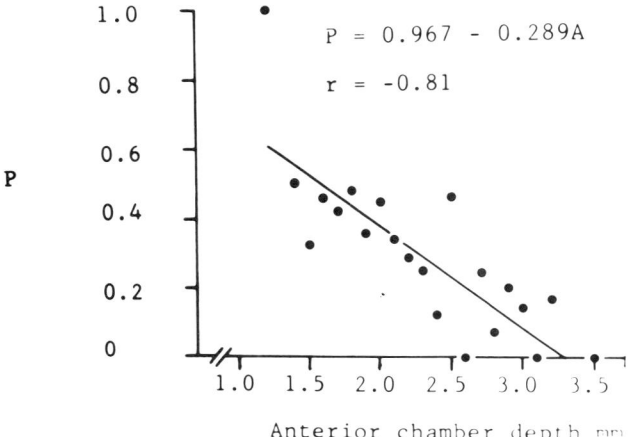

Fig. 12.1   A plot of the probability (P) of demonstrating an abnormal response to an oral glucose tolerance test against anterior chamber depth (A).

probability of an abnormal response and anterior chamber depth ($r = -0.81$, $p < 0.001$). Furthermore, there was no significant difference between the proportion of eyes with narrow angles, who developed an abnormal response, and the proportion in eyes with closed angle glaucoma. There does therefore appear to be an association between diabetes/impaired glucose tolerance and primary glaucoma/ocular hypertension but, the association is not with the disease, rather, it is with the anatomical dimensions of the anterior segment of the eye.

AUTONOMIC NEUROPATHY

Diabetes and autonomic neuropathy

One of the consequences of diabetes in man may be an autonomic neuropathy which was first adequately described by Rundles (1945). It is a multi-system disease capable of producing widespread signs and symptoms involving the cardiovascular, respiratory, gastrointestinal and urogenital systems together with involvement of sweat mechanisms and temperature control. Since its first description the literature has become voluminous and, during the past decade or so, attention has been directed to the diagnosis of this entity using simple, non-invasive bedside tests (Johnson & Spalding, 1974; Ewing, 1978; Hosking et al, 1978; Clarke et al, 1979).

All of the commonly used tests utilise cardiovascular reflexes and, if an abnormality is demonstrated, it is inferred that other parts of the autonomic nervous system are involved too. Each test depends upon a stimulus contrived by the clinician, this in turn is processed by the central nervous system and, the reflex response measured — either a change in heart rate or blood pressure.

Five tests are routinely used, in three of which the effect upon heart rate is measured and, in the other two, a change in blood pressure. If an abnormality is found in any one of the three tests which monitor heart rate (response to a Valsalva manoeuvre, to deep breathing and to a positional change from lying to standing) then a neuropathy involving the parasympathetic supply to the heart is inferred (Ewing, 1983). Conversely, if an abnormality is found in the blood pressure response to the remaining two tests (postural fall in blood pressure in response to standing, blood pressure response to a sustained hand grip) then a neuropathy involving the sympathetic innervation to blood pressure control mechanisms is inferred. Sufficient experience has now been obtained with these tests to indicate that autonomic neuropathy is more widespread in diabetics than symptoms would suggest (Ewing, 1983), with parasympathetic tests being more commonly abnormal than those involving the sympathetic. Ewing (1983) has shown that approximately one third of diabetic patients demonstrate a parasympathetic abnormality with a lesser involvement of the sympathetic. Furthermore autonomic function test responses deteriorate with time and, progress from parasympathetic damage to combined para- and sympathetic damage. They also have predictive value — the mortality rate is significantly increased during a 5 year period if the initial tests revealed an autonomic neuropathy.

Clark & Mapstone (1984) applied the same five tests of autonomic function to the sample of 316 patients described above (Fig. 12.1). They found that 60% of the patients demonstrated an abnormal response to one or more of the five tests. This contrasted with 7% in a control sample of 70 patients without primary glaucoma or ocular hypertension. The sample was therefore significantly different from normal, and showed a greater prevalence of autonomic neuropathy than is described in diabetic populations.

Denervation supersensitivity

In 1939 Cannon enunciated his law of denervation as follows "When in a series of afferent neurones, a unit is destroyed, an increased irritability to chemical agents develops in the isolated structure or structures, the effect being maximal in the part directly innervated". Two diseases of ophthalmological interest illustrate this phenomenon, namely, Horner's and Adie's syndrome. In the former (with a post-ganglionic lesion) a denervation supersensitivity to sympathomimetic amines has been clearly demonstrated (Thompson & Mensher, 1971) whereas, in the latter, $2\frac{1}{2}$% Mecholyl produces a marked sustained miosis (Scheie & Adler, 1940).

The cause of the supersensitivity is partly explained by considering the fate of noradrenaline. Endogenously released noradrenaline activates postsynaptic receptors, and is then removed from the synaptic cleft in one of two ways. The most important, uptake 1, is a "high affinity" process whereby noradrenaline re-enters adrenergic neurones and is incorporated into intracellular vesicles for future use. The second mechanism — uptake 2 — is particularly active when high levels of *plasma* noradrenaline appear. The recipient cells are non-neuronal and, because they contain no storage vesicles, the incorporated noradrenaline is destroyed.

When therefore a sympathetically innervated tissue is partially, or completely, denervated the sites available for uptake 1 will be reduced. Consequently endogenously released, or exogenously applied, sympathomimetic amines will 'hang around' in the synaptic cleft and produce a greater effect. If neurone depletion is a local phenomenon then the effects are necessarily restricted (e.g. in Horner's syndrome). But, if extensive neuropathy is present, then diffuse effects are to be expected (Robertson, 1979). Released acetylcholine does not participate in an uptake process for the reason that it is rapidly destroyed by acetylcholinesterase.

A second reason why supersensitivity may develop depends upon the relationship that exists between the number of postsynaptic adrenoceptors present in a tissue and their exposure to agonist drugs (Catt et al, 1979). In patients with phaeochromocytoma (and consequently increased levels of plasma noradrenaline) there is a decrease in the number of alpha receptors on platelets (Davies et al, 1981). Conversely, patients with widespread autonomic dysfunction (and low levels of plasma noradrenaline) demonstrate an increased number of platelet alpha receptors (Davies et al, 1982). It is to be expected therefore that a denervated tissue will have an increased number of receptors (and/or altered reactivity, Furchgott, 1964; Venter, 1980) so that exposure to an agonist drug may produce an enhanced response. Smith et al (1983) point out that the supersensitivity of the diabetic pupil to topically applied phenylephrine may depend upon some such mechanism as this because phenylephrine has a negligible affinity for a neuronal uptake mechanism (Burgen & Iverson, 1965).

Diabetes and the pupil

There are a number of diseases, both systemic and ocular, which are associated with damage to the autonomic nervous system and all demonstrate, in some degree, pupillary abnormalities.

Progressive autonomic failure, either alone, or with multiple system atrophy (Shy Drager syndrome) or with Parkinson's disease, demonstrate pupillary involvement — Horner's syndrome, alternating anisocoria or super-sensitivity to topically applied Methacholine (Bannister, 1983). Again, in amyloid disease, both primary and secondary there are reports of pupillary involvement manifest as abnormalities in size, shape and reactions to light and accommodation (DeNavasquez & Treble, 1938; Andrade, 1952; Juliao et al, 1974; Kito et al, 1973). The mechanism is uncertain but Duke & Paton (1965) correlated the changes with amyloid deposits in ciliary nerves whereas Okajima et al (1978) suggested that the sympathetic post ganglionic fibres were predominantly involved. Of interest too is the scalloped pupil seen in patients with familial amyloidosis (Andrade, 1952) which gives the appearance of multiple radial tears, ascribed by Lessell et al (1975) to amyloid infiltration of the terminal branches of the parasympathetic supply to the sphincter. It has been shown too that the pupil in patients with the Riley–Day syndrome is supersensitive to methacholine (Smith et al, 1965).

The most prevalent and investigated disease, however, is diabetes in which pupillary abnormalities have been recognised for a number of years (Rundles, 1945;

Martin, 1953) and characterised by Lowenstein & Loewenfeld (1969) as having a small rest diameter together with a sluggish response to light. Gunderson (1974) investigated this phenomenon and showed that the pupil of long term diabetics showed an absence of hippus together with small pupils and abnormalities of the light reflex. Findings which were confirmed by Smith et al (1978) who also demonstrated that the pupillary abnormalities were accompanied by signs of systemic autonomic neuropathy. Hreidarsson (1979) and Pfeifer et al (1982) looked at pupillary motility in diabetics of long standing and concluded that the pupillary response to light was no different from that of a control group, the implication being that the abnormalities were not a result of structural change but were rather, a consequence of an autonomic neuropathy involving predominantly the sympathetic innervation to the dilator muscle, with lesser involvement of the parasympathetic. So, electrophysiological studies suggest that, in insulin dependent diabetics of long standing, an abnormality involving both the sympathetic and parasympathetic innervation can be demonstrated.

In 1974, Sigsbee et al demonstrated in diabetics, a pupillary supersensitivity to topical methacholine which varied directly with the degree of peripheral neuropathy. Hayashi & Ishikawa (1978) investigated the response of diabetics with varying degrees of retinopathy to a number of different drugs, including methacholine and adrenaline. They concluded that their results signified a denervation supersensitivity to both sympathetic and parasympathetic agonists, with the sympathetic component more frequently involved. The sensitivity was greatest the greater the degree of retinopathy.

The evidence therefore seems compelling that the diabetic pupil is partly denervated and shows a supersensitivity to the action of exogenously applied autonomic agonists.

CLOSED ANGLE GLAUCOMA AND THE AUTONOMIC NERVOUS SYSTEM

Models of closed angle glaucoma

Provocative tests play an increasingly minor role in the clinical management of patients in whom it is thought that an angle closing mechanism may be operating. The reasons are various, but one is of fundamental importance. The theoretical and experimental base, upon which the commonly used provocative tests rest, is extremely tenuous. So, if a test result is classed positive then that provides no sufficient reason for asserting that the eye in question had, has, or will get any of the several problems to which an angle closing mechanism can lead. None-the-less it is of some relevance to examine, briefly, provocative test mechanisms.

With one exception (prone test) the commonly used provocative tests manipulate the autonomic nervous system. At the same time, varying degrees of pupillary inertia and wide dilatation are achieved by parasympathetic inhibition, or by sympathetic excitation. Differing rates of success are claimed by different investigators (Harris & Galin, 1972; Lichter & Anderson, 1977) but, the essence of a positive test is a pressure increase of 8 mmHg or more, accompanied by a gonioscopically verified closed angle—otherwise it is a 'false positive'. Apart from the fact that no longitudinal studies have been published, from which the predictive value of a test result can be deduced, there is one aspect of these tests which seems crucial to their use. That is the implicit acceptance that pupil dilation is a model of one of the mechanisms that can lead to closed angle glaucoma.

Mapstone (1984a) tested this assumption by looking at patients who had presented with a *unilateral* closed angle glaucoma. The fellow (unaffected) eye was provoked using a combination of pilocarpine and phenylephrine (Mapstone, 1981a). If the test was positive (that is, a pressure increase of 8 mmHg or more, together with closure of at least 90% of the angle and a reduction in outflow facility), it was reversed using a combination of thymoxamine and indentation with a Zeiss gonioprism. At least one week later the same eye was dilated using a parasympatholytic drug (tropicamide 1%), and not one of the 24 eyes investigated developed a closed angle glaucoma in the dilated position. Neither was closed angle glaucoma produced as the pupil moved down, past mid-dilation (Fig. 12.2). Another 42 fellow eyes, which had not developed closed angle glaucoma, were also dilated with tropicamide and two developed a positive test in the dilated position. From these results it necessarily follows that pupil dilation *can* produce a closed angle glaucoma but, it is so uncommon in eyes at great risk, that it cannot be regarded as a model of acute closed angle glaucoma. It is also of interest that no eye developed closed angle glaucoma as the pupil moved down past mid-dilation. Because all pupils were allowed to miose without the help of any added drug, it necessarily follows too that sphincter and dilator muscle contraction, with a power within the physiological range, does not produce closed angle glaucoma at, or around, mid-dilation.

Why then did pilocarpine and phenylephrine produce closed angle glaucoma in high risk eyes whereas pupillary dilation did not? The results (Fig. 12.2) suggest reasons. The pupils of eyes provoked with pilocarpine and phenylephrine moved to

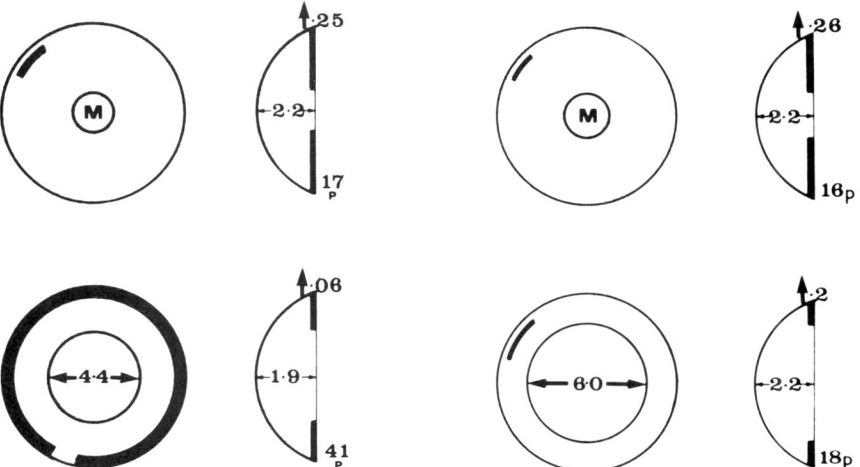

Fig. 12.2   The response of 24 fellow eyes to provocation with pilocarpine and phenylephrine and, their subsequent response to dilation with tropicamide. At the start of provocation with pilocarpine and phenylephrine (upper left) the pupil was mobile (M), mean outflow was 0.25 and mean pressure 17 mmHg. The mean anterior chamber depth (+ corneal thickness) was 2.2 mm. At the end of the test (Bottom left) the angle was largely closed and the pupillary diameter was fixed at a mean of 4.4 mm. At the same time outflow had fallen to 0.06, pressure increased to 41 mmHg and the anterior chamber depth decreased to 1.9 mm. Tropicamide (upper and lower right) had no effect on anterior chamber depth, outflow decreased and pressure increased a little but no eye developed a closed angle although pupillary diameter increased to 6.0 mm.

mid-dilation (mean 4.4mm), at which diameter pupil block is at a maximum (Mapstone, 1983). At the same time the anterior chamber shallowed from a mean of 2.2 mm to a mean of 1.9 mm. The same eyes dilated with tropicamide did not shallow at all and, for the reason that maximal shallowing depends upon the presence of a mid-dilation and increased autonomic activity (Mapstone, 1983). Neither of these requirements are met by a dilated pupil, *however* that may be achieved.

Diabetes and the aetiology of closed angle glaucoma

It seems therefore a reasonable working hypothesis that an experimental model of closed angle glaucoma must fulfil the following requirements:

1. A relatively immobile pupil at around mid-dilation which produces:
2. An increase in the pupil block force which, in turn produces:
3. A shallowing of the anterior chamber.

The sequence of events is illustrated in Figure 12.3 and all derive from a change in autonomic activity. The two small unlettered arrows represent the pupil block force

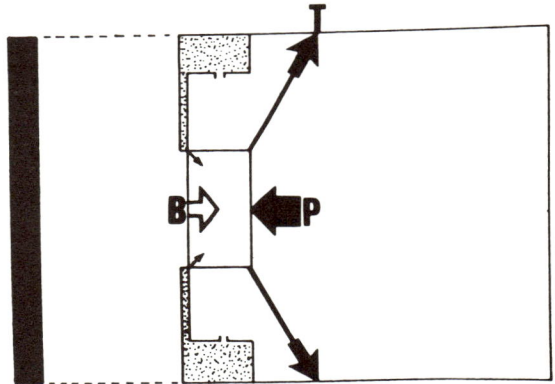

Fig. 12.3   Pupil block (the two small unlettered arrows) generate a force B which tends to push the lens backwards. Accumulated aqueous increases the pressure behind the iris/lens diaphragm and creates a force (P) which tends to push the lens forwards. The interplay of these two forces together with a force produced by zonular stretch (T) determines the depth of the anterior chamber, and whether or not an acute closed angle glaucoma results (Mapstone, 1981b).

apposing iris (stippled area) to lens. The sum of these forces is a net force (B) pushing the lens backwards (Fig. 12.4). At the same time aqueous escape from posterior to anterior chambers is impeded and, if pupil block is large enough, aqueous accumulates within the posterior chamber. The eye is now effectively two separate compartments, the area in front of, and the area behind, the iris/lens diaphragm. A new force (P) is therefore created which pushes or, tends to push, the iris *and* lens forwards. If B is greater than P the anterior chamber deepens; if P is greater than B the anterior chamber shallows until the movement of the iris/lens diaphragm is arrested by a contrary force (T) generated by zonular stretch. This is the essence of a pilocarpine phenylephrine provocative test (Mapstone, 1983).

A relatively immobile pupil is necessary and for the following reasons. The first stage of angle closure (Mapstone, 1983) involves the apposition of peripheral iris to peripheral cornea and this sequestrates a channel of aqueous between the iris

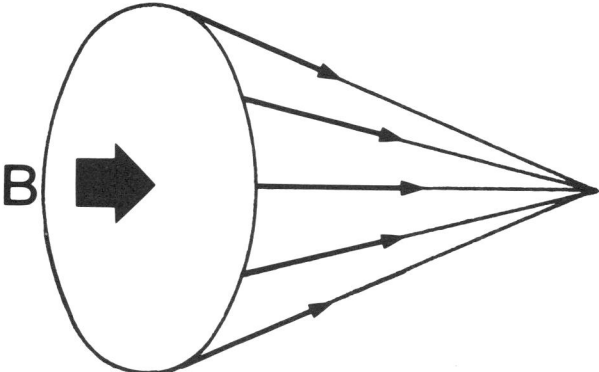

Fig. 12.4   The sphincter muscle apposes iris to lens (that is pupil block), and from each segment of its circumference the sum of these forces is a net force B which tends to push the lens backwards.

posteriorly and the cornea and trabecular meshwork anteriorly, effectively converting the anterior chamber into two separate compartments (Fig. 12.5). If assumptions are made about the dimensions of that sequestrated channel then the volume of aqueous contained therein is about $10 \mu l$. This aqueous has to drain away before the iris can come into contact with trabecular meshwork (so that the angle can become truly closed) and, if outflow is about $2 \mu l/min$ will take 5 minutes or so. In effect this means that one requirement for angle closure is an immobile pupil at mid-dilation. If the pupil were mobile then the sequestrated aqueous would be intermittently in contact with the rest of the anterior chamber and true angle closure would never occur (that is irido-trabecular apposition). A pupil demonstrating restricted movement (for whatever reason) is therefore one of the requirements for a closed angle to develop.

There are, theoretically, several reasons why diabetes/impaired glucose tolerance may be associated with eyes that have either a primary glaucoma or ocular hypertension, but the evidence described above (Fig. 12.1) suggests that the presence of a shallow anterior chamber is crucial.

If an eye already has a shallow anterior chamber then the displacement of the iris/lens diaphragm, required to close the angle, is less than in an eye with a deep anterior chamber. Because passive movement of the dilated pupil past mid-dilation did not precipitate closed angle glaucoma (see above), it necessarily follows that *the* requirement for closure is increased activity within the autonomic nervous system of

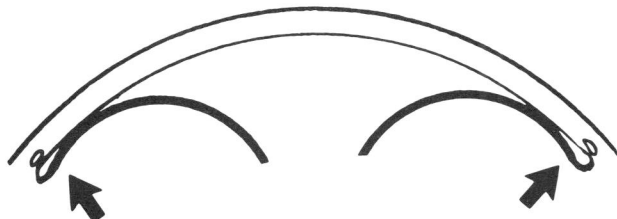

Fig. 12.5   The first stage of angle closure apposes peripheral iris to peripheral cornea, and converts the anterior chamber into two separate compartments. Before true angle closure can occur the circumferential channel of aqueous must escape through the trabecular meshwork so that iris can also become apposed to trabecular meshwork.

the anterior segment. This can be either in response to endogenously released, or to exogenously applied, autonomic agonists.

Pilocarpine 2% plus phenylephrine 10% precipitates closed angle glaucoma in 65% of *fellow* eyes (Mapstone, 1981a) but, if eyes with shallow anterior chambers only are provoked in a similar fashion then the figure drops to less than 5%. Furthermore, if the drug concentrations are reduced to pilocarpine 0.5% and phenylephrine 1% then closed angle glaucoma is readily produced in the *fellow* eye (Mapstone, 1984b).

It is clear therefore that a narrow angle, alone is neither a necessary (Mapstone, 1983) nor a sufficient (Mapstone, 1978) reason, for an eye so endowed, to develop closed angle glaucoma. Other factors are necessary, such as an autonomic neuropathy secondary to impaired glucose metabolism, which provide both pupillary inertia and a supersensitivity to autonomic agonist drugs. A narrow angle by itself is therefore of no particular significance but, associated with neuropathy, the combination predisposes to the development of glaucomatous change and this is one of the reasons for an association between diabetes and glaucoma.

Mixed mechanism pressure increase
Figure 12.1 shows that there is also an association between diabetes/impaired glucose tolerance and eyes with open angle glaucoma/ocular hypertension that happen to have a narrow angle. But, there is no association if the anterior chamber is deep.

The primary adult glaucomas are usually divided into closed and open angle types and regarded as the result of two distinct disease processes. There is, however, good reason to suppose that, occasionally, the two diseases may co-exist in the same patient, producing a combined mechanism or mixed glaucoma. If the two underlying mechanisms are independent, then the probability of any one patient exhibiting a combined mechanism pressure increase can be estimated. Hollows & Graham (1966) derive prevalence figures for open and closed angle glaucoma at 2.8/1000 and

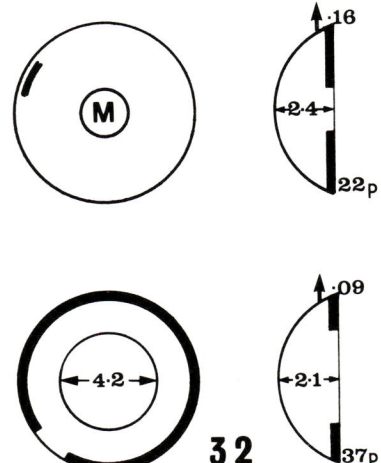

Fig. 12.6 Mean statistics of 32 eyes with ocular hypertension or open angle glaucoma provoked to angle closure with pilocarpine and phenylephrine. At the start of the test the pupil was mobile (M) anterior chamber depth (+ Cornea) was 2.4 mm, outflow 0.16 and intraocular pressure 22 mmHg. At termination the mean values are recorded in the bottom half of the figure.

0.9/1000 respectively; therefore the combined probability of their occurrence is about 2–3/1 000 000 patients. A clinician is therefore unlikely to have any patient with a mixed mechanism attending his/her clinic at any one time. Similar considerations apply to ocular hypertension, the prevalence of which is 86/1000 in the age group 40+ (Hollows & Graham, 1966). So, the probability of seeing an ocular hypertensive, who also has closed angle glaucoma, is about 7–8/100 000. Again, not a common occurrence, but more probable. Mapstone (1984a) described 32 patients with ocular hypertension or open angle glaucoma, in whom an acute closed angle glaucoma was produced by a pilocarpine phenylephrine provocative test (Fig. 12.6). In none was there any reason to suggest that they had developed an acute glaucoma in the past and the only reason for doing a provocative test was the presence of a raised pressure and a narrow angle. These results suggest that the rigid division of the primary glaucomas into open and closed angle types may obscure a common cause in some. They also suggest that if an eye has ocular hypertension and a narrow angle then that narrow angle may be involved in the pathogenesis of the disease process.

REFERENCES

Andrade C 1952 A peculiar form of peripheral neuropathy: familial atypical generalised amyloidosis with special involvement of peripheral nerves. Brain 75: 408–427

Armaly M F 1969 The visual field defect and ocular pressure level in open angle glaucoma. Investigative Ophthalmology 8: 105–124

Armstrong J R, Daily R K, Dobson H I, Gerard L J 1960 The incidence of glaucoma in diabetes mellitus. American Journal of Ophthalmology 50: 55–64

Bankes J L K 1967 Ocular tension and diabetes mellitus. British Journal of Ophthalmology 51: 551–561

Bannister R 1983 Autonomic failure, Oxford University Press, Oxford

Becker B 1967 In: Kimura S J, Caygill W M (eds) Vascular complications of diabetes mellitus, C V Mosby, New York

Becker B 1971 Diabetes mellitus and primary open angle glaucoma. American Journal of Ophthalmology 71: 1–16

Burgen A S V, Iversen L L 1965 The inhibition of noradrenaline uptake by sympathomimetic amines in the rat isolated heart. British Journal of Pharmacology 25: 34–49

Cannon W B, Rosenblueth A 1949 The supersensitivity of denervated structures. A law of denervation. Macmillan, New York

Catt K J, Harwood J P, Aguilera G, Dafau M L 1979 Hormal regulation of peptide receptors and target cell responses. Nature, London 280: 109–116

Clarke B F, Ewing D J, Campbell I W 1979 Diabetic autonomic neuropathy. Diabetologia 17: 195–212

Clark C V, Mapstone R 1984 Autonomic function tests in patients with glaucoma (in press)

Davies E W G 1980 Closed angle glaucoma in diabetic patients. Research and Clinical Forums 1: 85–88

Davies I B, Sever P S 1981 Endogenous agonist regulation of alpha-adrenoceptors in man. Clinical Science 61: Supplement 7

Davies I B, Sudera D, Sagnella G, Marchesi-Saviotti E, Mathias C, Bannister R, Sever P 1982 Increased number of alpha-receptors in sympathetic denervation super-sensitivity in man. Journal of Clinical Investigation 67: 1111–1118

DeNavasquez S, Treble H A 1938 A case of primary generalised amyloid disease with involvement of the nerves. Brain 61: 116–128

Duke J R, Paton D 1965 Primary familial amyloidosis: ocular manifestations with histopathologic observations. Transactions of the American Ophthalmological Society 63: 146–164

Ewing D J 1978 Cardiovascular reflexes and autonomic neuropathy. Clinical Science and Molecular Medicine 55: 321–327

Ewing D J 1983 Practical bedside investigation of diabetic autonomic failure. In: Bannister R (ed) Autonomic failure, Oxford University Press, Oxford

Furchgott R F 1964 Receptor mechanisms. Annual Review of Pharmacology 4: 21–50

Gundersen H J G 1974 An abnormality of the central autonomic nervous system in long term diabetics: absence of hippus. Diabetologia 10: 366

Hamman R F 1983 Diabetics in affluent societies. In: Mann J I, Pyorala K, Teuscher A (eds) Diabetes in epidemiological perspective, Churchill Livingstone, Edinburgh

Harris L S, Galin M A 1972 Prone provocative testing for narrow angle glaucoma. Archives of Ophthalmology 87: 493–496

Hayashi M, Ishikawa S 1978 Pharmacology of pupillary responses in diabetics-correlative study of the responses and grade of retinopathy. Japanese Journal of Ophthalmology 23: 65–72

Hollows F C, Graham P H 1966 The Ferndale glaucoma survey. In: Hunt L B (ed) Glaucoma, E & S Livingstone, Edinburgh

Hosking D J, Bennett T, Hampton J R 1978 Diabetic autonomic neuropathy. Diabetes 27: 1043–1054

Hreidarsson A B 1979 Pupil mobility in long-term diabetics. Diabetologia 17: 145–150

Johnson R H, Spalding J M K 1974 Disorders of the autonomic nervous system, Blackwell, Oxford

Juliao O F, Queirox L S, Lopes de Faria 1974 Portuguese type of familial amyloid polyneuropathy, anatomo-clinical study of a Brazilian family. European Neurology 11: 180–195

Keen H, Jarrett R J, Alberti K G M M 1979 Diabetes mellitus: a new look at diagnostic criteria. Diabetologia 16: 283–285

Kito S, Fujimori N, Yamamoto M 1973 A focus of familial polyneuropathy. Japanese Journal of Clinical Medicine. 31: 2325–2338

Klein B E K, Klein R 1984 Epidemiology of ocular hypertension in a population based study of diabetes. Proceedings 14 International meeting of the Israel Ophthalmological Society (in press)

Lessell S, Wolf P A, Benson M D, Cohen A S 1975 Scalloped pupils in familial amyloidosis. New England Journal of Medicine. 293: 914–915

Lichter P R, Anderson D R 1977 Discussions on glaucoma. Grune & Stratton, New York

Lieb W, Stark N, Jelinck M B, Malzi R 1967 Diabetes mellitus and glaucoma. Acta Ophthalmologica (Supplement 94)

Lowenstein O, Loewenfeld I 1969 The Pupil. In: Davidson H (ed) The Eye, volume 3. Academic Press, New York

Mapstone R 1978 Clinical significance of a narrow angle. Transactions of the Ophthalmological Societies of the United Kingdom 98: 216–218

Mapstone R 1981a The fellow eye. British Journal of Ophthalmology 65: 410–413

Mapstone R 1981b Acute shallowing of the anterior chamber. British Journal of Ophthalmology 65: 446–451

Mapstone R 1983 Glaucoma. In: Davidson S (ed) Recent advances in ophthalmology, Churchill Livingstone, Edinburgh

Mapstone R 1984a Mixed glaucoma. Proceedings 14 International meeting of the Israel Ophthalmological Society (in press)

Mapstone R 1984b Unpublished data

Mapstone R, Clark CV 1984 Diabetes Primary Glaucoma and Ocular Hypertension (in press)

Martin M M 1953 Diabetic neuropathy. Brain 76: 594–624

National Diabetes Data Group 1979 Classification and diagnosis of diabetes mellitus and other categories of glucose intolerance. Diabetes 28: 1039–1057

Nielsen N V 1983 The prevalence of glaucoma and ocular hypertension in Type 1 and 2 diabetes mellitus. Acta Ophthalmologica 61: 662–672

Okajima T, Nagata J, Hatamoto K, Kinoshita Y, Takaba Y, Tokuomi H 1978 Pharmacological studies of the pupils in familial amyloid polyneuropathy. Annals of Neurology 4: 80–84

Pfeifer M A, Cook D, Brodsky J, Tice D, Parrish D, Reenan A, Halter J B, Porte D 1982 Quantitative evaluation of Sympathetic and parasympathetic control of iris function. Diabetes Care 5: 518–528

Rundles R W 1945 Diabetic neuropathy: a general review with a report of 125 cases. Medicine, Baltimore 24: 111–160

Scheie H G, Adler F H 1940 Site of the disturbance of tonic pupils (Adies syndrome). Archives of Ophthalmology 24: 1041–1044

Robertson D 1979 Contraindication to the use of ocular phenylephrine in idiopathic orthostatic hypotension. American Journal of Ophthalmology 87: 819–822

Rundles R W 1945 Diabetic neuropathy: a general review with a report of 125 cases. Medicine, Baltimore 24: 111–160

Scheie H G, Adler F H 1940 Site of the disturbance of tonic pupils (Adies syndrome). Archives of Ophthalmology 24: 1041–1044

Sigsbee B, Torkelson R, Kadis G, Wright J W, Reeves A G 1974 Parasympathetic denervation of the iris in diabetes mellitus. Journal of Neurology, neurosurgery and Psychiatry 37: 1031–1035

Smith A A, Breinin G 1965 Ocular responses to autonomic drugs in familial dysautonomia. Investigative Ophthalmology 4: 458–462

Smith S E, Smith S A, Brown P M, Fox C, Sonksen P H 1978 Pupillary signs in diabetic autonomic neuropathy. British Medical Journal 2: 924–927

Smith S A, Smith S E 1983 Evidence for a neuropathic aetiology in the small pupil of diabetes mellitus. British Journal of Ophthalmology 67: 89–93

Thompson H S, Mensher J H 1971 Adrenergic mydriasis in Horners syndrome. American Journal of
  Ophthalmology 24: 1041–1044
Venter J C 1980 High efficiency coupling between beta-adrenergic receptors and cardiac contractility:
  direct evidence for spare beta-adrenergic receptors. Molecular Pharmacology 16: 429–440
WHO Expert Committee on Diabetes Mellitus. Second report. 1980. WHO Technical report series No 646
Wilensky J T, Podos S M, Becker B 1974 Prognostic indicators in ocular hypertension. Archives of
  Ophthalmology 91: 200–202
Zimmet P, Whitehouse S 1978 Bimodality of fasting and two hour glucose tolerance distributions in a
  Micronesian population. Diabetes 27: 793–800

13. Laser trabeculoplasty

J. B. Wise

EARLY ATTEMPTS AT LASER TRABECULO-PUNCTURE AND LASER TRABECULOTOMY

The first attempts to use laser energy in the treatment of open angle glaucoma were made by Krasnov (1973, 1974), who used Q-switched ruby laser energy to produce multiple perforations of the trabecular meshwork in one quadrant. Excellent and immediate results were obtained with pressures falling to normal in 70–80% of the cases. However, within a few weeks to a maximum of 6 months, nearly all of the pressures returned to the base line. About 35% of the patients ultimately required surgery, the remainder avoiding surgery by a combination of medical therapy and repeated laser trabecular perforations. Hager (1973) used argon laser burns of up to 3 seconds duration to produce 'pores' through the meshwork. Pupil distortion and peripheral anterior synechiae resulted, and very little control was obtained by this method. Hager also attempted to tighten the trabecular meshwork by treating the root of the iris 360 degrees with argon laser burns, not touching the meshwork directly, and achieved approximately 30% control by this indirect method. Worthen & Wickham (1974) performed 'laser trabeculotomy' in one quadrant using up to 150 laser burns of either continuous or pulsed argon laser energy. Their control rate was 33% at 3 months and 17% at 5 years, with 27% surgeries, and they ceased using this method in 1976 (Wickham & Worthen, 1979). Other attempts to produce trabecular puncture were made by Teichmann et al (1976), who utilised burns of up to 1 second and concluded 'the laser is not suitable for treatment of open angle glaucoma' and by Ticho & Zauberman (1976) who used 50 burns of 50 microns diameter at 0.1 second and 1000 mW in one quadrant, repeating the treatment in another quadrant in 55% of the eyes. They obtained a 20% control rate without medication and an additional 50% control rate with medication. Study of laser treatment of open angle glaucoma was almost totally aborted when Gaasterland & Kupfer (1974) demonstrated that confluent laser burns to the trabecular meshwork of the monkey would destroy the meshwork and cause very severe glaucoma. In 1976 the general opinion was that any trabecular perforations obtained would soon close, that scarring of the meshwork would be the only result of the application of laser energy, and that the usefulness of laser treatment of open angle glaucoma was probably very limited.

TRABECULAR RING EXPANSION AS A POSSIBLE CAUSE OF OPEN ANGLE GLAUCOMA

Numerous abnormalities of the trabecular meshwork have been described over the decades, including sclerosis and thickening of the trabecular lamellae, pigment deposits, cellular deposits, glycosaminoglycan deposits, collapse of the inter-trabecular spaces, and the collapse of Schlemm's canal. The latter two findings have been consistently noted since enucleated glaucomatous eyes were subjected to microscopic study a century ago, but have always been attributed to direct effects of the increased intraocular pressure possibly abetted by clogging of the meshwork from various deposits. No previous author, to my knowledge, has considered the possibility that the initial event in open angle glaucoma could be senile stretching of the trabecular tissues, resulting in expansion of the trabecular ring and collapse of the intertrabecular spaces and Schlemm's canal against the unyielding sclera. Because the trabecular meshwork is a ring, there is a fixed geometrical ratio between the circumference and the diameter, namely pi (3.1416 . . .). Any change in the trabecular circumference must necessarily result in corresponding change in the trabecular diameter. Because humans stretch all over as they age, it is quite likely that the tissues of the trabecular meshwork may stretch somewhat as well (Wise & Witter, 1979). A simplified mathematical model, which assumes that the meshwork is lying on the inside of a cylinder, (Tables 13.1 and 13.2) shows that with intertrabecular spaces of 0.5 microns, 0.17% stretch of the trabecular tissues will close all the intertrabecular spaces. With intertrabecular spaces of 6 microns and a Schlemm's canal width of 40 microns, 2.79% linear stretch of the meshwork will totally close the intertrabecular spaces and Schlemm's canal as well (Wise, 1982a). It must be obvious that long before

Table 13.1 Increase in trabecular circumference to collapse 0.5 micron intertrabecular spaces

Individual i-t space	0.5 micron
times	×
Number of spaces	20 spaces
times	×
Both sides of angle	2 sides
equals	=
Total width of i-t spaces	20 microns

$20\,\mu$ diameter $\times 3.1416 = 62.8\,\mu$ Circumference
Total Circumference = 36,000 microns
$62.8/36\,000 = 0.17\%$ increase in Circumference to increase the diameter 20 microns and collapse all the intertrabecular spaces.

Table 13.2 Amount of increase in trabecular circumference to collapse entire outflow system

Individual i-t space	6 microns
times	×
Number of spaces	20 spaces
times	×
Both sides of meshwork	2 sides
equals	=
Total width of i-t spaces	240 microns
plus	+
Both Schlemm's canals	80 microns
equals	=
Total width (i-t + Schlemm's)	320 microns

$320\,\mu$ diameter $\times 3.1416 = 1005\,\mu$ Circumference
$1005/36\,000 = 2.79\%$ increase in Circumference increases diameter enough to collapse both i-t spaces and Schlemm's.

total closure of these spaces has occurred, that serious outflow impairment would have occurred. It appears, therefore, that a small amount of senile stretching of the meshwork may by itself account for all the outflow abnormalities of open angle glaucoma, even though the other mechanisms of sclerosis and deposition may also be operating. If shrinkage in the trabecular meshwork could be induced, this would reduce the circumference of the trabecular ring, which would necessarily result in a corresponding reduction in ring diameter. This would pull open the intertrabecular spaces and Schlemm's canal, thus reversing this postulated basic mechanism of glaucoma (Wise & Witter, 1979; Wise, 1981b; Wise, 1983). Because the trabecular meshwork circumference is so very great in comparison to the total width of all the intertrabecular spaces plus Schlemm's canal, a small increase or reduction in trabecular circumference can have a profound effect on outflow. If one were to place 100 burns of 50 microns each around the trabecular meshwork, only 20% shrinkage at each burn would totally reverse complete collapse of Schlemm's canal and the intertrabecular spaces using the largest estimates (Table 13.3). This is the concept which is now termed laser trabeculoplasty. It must be re-emphasised that once one accepts the idea that the laser can cause shrinkage of trabecular tissues, reduction in ring circumference and diameter must necessarily follow. Dueker (1981) has demonstrated that argon laser treatment produces drastic and immediate shrinkage of the excised human trabecular meshwork. Laser trabeculoplasty alters outflow; it has no effect upon aqueous production (Brubaker & Leisegang, 1983).

Table 13.3 Amount of shrinkage at laser burns required to re-open both intertrabecular spaces and Schlemm's canal

Number of burns	100 burns
times	×
Burn diameter	50 microns
equals	=
Circumferential length	5000 microns
Circumference reduction	
needed to reverse collapse	1005 microns
divided by	÷
Circum. burn length	5000 microns
equals	=
% Shrinkage at each burn	20%

INITIAL METHOD OF TRABECULOPLASTY

The initial method of laser trabecular tightening or laser trabeculoplasty (Wise & Witter, 1979; Wise, 1981b) consisted of a single session of 100 laser burns of 50 microns each evenly spaced 360 degrees around the trabecular meshwork. Exposure time was 0.1 second. A power level was chosen which gave a small bubble or a small depigmented spot at the point of impact. This was usually 800–1200 mW. The majority of the eyes were treated with the spots placed in the middle of the pigmented trabecular band, directly over Schlemm's canal, although sometimes some of the spots were also placed behind the scleral spur in the ciliary body band or in the pigmented band just anterior to the scleral spur. Between 11 February 1976 and December 1981, 366 phakic eyes (patient age >39 years) were treated with 90 or more burns in one session (range 90–188). The control rate (20 mmHg or less, with or without medication), was 74.4% (221 of 297 eyes) at 2 years, and 67% (6 or 9 eyes) at 7 years. The control rate denominator includes all patients followed for the given duration, including those having surgery. The fall in IOP was accompanied by a reduced need for medical therapy (Wise, 1981a; Pollack et al, 1983). The overall failure rate (glaucoma surgery, late retreatment, or both) was 10.3% (38 of 366 eyes). Aphakic eyes do not have as high a success rate, with about 50% of those treated achieving control and all those controlled still requiring medical therapy (Wise & Witter, 1979). Pseudophakic eyes (pupil-supported and posterior chamber implants) have shown a success rate nearly as high as phakic eyes (Wise, 1982b). This method has been studied by Schwartz A. L. et al (1981), Wilensky & Jampol (1981), Thomas et al (1982), Schwartz & Kopelman (1983), and many others.

Complications
Complications have been few (Wise, 1981a; Thomas et al, 1982a,b; Hoskins et al, 1983), particularly considering the alternatives of debilitating medical therapy (Van Buskirk, 1982; Schwartz et al, 1983), medically uncontrolled glaucoma, and glaucoma surgery. They have included angle closure glaucoma after discontinuing miotics, peripheral anterior synechiae in shallow angles, ischaemic uveitis from subconjunctival lidocaine with epinephrine, corneal endothelial burns in argyrosis and corneal bloodstaining, small corneal epithelial burns (common), small oozes of blood from the trabecular meshwork, mild degrees of redness and iritis, and occasional syncope during therapy. The principal problem, however, is pressure elevations in the post-laser period. Most eyes show a profound drop in pressure the next day, and the majority of the remainder will show little pressure change for 2–4 weeks and then a marked decrease. A few eyes, however, can develop IOP rises up to the level of 50–60 mmHg after treatment with 80 or more burns in one session.

Two session laser treatment
Because of the uncommon but real phenomenon of severe pressure rise after single-session laser trabeculoplasty, Thomas et al (1982) began to treat one-half of the angle with 50 burns, treating the other 180 degrees a few weeks later with another 50 burns. They showed that the pressure decreases obtained were as large as those of 100 burns in one session and that while pressure elevations occurred just as often, the rises were not so high and were all controllable. Schwartz L. W. et al (1983) and Wilensky & Weinreb (1983) confirmed this finding. Because occasional severe pressure rises are essentially the only important complication of laser trabeculoplasty, it has become the practice of most laser surgeons including this author to split the treatment into two sessions of approximately 50 burns with an interval of 4–6 weeks between the sessions. Even this method is not absolutely free of post-laser pressure rises, but IOP levels have not exceeded 40 mmHg, all of these pressure rises were controllable with subconjunctival dexamethasone plus increased medical therapy, and none have forced prompt filtering surgery.

While in theory and in practice, two session therapy is superior to one session therapy, the method is subject to the problem of failure to do the second session. Patients object to the additional time and expense, and laser surgeons object to the additional trouble. Unless the patient is carefully instructed, he may well fail to have the second session performed. When the patient is treated with only 50 or 60 burns, either 180 or 360 degrees, the pressure can come down quite substantially. However, the trabecular tightening thus obtained may not be adequate for long term control, so that the pressure will eventually rise again. If the patient has been lost to follow-up, severe damage can occur. Furthermore, there is a serious question as to whether two sessions of 50 burns, a year or more apart, will produce the same result as two sessions close together.

CLASSIFICATION OF PRESSURE RISES AFTER LASER TRABECULOPLASTY

These pressure rises can be immediate (0–24 hours), intermediate (1–28 days), or late (after 28 days). Their significance and treatment are entirely different.

Immediate pressure rises have been noted by a number of authors (Hoskins et al, 1983; Weinreb et al, 1983b) and occur in 40–50% of the laser treated eyes. The usual occurrence is an elevation of 5–15 mmHg beginning within 20 minutes after LTP and lasting from 2–6 hours. These rises should be minimised because of the possibility of vascular occlusion or damage to an extremely deteriorated optic nerve with loss of a tiny central visual field (Thomas et al, 1982), but they do not influence the long term result. Shirato et al (1982) have shown they are not influenced by retrobulbar anaesthesia, topical steroids, or topical indomethacin. Hotchkiss et al (1983) found little effect from topical flubiprofen. Subconjunctival dexamethasone did not prevent the immediate rises, but instead made them worse (Table 13.4). Use of an ice bag over the eye for 3 hours post LTP does considerably reduce the immediate IOP rise (Table 13.5). While not necessary for all eyes, those with serious glaucoma disc damage or IOP over 30 mmHg prior to laser treatment should have an ice bag placed over them for 15 minutes before and 3 or 4 hours after laser trabeculoplasty. For very severely damaged discs, pretreatment with miotics and/or oral glycerol may

Table 13.4 Effect of 4 mg subconjunctival dexamethasone upon early IOP change after laser trabeculoplasty. Identical laser treatment each eye, subconjunctival lidocaine each eye, sub-conjunctival steroid in right eye of each patient

	1 h	2 h	3 h	18 h
Average steroid eye IOP change	+13.2	+11.3	+9.3	−5.4
Average control eye IOP change	+5.9	+6.5	+5.4	−6.6
# Steroid eyes, IOP > 39	4	3	2	0
# Control eyes, IOP > 39	2	3	2	0

Table 13.5 Effect of ice-bag upon early IOP change after laser trabeculoplasty. Fifteen eyes had identical laser treatment. Ice-bag over one eye

	1 h	2 h	3 h
Average ice-bag IOP change	+3.3	+3.3	+2.0
Average control IOP change	+9.6	+8.3	+5.8
# Ice-bag eyes, IOP > 39	0	0	1
# Control eyes, IOP > 39	5	5	1

be used as well. The IOP should be measured hourly for at least 4 hours, and also the next day.

Intermediate pressure rises (1–21 days) are due to uveitis and trabecular swelling or plugging. They should be treated with subconjunctival dexamethasone, carbonic anhydrase inhibitors, osmotic agents, timolol, and weak miotics. Most eyes (75%) will respond within 24 hours. The ultimate result in these eyes is not as successful as in eyes without such IOP rises. In 50 eyes with a 10 mmHg or more rise in the 1–21 day period post-laser, only 48% were controlled (IOP <21 mmHg) at 6 months and 32% had required surgery (Wise, unpublished). These rises are quite unpredictable, occurring in blue, brown, and Negro eyes, but there is some association with plethoric complexions and high (>30 mmHg) prelaser IOP. These are the dangerous rises. They can cause additional field loss (Schwartz et al, 1983) and loss of a central visual island (Thomas et al, 1982), and can force emergency filtering surgery. As noted, two-session therapy greatly reduces their intensity.

Late pressure rises (after 28 days), particularly if severe, usually imply failure. This can occur when unfavourable eyes (aphakia, uveitis) have been treated with fairly high power levels during laser trabeculoplasty. Apparently temporary trabecular perforation can occur with immediate and marked drops in pressure (as in Krasnov's work) but when these perforations close the previously obstructed trabecular meshwork will not respond to the tightening effect of the laser, and filtering surgery must be done.

Modifications of technique
The principle modification has been the advent of two session laser therapy as discussed above. Another inadvertant modification has been the use of spot sizes substantially larger than 50 microns, which has resulted in iritis, synechiae, and pressure rises in the hands of some investigators (Levy & Bonney, 1982). Other modifications include laser focusing, spot location, power levels, exposure duration, and burn number.

LASER FOCUS

In testing the 18 argon lasers at the 1982 meeting of the American Academy of Ophthalmology plus nine other lasers, I found (Wise, 1984) that only four (14%) of these instruments produced a spot diameter of 50 or 60 microns with the eyepieces set on zero, all others giving spots of 70 microns or more. With the eyepieces properly focused (see below) 56% of the lasers gave a 50 or 60 micron spot size, but 44% gave a minimum spot of 70 microns (double the area of a 50 micron spot) or more. The laser produces a converging beam of light which has an aerial focal point in front of the instrument. It is necessary to focus the eye pieces of the biomicroscope at the same point as the laser, so that when the trabecular meshwork is in focus, the laser will also be in focus at that point. This is achieved by placing a soft-textured orange or red paper in front of the laser, at the same location that a patient's eye would be. The eyepieces are placed on the various settings from maximum plus to maximum minus. At each eyepiece setting, the biomicroscope is focused on the fibres of the paper, and burns are made with the laser set on 50 microns and enough power to burn half-way through the paper. The eyepiece setting giving the smallest burn, regardless of the numerical setting, should be used for treatment of patients. In the various lasers tested the smallest spot was obtained with the eyepieces anywhere from +5 to −5 eye-piece setting.

Minimum spot diameter
Even more disturbing than the lack of correlation between eyepiece setting and laser focus was the finding that only 11 of the 27 lasers tested would produce a true 50 micron spot when the burns on the paper were measured with a microscope, measuring the smallest spots obtained from a given laser at the proper eyepiece setting. The majority of the lasers tested would not produce a 50 micron spot at all. Surgeons using such lasers would be burning a substantially larger area of trabecular meshwork than they realised. For example, a 100 micron spot has four times the area of a true 50 micron spot. A surgeon using a laser to apply 100 spots of 100 microns each would be delivering the equivalent of 400 spots of true 50 microns, which would certainly be excessive treatment. The fact that so few lasers produce their advertised spot size, and that most of them do not do it with the eyepiece set at zero, means that the great majority of laser surgeons may well be unwittingly over-treating the trabecular meshworks of their patients. Each laser surgeon must check the focusing of each individual laser that he uses, and measure the minimum burn on the paper with microscope, to ascertain the actual minimum spot size of that laser. Only in this way can discussions of the proper spot numbers for laser trabeculoplasty be reduced to a rational basis.

ASSOCIATED ANGLE CLOSURE

Perhaps 25% of the referral patients which I see have partial or total angle closure. While partial angle closure can be temporarily relieved by flattening the peripheral iris with low-power 200 micron laser burns of 0.2 second duration (peripheral laser iridoplasty), this does not relieve the underlying pupillary block component and the angle can again became shallow later on. Argon laser iridectomy by the chipping technique through the Abraham lens (0.05 or 0.02 second burns, without using 'stretch burns') has been very reliable and produced very little iritis in my hands. In eyes with shallow angles, 30 or 40 burns are applied to the accessible trabecular meshwork and then a laser iridectomy is done. The rest of the 100 burns to the meshwork are given a month later. In this way the patient is adequately treated in a two session treatment with no increase in complications. If severe angle closure is present, then laser iridectomy alone is done, doing trabeculoplasty later if indicated. Squeezing laser burns into the trabecular meshwork through a slit angle is dangerous, as further pupillary block from the mild laser-induced iritis can lead to complete angle closure and extensive peripheral anterior synechiae. If enough iris bowing is present to cause consideration of laser iridectomy, then the iridectomy should almost always be done, to avoid problems with progressive angle closure in the future. Laser iridectomy should always be done first in black patients with plateau iris, as peripheral anterior synechiae are very apt to occur if LTP alone is done.

NUMBER OF BURNS

The technical point most debated in laser trabeculoplasty is the number of burns to be used, their distribution (180 degrees versus 360 degrees), and the timing of their application. In the early attempts at laser trabeculopuncture and laser trabeculotomy, burn numbers varied from the three or four burns, each of 3 seconds duration, placed in one quadrant by Hager, to the 150 Britt laser burns placed in one quadrant by Worthen. In the original laser trabeculoplasty protocol, 100 burns were distributed 360 degrees in one session (Wise & Witter, 1979; Wise, 1981b). Subsequently, Thomas et al (1982) recommended 50 burns into 180 degrees of the meshwork, followed a month later by 50 burns in the other 180 degrees. Schwartz L. W. et al (1983) compared burn numbers from 25 burns in one quadrant up to 100 burns in four quadrants. There was little response to 25 burns, but nearly as much response to 50 burns in 180 degrees as to 100 burns in 360 degrees. They noted little difference between pulsed and continuous wave lasers in this study. Weinreb et al (1983a) reported that 50 burns in 180 degrees produced results nearly as good as 100 burns at 360 degrees, and advocated treating only 180 degrees, with the second 180 degrees to be done only if the first treatment has not produced adequate control. Wilensky & Weinreb (1983) tried 25 burns into one quadrant, then 25 burns into a second quadrant. An anonymous laser surgeon, as reported by Spaeth, applied 250 burns 360 degrees in one session to each eye of the same patient, who was aphakic, and 10 days later the patient developed 360 degree peripheral anterior synechiae in each eye, with a pressure of 60 mmHg in each eye. None of the above authors have published measurements of their spot size, which as discussed above can considerably influence the required number of burns. Because lasers and laser surgeons are not interchangeable, it does appear that to some extent each laser surgeon will have to determine the optimum number of burns required in his hands with his equipment.

DURATION OF EFFECT OF VARIOUS BURN NUMBERS

As glaucoma is a lifelong disease, the duration of effect of a given number of laser burns in either 180 or 360 degrees is just as important as the immediate effect. To investigate this, I performed a computer study on the 1500 eyes which I have treated with laser trabeculoplasty. The computer was used to retrieve groups of patients who were phakic, 40 years or more, had no complicating eye diseases, and who had a pre-laser IOP from 26–30 mmHg. The groups of patients were retrieved by the number of single session burns applied, such as 46–55 (average of 50), 56–65 (average of 60), etc. The average pressure drop and change in medications score was tabulated for the 6 months follow-up interval and for the 2 year follow-up interval. Because so many of the patients treated with the smaller numbers of burns had required a second treatment before the 2 year time interval, the computer was also used to retrieve patients who had a second laser trabeculoplasty more than 13 weeks after the first (to eliminate patients with planned two-stage treatments), and patients who had surgery within 3 months. The 'two-year IOP' for the re-treated patients was the IOP immediately before the laser re-treatment. The largest IOP reduction at 6 months occurred with 140 burns and at 2 years with 110 burns of true 50 micron size (Table 13.6). The incidence of filtering surgery and repeat trabeculoplasty declined with increasing burn numbers, on a parabolic curve (Fig. 13.1). The laser used for these studies produces a true 50 microns spot. Lasers producing somewhat larger spots may not need to use this large a number of laser burns.

Table 13.6 IOP response to various number of single-session laser burns spaced 360 degrees. All eyes were phakic and had a pre-laser IOP of 26–30 mmHg. Patient age >39 years

# Burns	# Eyes	IOP drop at 3 months (mmHg)	IOP drop at 24 months (mmHg)	IOP rise over 10 mmHg (1 to 21 days)
50	14	9.0	6.5	1/14
60	30	8.9	8.3	2/30
70	11	9.7	7.0	0/11
80	13	10.9	8.4	1/13
90	14	10.1	8.7	1/14
100	34	10.7	9.4	1/30
110	33	11.6	11.1	2/33
120	21	10.2	9.4	0/21
130	8	12.0	8.7	0/8
140	6	12.5	10.3	0/6

Total eyes = 184. Total with IOP rise 8/184 = 4.3%

The two principal reasons that 180 degree treatment with smaller numbers of burns has been advocated are to minimise post-laser pressure rises and to have the other 180 degrees of the angle available for future treatment if necessary. While these are desirable objectives, in the long run the most important objective of glaucoma therapy is to control the glaucoma, the leading cause of blindness. The computer studies presented above indicate that initial good results can be obtained from small numbers of burns (50 or 60) applied over either 180 or 360 degrees, but that these good results can later deteriorate. The results of late retreatment of eyes that have had failure of the first treatment have not been as satisfactory as the results in eyes which were treated 360 degrees in one session or in two sessions 4–6 weeks apart. Adequate trabeculoplasty pulls the meshwork wide open, relieving the aqueous pressure upon it and allowing debris in the aqueous to pass through the meshwork (when one-half of the mesh has been treated, it becomes depigmented relative to the untreated half). There is a real possibility that return of the elevated pressure after inadequate laser trabeculoplasty

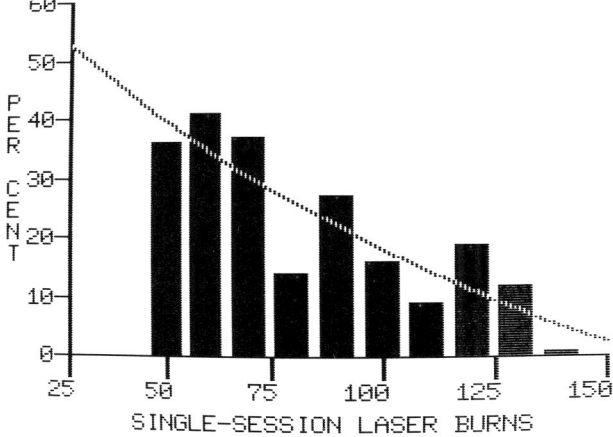

Fig. 13.1 Rate of late re-laser or filter after various numbers of burns (parabolic curve fitted).

may represent recurrent collapse and plugging of the meshwork, so that a second limited number of burns will have no more effect or duration of effect than the first inadequate treatment did, ultimately resulting in the eye becoming refractory to additional laser treatment and requiring filtering surgery. Because glaucoma is a lifetime disease, and because 100 laser burns spaced 360 degrees have now shown good control rates for 6 and 7 years, I believe that the patient should be treated to a total of 100–110 burns placed in two sessions of 50–55 burns in 180 degrees, 4–6 weeks apart. The only exception would be the rare patient who shows a dramatic response to the first 180 degree treatment with a fall of intraocular pressure to the low teens on little or no medication. The authors advocating half-angle treatment with 50 burns must present long term follow-up of their data, before they can justify general adoption of their modification.

The use of inadequate half-angle trabeculoplasty may ultimately result in the loss of more eyes than if the eyes had been treated with single-session LTP, with the rare uncontrollable pressure rises treated with filtering surgery, which was necessary in only 5/366 (1.4%) of the patients treated in the single session protocol. Patients and laser surgeons must understand the necessity for adequate laser trabeculoplasty, either in a single session or preferably in two sessions not separated by more than 4–6 weeks, in order to widely open the meshwork and obtain long term control. In 24 hour follow-up, glaucomatous eyes can vary as much as 13 mmHg between high and low pressures on the same day (Drance, 1960). In the great majority of eyes receiving LTP, any IOP rises are of the same magnitude as those of natural diurnal variation and those of missed medications. The philosophy of LTP must be directed toward maximal control of Glaucoma, not maximal avoidance of temporary IOP rises. The arguments of Watson (1981) and Cairns (1982), who advocate early surgical trabeculectomy in glaucoma, highlight the long term dangers of inadequate pressure lowering by medical therapy and by inadequate trabeculoplasty. The discussion of blindness from glaucoma by Grant & Burke (1982) should be read by all who treat this disease.

LOCATION OF BURNS

The original study of laser trabeculoplasty utilised laser burns in the middle of the pigmented trabecular band, with some burns placed in the posterior half of the band just anterior to the scleral spur, and a few burns placed posterior to this scleral spur in the ciliary body band (Wise & Witter, 1979). Subsequent studies (Schwartz L. W. et al, 1983) have indicated that equally good results are obtained by placing the burns in the anterior half of the pigmented trabecular band, with less tendency toward iritis and post-laser pressure rises. Shirato et al (1982), treating Japanese patients, applied laser burns posterior to the scleral spur, into the ciliary body band, using 0.2 second exposure times. This method results in a high incidence of iritis and post-laser pressure rises, with a reduced percentage of control compared to more anterior burn placement.

The geometry of the outflow system may clarify the optimum point for placing the laser burns. The trabecular meshwork does not lie on the inside of a cylinder, but on the inside of the cone described by imaginary lines tangential to the limbus, which meet at an imaginary point anterior to the corneal apex. If the trabecular tissues stretch with age, the circumference of the trabecular ring will increase. The corneo-scleral meshwork will then move not only outward against the sclera, but also posteriorly into the area bounded by the sclera and the scleral spur. This reduces the tension of the scleral spur upon the corneal scleral meshwork, reducing the effectiveness of the normal tensioning of the meshwork induced by posterior pulling of the scleral spur by the ciliary muscle. If a ring of laser burns is placed in the meshwork anywhere anterior to the scleral spur, the resulting contraction ring will not only move toward the anterior chamber, but also upward toward the apex of the cornea, pulling the opposite way from the scleral spur and thus creating a two way pull on the trabecular tissues (Wise, 1983). In theory it would make little difference where the burns were placed, provided only that they were placed anterior to the scleral spur. The various experimental studies confirm this, showing that all patterns placed anterior to this scleral spur produced approximately equivalent results, and that the only difference is the reduction of iritis and adhesions with more anterior placement of the burns. At the present time placement of the burns in the anterior margin of the pigmented trabecular band appears to give the best absorption of the laser energy and contraction of the trabecular tissues, without being so far anterior as to endanger the corneal endothelium and result in corneal endothelial growth on the meshwork (Rodrigues et al, 1982). Placement on or posterior to the scleral spur should be avoided, as this does not produce the anterior contraction ring pulling against the scleral spur, and does produce an undue amount of iritis and synechiae.

DURATION

The early studies on 'laser trabeculotomy' used burn durations from 0.02 up to 3 seconds. None of those authors using burn durations longer than 0.1 second obtained good results. A burn duration of 0.1 second has been used in nearly all studies of laser trabeculoplasty. Ritch (1983) has orally reported improved results in refractory aphakic glaucomas by using burn durations of 0.2 seconds, but no controlled study of 0.1 second versus 0.2 second burn durations has so far been done. As can be observed by anyone treating the retina or iris with the laser, a 0.2 second burn duration produces a considerably larger burn than a 0.1 second burn at the same power setting. Furthermore, involuntary eye movements occur in the interval between 0.1 and 0.2 seconds, so that 0.1 second burns are small and discrete, while 0.2 second burns can frequently be comet shaped or linear. The 0.2 second burn is therefore a much less standardised burn than a 0.1 second burn because of the factor of patient eye motion. Use of 0.2 second and longer burns is therefore not recommended at this time.

Experience with laser iridectomies suggests that burn durations shorter than 0.1 second produce less iris shrinkage and more of an excavating effect than 0.1 second burns. As laser trabeculoplasty produces its effect principally by immediate collagen shrinkage of the trabecular tissues, the shorter duration burns should produce less shrinkage and less effect. Short burns will also be shallow and will not shrink and tighten the important justa-canalicular area. The Britt laser should always be used in the thermal mode to achieve trabecular shrinkage, rather than the 'cool' mode which produces little shrinkage and little effect, (John Lynn, personal communication). Until controlled studies have been done to compare other burn durations with the 0.1 second burn, all trabeculoplasties should use this duration.

POWER

The original attempts to treat open angle glaucoma with the laser involved a great deal of power, for example the three second high intensity burns of Hager (1973) and of Teichmann (1976), attempting to burn holes in the meshwork. The principal result of this type of treatment was extensive pupil distortion and synechia formation. In the original trabeculoplasty protocol, a power was recommended which would produce a visible trabecular reaction, either a small depigmented spot or a small bubble. Other studies have utilised even smaller power levels which produced only an occasional visible reaction. In my experience, however, lack of visible reaction has frequently been associated with poor results. The principle barrier to outflow resides at the juxta-canalicular area, deep in the meshwork. It is possible that inadequate power level (or over-sized spots with low power density) will tend to sear the surface of the meshwork without tightening the important deep layers. To reach these deep layers, especially in densely pigmented meshworks, one should use a power level producing a visible reaction, preferably a small bubble. In histological study of successful LTP performed using these power levels, the burns ablate the superficial layers, tighten the deep layers, and do not perforate or close Schlemm's canal (Fig. 13.2). The spectacular results obtained in this case suggest this burn power as ideal.

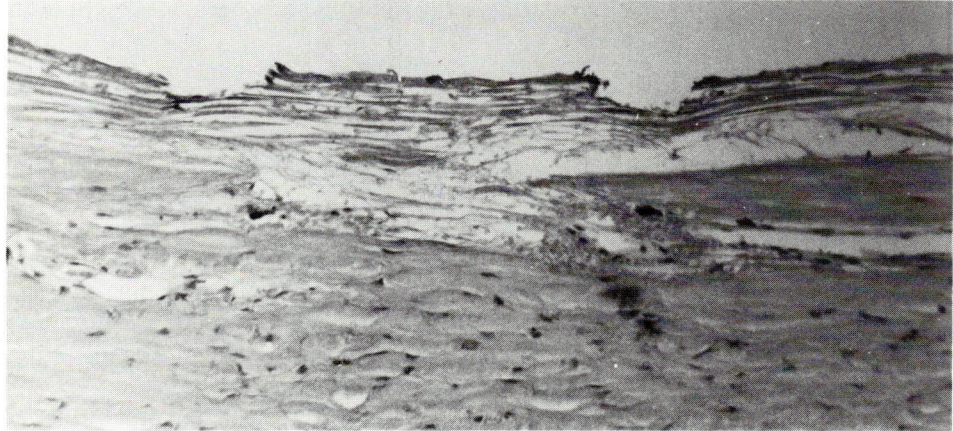

Fig. 13.2   Frontal section of trabecular meshwork of an eye which went from a pre-laser IOP of 38 mmHg on 4% pilocarpine therapy to a post-laser IOP of 12 mmHg on no therapy, remaining at this level for the 21 months prior to the patient's death.

LATE FAILURE

The original protocol of 100–120 laser burns placed 360 degrees in one session has produced a large number of long term good results. However, some patients do show a gradual deterioration of control ultimately resulting in a need for repeat laser treatment or filtering surgery. Alverado & Polansky (1983) have demonstrated a marked reduction in the cell population of the superficial trabecular layers in glaucoma, indicating that there is a true abnormality of the trabecular meshwork itself rather than only passive plugging or stretching. It is possible that the late failures represent a continuation of the natural history of glaucoma, which is a progressive disease. All patients treated with laser trabeculoplasty should therefore have regular follow-ups for life to detect any deterioration of results. This is of course true of patients treated with filtering surgery as well, as they can also show elevations of pressure after years of successful control by either trabeculectomy or by full thickness procedures.

There are no indications at the present time that primary open angle glaucoma properly treated with laser trabeculoplasty will ultimately fail and have a higher pressure than if the patient had been treated with heavy medical therapy alone, but this possibility does make it advisable to restrict laser trabeculoplasty to patients whose glaucoma is not controlled by tolerated medical therapy, as such patients are at risk from their disease and many would be considered surgical candidates if the laser were not available. Patients with pseudoexfoliation represent a special group, as they show excellent initial responses to the laser but have in a few cases shown late rise in pressure months or years later (Ritch, 1983). Patients with this type of glaucoma should therefore be followed at somewhat closer than patients with uncomplicated primary open angle glaucoma treated with laser trabeculoplasty. Eyes with secondary and complicated forms of glaucoma are also more prone to have late failure and should be followed more closely. However, as noted above as many as 6 (Wise, 1982b), 7, and even 8 year follow-ups of laser trabeculoplasty are now available and the procedure is certainly capable of producing excellent long term results in a large percentage of the patients treated.

ACKNOWLEDGEMENTS

Gail Toumbs gave technical assistance. Ray Lynch Jr obtained follow-up data and maintained the computer database. Elizabeth Homans gave secretarial assistance. Tom Hewett MD prepared the photomicrograph.

REFERENCES

Alverado J A, Polansky J R 1983 The trabecular meshwork endothelium in glaucoma. Presented at the American Academy of Ophthalmology, Chicago, Nov 3, 1983
Brubaker R F, Liesegang T J 1983 Effects of trabecular photocoagulation on the aqueous humor dynamics of the human eye. American Journal of Ophthalmology 96: 139–147
Cairns J E 1982 The case for early surgery in primary open-angle glaucoma. Glaucoma 4: 7–9
Drance S M 1960 Significance of the diurnal tension variations in normal and glaucomatous eyes. Archives of Ophthalmology 64: 494
Dueker D 1981 Presented at the Annual Meeting of the American Academy of Ophthalmology, Atlanta, Georgia
Gaasterland D, Kupfer C 1974 Experimental glaucoma in the Rhesus monkey. Investigative Ophthalmology 13: 455–457
Grant W M, Burke J F 1982 Why do some people go blind from glaucoma? Ophthalmology 89: 991–998
Hager H 1973 Besondere mikrochirurgische Eingriff. 2. Teil. Erste Erfahrunger mit dem Argon-Laser-Gerat 800. Klin Monatsbl Augenheilkd 162: 437–450
Hoskins H D, Hetherington J, Minckler D S, Lieberman M F, Shaffer R N 1983 Complications of laser trabeculoplasty. Ophthalmology 90: 796–799
Hotchkiss M L, Pollack I P, Robin A L 1983 Non-steroidal anti-inflammatory agents after argon laser trabeculoplasty: A trial with flubiprofen and indomethacin. Presented at the American Academy of Ophthalmology, Chicago, Nov 1, 1983
Krasnov M M 1973 Laseropuncture of anterior chamber angle in glaucoma. American Journal of Ophthalmology 75: 674–678

Krasnov M M 1974 Q-switched laser goniopuncture. Archives of Ophthalmology 92: 37–41

Levy N S, Bonney R C 1982 Argon laser therapy in advanced open-angle glaucoma. Glaucoma 4: 25–29

Pollack I P, Robin A L, Sax H 1983 The effect of argon laser trabeculoplasty on the medical control of primary open-angle glaucoma. Ophthalmology 90: 785–789

Rodrigues M M, Spaeth G L, Donohoo P 1982 Electron microscopy of argon laser therapy in phakic open-angle glaucoma. Ophthalmology 89: 198–210

Ritch R 1983 Presented at 5th International Medical Laser Congress, Detroit, 6 Oct, 1983

Schwartz A L, Kopelman J 1983 Four year experience with argon laser trabecular surgery in uncontrolled open-angle glaucoma. Ophthalmology 90: 771–780

Schwartz A L, Whitten M E, Bleiman B, Martin D 1981 Argon laser trabecular surgery in uncontrolled phakic open-angle glaucoma. Ophthalmology 88: 203–212

Schwartz L W, Spaeth G L, Brown G 1983 Laser Therapy of the Anterior Segment. A Practical Approach. SLACK Incorporated, Thorofare NJ, USA. P 2, 63–65

Schwartz L W, Spaeth G L, Traverso C, Greenidge K C 1983 Variation of techniques on the results of argon laser trabeculoplasty. Ophthalmology 90: 781–784

Shirato S, Yamamoto T, Kitazawa Y 1982 Argon laser trabeculoplasty in open-angle glaucoma. Japanese Journal of Ophthalmology 26: 374–386

Teichmann I, Teichmann K D, Fechner P U 1976 Eye Ear Nose Throat Monthly 55: 209–211

Thomas J V, Simmons R J, Belcher C D III 1982a Argon laser trabeculoplasty in the presurgical glaucoma patient. Ophthalmology 89: 187–197

Thomas J V, Simmons R J, Belcher C D III 1982b Complications of argon laser trabeculoplasty. Glaucoma 4: 50–52

Ticho U, Zauberman H 1976 Argon laser application to the angle structures in the glaucomas. Archives of Ophthalmology 94: 61–64

Van Buskirk E M 1982 Hazards of medical glaucoma therapy in the cataract patient. Ophthalmology 89: 238–241

Watson P G, Grierson I 1981 The place of trabeculectomy in the treatment of glaucoma. Ophthalmology 88: 175–196

Weinreb R N, Ruderman J, Juster R, Wilensky J T 1983 Influence of the number of laser burns on the early results of argon laser trabeculoplasty. American Journal of Ophthalmology 95: 287–292

Weinreb R N, Ruderman J, Juster R, Zweig K 1983 Immediate intraocular pressure response to argon laser trabeculoplasty. American Journal of Ophthalmology 95: 279–286

Wickham M G, Worthen D M 1979 Argon laser trabeculotomy: long-term follow-up. Ophthalmology 86: 495–503

Wilensky J T, Jampol L M 1981 Laser therapy for open angle glaucoma. Ophthalmology 88: 213–217

Wilensky J T, Weinreb R N 1983 Low-dose trabeculoplasty. American Journal of Ophthalmology 94: 423–426

Wise J B 1981a Long-term control of adult open angle glucoma by argon laser treatment. Ophthalmology 88: 197–202

Wise J B 1981b Glaucoma treatment by trabecular tightening with the argon laser. International Ophthalmology Clinics 21: 69–78

Wise J B 1982a Laser burns around trabecular edge can reverse glaucoma process. Ophthalmology Times 7(1): January 1982

Wise J B 1982b Long term results of laser trabeculoplasty. Presented at the America Academy of Ophthalmology, San Francisco, November 1982

Wise J B 1983 Interview with B F Boyd, MD. Highlights of Ophthalmology 11(7): 1–8, 11(8): 1–8

Wise J B 1984 Errors in laser spot size in laser trabeculoplasty. Ophthalmology (in press)

Wise J B, Witter S L 1979 Argon laser therapy for open-angle glaucoma; a pilot study. Archives of Ophthalmology 97: 319–322

Worthen D M, Wickham M G 1974 Argon laser trabeculotomy. Transactions of the American Academy of Ophthalmology and Otolaryngology 78: 371–375

Index